VOICE THERAPY:

CLINICAL STUDIES

Voice Therapy: Clinical Studies

Joseph C. Stemple, Ph.D.
Voice Pathologist
Institute for Voice Analysis and Rehabilitation
Dayton, Ohio

**Mosby
Year Book**

St. Louis   Baltimore   Boston   Chicago   London   Philadelphia   Sydney   Toronto

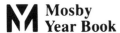

Mosby
Year Book

Dedicated to Publishing Excellence

Sponsoring Editor: David K. Marshall
Developmental Editor: Julie Tryboski
Associate Managing Editor, Manuscript Services: Deborah Thorp
Production Supervisor: Kathryn Solt
Proofroom Manager: Barbara M. Kelly

1 2 3 4 5 6 7 8 9 0   GW/MV 97 96 95 94 93

Library of Congress Cataloging-in-Publication Data

Stemple, Joseph C.
    Voice therapy : clinical case studies / Joseph C.
Stemple.
        p.   cm.
    Includes bibliographical references and index.
    ISBN 0-8016-4763-0
    1. Voice disorders — treatment.   I. Title.
    [DNLM: 1. Voice Disorders — therapy.   WV 500
S824v]
    RF510.S743   1992
    616.85'506 — dc20
    DNLM/DLC   92-49999
    for Library of Congress   CIP

To the son I finally have.

CONTRIBUTORS

Moya Andrews, Ph.D.
Professor of Speech and Hearing Sciences
Indiana University
Bloomington, Indiana

Andrew Blitzer, M.D., D.D.S.
Professor of Clinical Otolaryngology
Acting Chairman
College of Physicians and Surgeons
Columbia University, New York City

Gordon W. Blood, Ph.D.
Professor
Department of Communication Disorders
Pennsylvania State University
University Park, Pennsylvania

Eva I. Carlson, M.Sc.
Member, College of Speech and Language
   Therapists
London, England

James L. Case, Ph.D.
Associate Professor
Director of Clinical Services
Department of Speech and Hearing Science
Arizona State University
Tempe, Arizona

Janina K. Casper, Ph.D.
Associate Professor
State University of New York Science Center at
   Syracuse
Syracuse, New York

Bernice S. Gerdeman, Ph.D.
Institute for Voice Analysis and Rehabilitation
Dayton, Ohio

Leslie E. Glaze, Ph.D.
Midwest Voice and Speech Institute
St. Paul, Minnesota

Jack L. Gluckman, M.D.
Professor and Chairman
Department of Otolaryngology-Head and Neck
   Surgery
University of Cincinnati Medical Center
Cincinnati, Ohio

Jon Hufnagle, Ph.D.
Associate Professor
Department of Speech Pathology and Audiology
Illinois State University
Normal, Illinois

Krzytof Izdebski, F.K., M.A., Ph.D., C.C.C.
Director, Pacific Voice Care
San Francisco, California

Barbara H. Jacobson, Ph.D.
Speech-Language Sciences and Disorders
Henry Ford Hospital
Detroit, Michigan

Thomas J. Kereiakes, M.D.
Department of Otolaryngology and Head and
   Neck Surgery
Christ Hospital
Professional Voice Center of Greater Cincinnati
Medical Director
Cincinnati, Ohio

Danna Koschkee, M.A.
Department of Surgery
Division of Otolaryngology
University of Wisconsion
Madison, Wisconsin

William L. Kramer, Ph.D.
Speech Pathology and Audiology Department
Ball State University
Muncie, Indiana

Ann W. Kummer, Ph.D.
Director, Speech Pathology Department
Children's Hospital Medical Center
Cincinnati, Ohio

Linda Lee, Ph.D.
Associate Professor
Department of Communication Sciences and
   Disorders
University of Cincinnati
Cincinnati, Ohio

Dawn B. Lowery, Ph.D.
Voice Disorders Center
Ear, Nose, Throat, and Head and Neck Surgeons
Columbus, Ohio

Robert C. Peppard, Ph.D.
Assistant Professor
Department of Speech/Language Pathology and
   Audiology
Northeastern University
Boston, Massachusetts

Bonnie N. Raphael, Ph.D.
Voice, Speech, Dialects and Text Coach
American Repertory Theatre and Institute
Cambridge, Massachusetts

Robert Thayre Sataloff, M.D., D.M.A.
Professor of Otolaryngology
Thomas Jefferson University
Chairman, The Voice Foundation
Philadelphia, Pennsylvania

Susan Shulman, M.S., C.C.C., Sp/A
Private Practice
Dallas, Texas

Joseph C. Stemple, Ph.D.
Voice Pathologist
Institute for Voice Analysis and Rehabilitation
Dayton, Ohio

R.E. (Ed) Stone, Jr., Ph.D.
Associate Professor
Vanderbilt Voice Center
Department of Otolaryngology
Vanderbilt University Medical Center
Nashville, Tennessee

Celia Stewart, M.D.
Senior Speech-Language Pathologist
College of Physicians and Surgeons
Columbia University
New York, New York

FOREWORD

This book is overdue; it will undoubtedly contribute importantly to the treatment of voice disorders. Many who will read *Voice Therapy: Clinical Studies* and study it are already familiar with the field of speech and language pathology and know that one major division of the field is directed toward the management of voice disorders. Traditionally, introductory texts are obligated to survey the many communication disorders and are consequently limited in the depth of treatment of each, including voice disorders. The basic books usually classify deviant voices and briefly describe diseases, structural abnormalities, emotional problems, and behavioral variations that cause the vocal disorders. These texts also customarily recommend general remedial measures for recognized voice problems; however, the authors of those books never intended their limited presentations to prepare the speech clinician, or speech pathologist, to manage remedial programs expertly. Furthermore, even after advanced study, many clinicians find themselves unprepared to handle voice problems. They usually understand much about voice production and deviations, but they express weakness where it counts: at the patient or client level, and in proceeding with the actual therapy. For example, they are apt to be unprepared to assist the teacher who has developed vocal nodules, how to guide a remedial program for a businessman who has hoarseness and a chronic laryngitis, how to help a child with a hoarse voice, or how to refer and guide a minister with spasmodic dysphonia. This simply means that many of the advanced students and practicing speech pathologists have not received sufficient training in the most important and difficult phase of our work, the application of remedial procedures that enable a specific patient (or client, if you prefer) to alleviate problems and develop a satisfactory voice.

This book confronts the fundamental problem squarely. It is a type of casebook in which 25 experienced speech pathologists, teachers of voice, and medical doctors, individually and in cooperation, present detailed reports of how they managed some of their cases. Remedial programs are described explicitly and therapeutic principles are illustrated realistically. There is great diversity in methodology, which demonstrates that there can be many effective approaches to similar types of voice problems. Nine experts in the management of hyperfunctional voice problems present illustrative cases, five individually describe their management of hypofunctional voice and resonation disorders, three reveal how they manage functional voice problems in patients, three describe how they manage spasmodic dysphonia, and four detail their management of the disorders of the professional voice. The major author and editor initially points the way and later analyzes and summarizes the offerings.

It is refreshing to note the acknowledgement that not all remedial programs restore voices to normal; realistic limitations and expectations are discussed and clinical mistakes, as well as remarkable restorations, are described. The case presentations provide useful methods and insights, but not recipes. Each vocal problem is unique and the therapy is designed for the individual patient (or client). Persons who have the privilege of managing remedial programs for voice disorders will find guidance and inspiration in this book.

G. PAUL MOORE, PH.D.
Distinguished Service Professor Emeritus
Institute for Advanced Study of the
Communication Processes
Gainesville, Florida

PREFACE

Our knowledge and understanding of clinical voice disorders has taken a giant leap in the last ten years. Indeed, the science of voice production as well as the evaluation and management of its disorders has become a formidable specialty within the professions of speech pathology and otolaryngology. One of the most exciting aspects of this development has been the encouragement of the interdisciplinary team approach to the care of patients with voice disorders. The *basic scientist* has greatly advanced our techniques for objectively evaluating voice production, which aids in planning appropriate management approaches. *Laryngologists* are concerned with the medical management of voice disorders and utilize appropriate surgeries and pharmacological treatments to aid the voice-disordered patient. *Voice pathologists* are concerned with discovering the causes of the voice problem and eliminating and modifying these causes to improve overall voice production. Finally, other specialists such as *vocal coaches* and *singing instructors* are concerned with maximizing use of the performance voice. *Voice laboratories* developed within the past several years utilize many or all of these professionals in a multidisciplinary team approach for management of clinical voice disorders.

As the knowledge of voice production has expanded, so too have the publications dedicated to describing this knowledge. There are currently excellent texts and journals dedicated to describing the scientific understanding of voice. Other publications are presented to help prepare students to evaluate and manage clinical voice disorders. By necessity, these texts must include great quantities of didactic

information so that the student not only learns "how," but "why." To utilize a management approach without understanding the underlying basis of the approach is totally inappropriate. However, because of the breadth of material necessary, therapeutic methods that are available for the treatment of voice disorders often receive an "overview" type of treatment.

The purpose of this text is to provide the working clinician and student with a broad sampling of evaluation and management strategies culled from previous literature, current expert voice clinicians, and my own personal clinical experience. The text is meant to serve as a practical adjunct to the more didactive publications.

Utilizing the format of actual case studies, complete descriptions of diagnostic and therapeutic methods are provided for a full array of voice disorders. Chapter 1 includes information on the various philosophies of treatment. With the expansion of our knowledge of voice, different schools of thought have evolved regarding treatment designs. These philosophical orientations include symptomatic, psychogenic, etiological, physiological, and eclectic orientations. Each orientation is discussed and illustrated with a representative case study.

Chapter 2 describes various evaluation techniques utilized by voice clinicians. These techniques include the formal questionnaire, the patient interview, and subjective and objective voice analyses. The role of the evaluation process as a part of the overall management plan is also discussed.

Chapter 3 discusses treatment approaches for problems caused by laryngeal hyperadduction and provides information regarding the types of behaviors that lead to the development of common laryngeal pathologies. Management approaches illustrating various treatment philosophies are presented in case study format.

Treatment of laryngeal hypoadduction and resonation disorders are described in Chapter 4. Management of laryngeal myasthenia, bowed vocal folds, and vocal fold paralysis is presented, utilizing both direct therapy and surgical intervention. Functional and organic disturbances are also discussed, along with management suggestions.

Chapter 5 presents management approaches for various functional voice disorders. Descriptions of these disorders as well as case study presentations are aimed at making the clinician more comfortable in dealing with what are often easily remediated symptoms demonstrated by emotionally difficult individuals.

Spasmodic dysphonia has been afforded a special chapter in this text. Though the incidence of this disorder is quite low, the impact it has on those who suffer with the disorder is immeasurable. Chapter 6, therefore, is devoted to describing current knowledge of etiology and management approaches. Again, case studies are utilized to describe suggested management approaches.

Chapter 7 is devoted to the special problems of the professional voice user. It must be understood that while many of the suggestions made to individuals with voice disorders apply just as well to the professional voice user, the fact remains that most often "the show must go on!" The realities associated with this special group of voice users and various management approaches are described.

The final chapter, Chapter 8, is devoted to the pitfalls of voice therapy. What makes therapy successful or unsuccessful? This chapter attempts to suggest some answers to these questions.

The most exciting element in the preparation of this text was the support received from the individual clinical experts who graciously submitted case studies. I consider these individuals some of the most accomplished voice care professionals in practice today. They are in the clinical "trenches," see numbers of patients on a daily basis, and know through experience which management approaches work and when and how to apply treatment. I am indebted to them all and proudly offer their expertise. I am sure that you will benefit from their vast clinical experiences.

Beyond the contributors to this text, I am greatly indebted to many individuals who helped to prepare me to prepare this text. They include the late Vernon Stroud, who piqued my interest in voice disorders when I was a student at the University of Cincinnati; my old friends Bob Peppard, Linda Lee, and Gordon Blood, who have constantly reinforced my own professional goals; my partners and colleagues in both the Dayton and Cincinnati voice laboratories; and Diane Bless, whom I consider to be a long-distance mentor, who more than anyone, has helped me to bridge the science to the art, which is the management of voice disorders.

The actual text preparation would not have been possible without the expert assistance of David Marshall and Julie Tryboski of Mosby–Year Book. Their expert consultation, support, and encouragement are greatly appreciated. I am also indebted to Peggy Eitzen for her invaluable assistance in manuscript preparation. Finally, I wish to thank my wife, Candy, for once again living through my "writing moods." I hope that you learn as much reading this text as I learned in preparing it.

JOSEPH C. STEMPLE, PH.D.

CONTENTS

CHAPTER 1

Principles of Voice Therapy

In reviewing the literature on voice therapy of the past 60 years, one theme became apparent: the more things change, the more they appear to stay the same. The past 10 to 15 years have yielded tremendous growth in our knowledge and understanding of laryngeal anatomy and physiology. Computer models of phonation (Titze, 1981), histologic studies of the vocal folds (Kahane, 1983), and the vocal fold cover theory (Hirano, 1981) are but a few of the many advances in voice science. Further, consider the rapidly evolving ability to measure and describe normal and pathologic voice function objectively through sophisticated acoustic and aerodynamic instrumentation. Through all of these scientific advancements, however, the principles of voice therapy have remained basically the same.

The historical sameness of voice therapy techniques is not an indictment of present-day voice therapy. It is, rather, a statement of strong appreciation and admiration for the scientists and clinicians of earlier days. The accuracy of their empirical observations regarding voice function has proved to be uncanny. Though many traditional voice therapy techniques are now being tested with computerized instrumentation, the ultimate proof of the worthiness of these techniques has been well established by the clinical results of skilled voice pathologists.

The major difference in voice therapy today compared with even 10 to 15 years ago, is the ability to diagnose a problem more quickly and accurately and to confirm the efficacy of our management approaches through objective measures. These objective measures may also be utilized as patient feedback during the therapeutic process. While our management approaches have remained rather constant, voice therapy has truly become a blend of "art" with "science."

The artistic nature of voice therapy is dependent on the human interaction skills of the clinician. Compassion, understanding, empathy, and projection of credibility, together with listening, counseling, and motivational skills are essential attributes of the successful voice clinician. Philosophically we might give this description of the artistic nature of voice:

- When considering the voice, we must consider the whole person.
- To examine a voice disorder is to examine that unique individual.
- The way that individual feels, both physically and emotionally, may be directly reflected in the voice.
- To remediate a voice disorder, we must have the skills to counsel and motivate and to remember that the voice is a mirror of the soul (Murphy, 1964; Aronson, 1990; Stemple, 1984; Stemple and Holcomb, 1989).

The scientific nature of voice therapy involves the clinician's knowledge of several important areas of study. These areas include the anatomy and physiology of normal and pathologic voice production; the nuances of laryngeal pathologic conditions; the acoustics and aerodynamics of voice production; and the etiologic correlates of voice disorders, including patient behaviors, medical causes, and psychological contributions.

- When considering the voice, we are considering the most widely used instrument on earth.
- To understand a voice disorder, we must understand the instrument's physical structure and functional components.
- We must have the skills to measure these components objectively and to relate these measures to our management choices.
- In addition, we must possess a broad knowledge of the common causes of voice disorders and the nuances of laryngeal pathologic conditions (Murphy, 1964; Stemple, 1984).

The successful voice clinician will combine attributes of the artistic approaches toward voice therapy with the objective scientific bases to identify the problem and then to plan and carry out appropriate management strategies. However, possession of a solid base of didactic information cannot replace experience. Experience continues to teach even the masters. It is hoped that the experiences of others provided in this text will prove helpful in the development of superior voice clinicians.

HISTORICAL PERSPECTIVE

In examining the evolution of the treatment of voice disorders, we find that it was not until around 1930 that a few laryngologists, singing teachers, instructors in the speech arts, and a fledgling group of speech correctionists became interested in retraining individuals with voice disorders. This group used drills and exercises borrowed from voice and diction manuals designed for the normal voice in attempts to modify disordered voice production. Many of these rehabilitation techniques were and remain creative and effective, but were not necessarily based on scientific principles. Indeed, the "artistic" portion of voice treatment was the strong point of the early clinician.

Out of this artistic mix came the general treatment suggestions of (1) ear training, (2) breathing exercises, (3) relaxation training, (4) articulatory compensations, (5) emotional retraining, and (5) special drills for cleft palate and velopharyngeal insufficiency (West et al., 1937; Van Riper, 1939). These treatment suggestions became the foundation of vocal rehabilitation.

From the early foundation of voice rehabilitation have arisen several general management philosophies. These philosophical orientations are based primarily on the clinician's mindset regarding the voice disorder which directs the management focus. For the sake of discussion, we will classify these philosophies as

- Symptomatic voice therapy
- Psychogenic voice therapy
- Etiologic voice therapy
- Physiologic voice therapy
- Eclectic voice therapy.

In short, symptomatic voice therapy focuses on modification of the deviant vocal symptoms identified by the voice pathologist — such as breathiness, low pitch, glottal attacks, and so on. The focus of psychogenic voice therapy is on the emotional and psychosocial status of the patient which led to and maintained the voice disorder. Etiologic voice therapy concentrates on discovering the causes of the voice disorder and modification/elimination of these causes. The physiologic orientation of voice therapy focuses on directly modifying and improving the balance of laryngeal muscle effort to the supportive airflow as well as the correct focus of the laryngeal tone. Finally, the eclectic approach to voice therapy is the combination of any and all of the previous voice therapy orientations. Indeed, none of these philosophic orientations is pure. Much overlap is present, often leading, of course, to the use of eclectic voice therapy. With this in mind, let us examine the philosophies of voice therapy in greater detail.

SYMPTOMATIC VOICE THERAPY

The term symptomatic voice therapy was introduced by Daniel Boone (1971). This voice management approach was based on the premise that most voice disorders are caused by the functional misuse or abuse of the voice components including pitch, loudness, respiration, and so on. Once identified, the misuses were eliminated or reduced through various voice therapy **facilitating** techniques.

In the voice clinician's attempt to aid the patient in finding and using his best voice production, it is necessary to probe continually within the patient's existing repertoire to find that one voice which sounds "good" and which he is able to produce with relatively little effort. A **voice therapy facilitating technique** is that technique which, when used by a particular patient, enables him easily to produce a good voice. Once discovered, the facilitating technique and resulting phonation become the symptomatic focus of therapy. . . . This use of a facilitating technique to produce a good phonation is the core of what we do in symptomatic voice therapy for the reduction of hyperfunctional voice disorders. (Boone, 1971, p. 11)

Boone's (1971) original facilitating approaches included

1. Altering tongue position.
2. Change of loudness.
3. Chewing exercises.
4. Digital manipulation.
5. Ear training.
6. Elimination of abuses.
7. Elimination of hard glottal attack.
8. Establish new pitch.
9. Explanation of problem.
10. Feedback.
11. Hierarchy analysis.
12. Negative practice.
13. Open mouth exercises.
14. Pitch inflections.
15. Pushing approach.
16. Relaxation.
17. Respiration training.
18. Target voice models.
19. Voice rest.
20. Yawn-sigh approach.

Many, if not all of these facilitators remain useful and popular in the treatment of voice disorders and are described in greater detail later in this text.

The main focus of symptomatic voice therapy is direct modification of the vocal symptoms. For example, if a patient presents with a voice quality characterized by low pitch, breathiness, and hard glottal attacks, then the main focus of therapy is to directly modify these symptoms. The facilitating approaches used to modify these symptoms might include items 9, 5, 8, 7, and 17 (as listed above). The voice therapist constantly probes for the "best" voice and then attempts to stabilize that voice with the various appropriate facilitating techniques. Symptomatic voice therapy assumes voice improvement through direct symptom modification.

PSYCHOGENIC VOICE THERAPY

Early in the study of voice disorders, the relationship of emotions to voice production was well recognized. As early as the mid-1800s, journal articles discussed hysteric aphonia (Russell, 1864; Ward, 1877; Goss, 1878). West et al. (1937) and Van Riper (1939) discussed the need for emotional retraining in voice therapy. Murphy (1964) presented an excellent discussion of the psychodynamics of voice. Freidrich Brodnitz (1971) was, as an otolaryngologist, uniquely sensitive to the relationship of emotions to voice. These early readings are most interesting and remain very informative for those treating voice disorders.

Our understanding of psychogenic voice therapy was further expanded by Aronson (1990), Case (1984), Stemple (1984), and Colton and Casper (1990). These authors discuss the need for determining the emotional dynamics of the voice disturbance. Psychogenic voice therapy focuses on identification and modification of the emotional and psychosocial disturbances associated with the onset and maintenance of the voice problem. Pure psychogenic voice therapy is based on the assumption of underlying emotional causes. Voice clinicians, therefore, must develop and possess superior interview skills, counseling skills, and the skill to know when the emotional/psychosocial problem is beyond the realm of their skills. A referral system of support professionals must be readily available.

ETIOLOGIC VOICE THERAPY

Etiologic voice therapy is based on the premise that identification and modification/elimination of the causes of the voice disturbance, should be the primary focus of therapy

(Stemple, 1984). Much effort is focused on identifying the direct causes of the voice disorder. The voice clinician must, therefore, understand the many etiologic factors contributing to voice disorders, including abuse/misuse, medically related causes, and personality related causes. The therapist must understand laryngeal anatomy and physiology as well as the causes and symptoms of the common laryngeal disorders. Etiologic voice therapy, through systematic information gathering during the initial patient interview, determines whether the precipitating causes are still a consideration for maintaining the voice problem. If so, the cause is modified or eliminated. If the precipitating cause is no longer a factor, the maintenance causes are identified and then modified.

Once the etiologic factors are treated, the vocal symptoms often improve without direct voice manipulations. Direct symptom modification is a secondary consideration. For example, we may expect that various laryngeal disorders will cause specific vocal symptoms. Vocal nodules may cause breathiness, pitch modification, and laryngeal/neck tension. Utilizing an etiologic approach, therapy would focus on identifying and modifying/eliminating the abuses that caused the vocal symptoms. Therapy would not focus directly on the symptoms. Therefore, facilitating techniques for pitch modification, muscle tension, and breathiness would not be chosen as the first line of management. However, should the inappropriate use of pitch, laryngeal muscle posture, and so on be identified as the primary causes of the voice disorder, then direct symptom modification would be deemed necessary.

Etiologic voice therapy presumes that every voice disorder has a cause. If that cause can be identified and modified/eliminated, then the voice quality should improve.

PHYSIOLOGIC VOICE THERAPY

The ability to measure the acoustics and aerodynamics of vocal function objectively, together with the ability to observe the vocal fold vibratory patterns through stroboscopy, has given rise to a management approach we will call physiologic voice therapy. Physiologic voice therapy utilizes objective data regarding the patient's laryngeal function to directly modify the function of the laryngeal musculature and the respiratory support of voice production. Normal voicing is dependent on a dynamic balance of airflow through the vocal folds and the muscular activities and adjustments of both the intrinsic and extrinsic laryngeal musculature. Any disturbance in the balance will lead to a vocal symptom. These disturbances may be in laryngeal muscle strength, tone, mass, stiffness, flexibility, and approximation. Disturbances may also manifest in respiratory volume, power, pressure, and flow. The overall causes of these disturbances may be mechanical, neurologic, or psychological. Whatever the cause, the management approach is direct modification of the inappropriate physiologic activity through direct exercise and manipulation.

For many years, this author has been interested in voice therapy techniques involving direct exercise or physical manipulation of the laryngeal musculature. The laryngeal musculature is similar to other muscle systems in the body; it may become strained, weakened, and imbalanced in its function as a result of the mechanical, psychological, or neurologic disturbances previously mentioned. Various direct exercises such as glottal attack exercises, dynamic range exercises, and digital manipulation (all described in later case studies) have been used to modify laryngeal muscle activity directly. While addressing closure, adductory strength, and laryngeal muscle tension problems, these exercises neglected the role of airflow as related to the muscular activity. A physiologic voice therapy program we call **Vocal Function Exercise** that addresses the problems of both airflow and laryngeal muscle strength and tone is introduced later in this chapter. As you can see, physiologic voice therapy presumes that a measurable voice disturbance is present which can be directly modified and monitored through physical exercise of the laryngeal and respiratory systems.

ECLECTIC VOICE THERAPY

Only the narrow-minded, less experienced, or foolish voice therapist would adhere to one philosophic orientation toward voice therapy.

Indeed, successful voice therapy depends on utilization of any approach that happens to work for the therapist and the individual patient. The more management approaches understood and mastered by the clinician, the greater the likelihood for success. Management techniques that prove successful for one patient may not be successful for a similar patient. The clinician, therefore, must possess the knowledge to adjust the management approach.

On the other hand, some techniques that work well for one therapist may prove to be difficult for another. In whatever management approach you choose, you must have supreme confidence in your understanding of the technique and your ability to make that approach work successfully. Your confidence will determine the success or failure of therapy. Utilizing a typical case, let us examine how each therapy orientation might be used to treat the vocal difficulties of this composite patient.

CASE STUDY: PATIENT A

Patient A, a 52-year-old woman, was referred by her laryngologist to the voice center for postsurgical evaluation and treatment. Large bilateral draping polyps were first identified by an anesthesiologist while intubating the patient for a laminectomy 6 months prior to her voice evaluation. Because of the large polyps, intubation had been difficult. The problem was reported to her family physician, who in turn referred the patient for a laryngological examination.

Indirect laryngoscopy revealed bilateral polypoid degeneration, worse on the left than the right. Audible inspiratory stridor was noted by the physician, and patient A reported shortness of breath during even limited physical exertion. Two surgeries were therefore scheduled 6 weeks apart for aspiration of fluid and laser vaporization of redundant tissue. The surgeries were performed without complication, and the patient was seen for voice evaluation 5 weeks after the second surgery.

History of the Problem

The patient reported that she had always had a "deep" voice, which had lowered even more over the past several years. Her presurgical voice quality, however, had not been a concern to her. Rather, the shortness of breath led her to agree to surgery. She reported that voice quality following the first surgery (left fold) was a little "hazy" but returned to "normal" within 1 week. The second surgery left her with significant, bothersome hoarseness that made her "wish I had never had surgery."

Medical History

The patient reported undergoing two previous surgeries: removal of her gallbladder 10 years earlier, and the laminectomy performed earlier this year. Even with the difficult intubation and the risks inherent in laminectomy, her presurgical voice quality was maintained. In addition to surgeries, she had been hospitalized 3 years previously for 3 weeks and treated for chronic depression.

Chronic medical disorders included frequent upper respiratory infections, including bronchitis; high blood pressure; circulatory problems in her legs; elevated blood sugar, and chronic neck and back pain. Daily medications were taken for blood pressure, chronic pain, depression, and sleep. She continued a 30-year history of smoking 1½ to 2 packs of cigarettes per day. Her liquid intake consisted mostly of five to six cups of caffeinated coffee per day. Chronic throat clearing and a persistent cough were noted throughout the evaluation.

Social History

Patient A was married for 12 years to her second husband, following a first marriage of 18 years and divorce. She had two adult children from her previous marriage. Her elderly mother-in-law lived with the patient and her husband, a situation that often caused friction and conflict in her marriage. Indeed, she was not shy in reporting her unhappiness with her marital relationship. This unhappiness was said to be a major factor in her history of depression.

Both the patient and her husband were employed by the local automobile assembly plant. She had worked as an assembler for 14 years in an environment described as "noisy, dusty, and full of fumes," and was on a temporary medical disability because her back problems precluded her working in the plant. Present activities included shopping with her daughter, talking on the telephone, caring for her home (back permitting), watching daytime television "talk" shows, and bowling two nights per week in two different leagues. The latter activity appeared somewhat inconsistent with her report of current back problems.

Vocal Evaluation

Perceptually, the patient's voice quality was described as moderately dysphonic—characterized by low pitch, inappropriate loudness, strained raspiness, and intermittent glottal fry phonation. Acoustic and aerodynamic analyses revealed the following:

- Fundamental frequency = 150 Hz
- Frequency range = 118 to 290 Hz
- Jitter: vowels $\overline{X}$ = 1.18 Hz; conversation = 3.67 Hz
- Intensity (habitual) = 76 dB
- Air flow volume = 2,300 mL H_2O
- Air flow rate = < 80 mL H_2O/sec, all pitch levels
- Phonation time = < 12 seconds, all pitch levels.

Laryngeal videostroboscopic observation revealed mild to moderate bilateral vocal fold edema and erythema. Glottic closure demonstrated an irregular glottal chink with a moderate ventricular fold compression. The edges of the vocal folds were rough and irregular, worse on the left than the right. The amplitude of vibration was severely decreased bilaterally. The mucosal waves were barely perceptible. The closed phase of the vibratory cycle was strongly dominant, while the symmetry of vibration was generally irregular. No mass lesions, paresis, or paralysis was evident. In short, the patient had an edematous, stiff, hyperfunctioning vocal fold system.

Impressions

Patient A presented with a voice disorder which derived from the following possible causal factors:

- Cigarette smoking
- Harsh employment environment
- Talking over noise at work
- Large caffeine intake
- Frequent upper respiratory infections
- Prescription medications
- Coughing and throat clearing
- Emotional instability
- Talking too loudly (suggesting possible hearing loss, which later proved not to be present)
- Using a low pitch
- Laryngeal muscle tension.

Recommendations

Symptomatic Voice Therapy

General focus would use facilitating techniques to

1. Raise pitch
2. Reduce loudness
3. Reduce laryngeal area tension and effort.

This direct symptom modification would follow an explanation of the problem and would run concurrently with modification of vocally abusive behaviors, including

1. Smoking
2. Caffeine intake
3. Coughing and throat clearing.

Psychogenic Voice Therapy

General focus would explore the psychodynamics of the voice disorder. Techniques would include

1. Detailed interview with the patient to determine the cause and effects of depression
2. Determination of the relationship of emotional problems and voice problem
3. Counseling the patient regarding the effects of emotions on voice production
4. Reduction of the musculoskeletal tension caused by emotional upheaval
5. Referral for marital counseling as deemed appropriate.

Secondary focus would deal with modification/elimination of the abusive behaviors including

1. Smoking
2. Caffeine and medications
3. Coughing and throat clearing.

Inappropriate use of pitch and loudness would most likely be viewed as obvious symptoms of the problem. These symptoms would likely improve as the psychodynamics were improved.

Etiologic Voice Therapy

The general focus would be to identify the primary and secondary causes of the voice disorder and then to modify or eliminate these causes. The primary etiologic correlates would include

1. Smoking
2. Laryngeal dehydration from caffeine and drugs
3. Voice abuse, such as coughing, throat clearing, and talking loudly over noise at work.

Secondary precipitating factors that result from the pathologic condition include

1. Laryngeal area muscle tension and hyperfunction due to stiffness
2. Low pitch due to increased mass
3. Increased loudness due to effort to force stiff vocal folds to vibrate.

Therapy would focus on modification or elimination of the primary causes. The patient would be aided in her attempt to stop smoking, encouraged to begin a hydration program, and given vocal hygiene counseling to aid in elimination or reduction of vocally abusive behaviors. The secondary causes would most likely spontaneously improve as the primary causes were modified and the vocal fold condition improved.

Physiologic Voice Therapy

The general focus would be in evaluating the present physiologic condition of the patient's voice production and developing direct physical exercises to improve that condition. The patient had presented with extreme laryngeal tension. Irregular vocal fold edges caused a glottal chink. In addition, her vocal folds were extremely stiff both in muscular amplitude and mucosal tissue wave.

Normal voicing is dependent on near total closure of the vocal folds, permitting air pressure to build below the folds. As the pressure builds, it eventually overcomes the resistance of the approximated folds, permitting the release of one puff of air. As the air rushes between the vocal folds, the Bernoullli effect, together with the static position of the folds, draws them back together, completing one vibratory cycle. Air gaps, or glottal chinks, change the physical dynamics of vocal fold vibration, requiring a greater buildup of air pressure. Patients such as this woman often make physical adjustments in an attempt to push out the "best voice" by hyperfunctioning the supraglottic structures. Add vocal fold muscular and mucosal stiffness to this mix and the patient presents with a significant vocal hyperfunction with associated respiratory abnormalities. This patient's hyperfunctional laryngeal activity had decreased her airflow rate to abnormally low levels.

Direct physiologic voice therapy would focus on Vocal Function Exercises for restrengthening and balancing the laryngeal musculature, improving vocal fold flexibility and movement, and rebalancing airflow to muscular activity. The techniques chosen to treat these problems would be digital massage (see Chapter 4) and vocal function exercises. A rather simple, four-part exercise program described by Barnes (1977) and modified by Stemple (1984) was used to accomplish the latter task. The following explanation was stated to the patient.

"The vocal fold system is very similar to other muscle systems in the body. It may become strained, weakened, stiff and imbalanced in its function. Indeed, we might say that it is very similar to your knee. Just like your knee, the voice box, or larynx, is made of many muscles, cartilages, and connective tissues.

"When the knee is injured, it often requires surgery or physical therapy, or both. When surgery is required, the knee is immobilized to permit swelling to subside. Limited activity is then permitted followed by vigorous directed physical therapy with the purpose of restrengthening and balancing the muscles above, below, behind, and beside the knee to again make it a solid joint system.

"The vocal fold system, after injury or surgery, requires similar "physical therapy." Following surgery, the patient is placed on a brief voice rest to permit acute healing to take place. Direct exercises, similar to physical therapy, are then required to restrengthen, to balance, and to return flexibility to the laryngeal musculature.

"Just walking does not systematically work out all the muscles of the knee. Healing will therefore most likely not be complete. Just talking does not work out all the laryngeal muscles, thus the voice disturbance may persist. Direct, systematic laryngeal muscle exercise is required."

Vocal Function Exercises involve four parts: a warm-up, stretching exercises, contracting exercises, and a power exercise. They require the use of a C-scale pitch pipe or keyboard and a stopwatch. The exercises are as follows:

1. **Warm-up.** Sustain the musical note F (above middle C for a woman or child; F below middle C for a man) for as long as possible on the vowel "E." The goal = _____ seconds. The amount of time depends on patient's airflow volume, which is calculated as follows:

Flow volume, mL H_2O/100 mL H_2O = _____ seconds

2. **Stretching:** Glide from your very lowest note to your very highest note on the vowel "O." The goal is to perform the exercise without voice breaks. (Continue the exercise even if the voice does break. The vocal folds will continue to lengthen in the absence of phonation.)

3. **Contraction.** Glide from your very highest note to your very lowest note on the vowel "O," again without voice breaks. (Do not permit the voice to fry or growl on the lower end.)

4. **Adductory Power Exercises.** Sustain the musical notes middle C–D–E–F–G (for a woman or child; one octave lower for a man) for as long as possible on the vowel "O." The goal is the same as 1.

Each exercise should be done twice in a row, two times per day, (preferably in the morning and evening). All exercises are to be done as softly as possible, increasing the muscular and respiratory effort and control to maintain phonation. The patient is taught to utilize extreme frontal focus and easy onsets of the "E" and "O" vowels, thus decreasing laryngeal muscle tension and impact. Progress may be plotted by keeping track of phonation times. Adjustments are made in the musical notes used (up or down) as dictated by the pathologic voice range.

Patient A presented with extreme stiffness and vocal hyperfunction. Her airflow rates were all very low, yet she could only sustain for a maximum of 12 seconds. Her goal for exercises 1 and 4 was 26 seconds based on 2,600 mL H_2O divided by 100 mL H_2O. The musical range had to be adjusted down by two notes for her deeper voice.

Vocal function exercises appear to be effective because

1. Patients readily understand the concept of physical exercise
2. Exercise is systematic and permits plotting of progress
3. Patients must "think" of voice at least twice daily
4. Exercises improve phonation time and pitch range
5. Exercises improve voice quality.

Clinically, vocal function exercises are a means of breaking the hyperfunctional cycle and helps to focus the laryngeal tone to optimize more efficient conversion of aerodynamic power to acoustic power. In addition, the exercises appear to train a more appropriate (minimum) subglottic air pressure necessary to drive the vocal folds.

Eclectic Voice Therapy

Hopefully in our review of the philosophic orientations of voice therapy you have seen the various strengths of each management orientation as well as the folly of subscribing to any one philosophy. The patient described, or any patient, will be best treated by a therapist with knowledge and understanding of all possible management strategies and alternatives. As you read and study the many case presentations of this text, it is helpful to evaluate the philosophy behind the treatment approach as a means of better understanding the reasons for the approach. But the successful voice pathologist is an artistic scientist with an eclectic point of view. Therapy for patient A should focus on

1. Symptom modification
2. Elimination of causes
3. Attention to the psychodynamics of the problem
4. Direct vocal function exercise.

Voice Care

Thus far we have discussed the treatment of voice disorders in terms of direct voice therapy. Voice care, however, is a shared province, with contributions from the primary care physician, laryngologist, neurologist, speech pathologist, psychologist, vocal coach, singing instructor, and others. Case studies presented in all chapters of this text describe the unique, complimentary relationships of each of these professionals with their patients.

REFERENCES

Aronson A: *Clinical voice disorders*, ed 3, New York, 1990, Thieme.

Barnes J: Briess exercises, Workshop presented for the Southwestern Ohio Speech and Hearing Association, Cincinnati, 1977.

Boone D: *The voice and voice therapy*, Englewood Cliffs, N.J., 1971, Prentice-Hall.

Brodnitz F: *Vocal rehabilitation*, Rochester, NY, 1971, American Academy of Ophthalmalogy and Otolaryngology.

Case J: *Clinical management of voice disorders*, Rockville, Md, 1984, Aspen.

Colton R, Casper J: *Understanding voice problems*, Baltimore, 1990, Williams & Wilkins.

Goss F: Hysterical aphonia. *Boston Med Surg J* 99:215–222, 1878.

Hirano M: *Clinical examination of voice*, Vienna, 1981, Springer-Verlag.

Kahane J: Postnatal development and aging of the human larynx. *Semin Speech Lang* 4:189–204, 1983.

Murphy A: *Functional voice disorders*, Englewood Cliffs, N.J., 1964, Prentice-Hall.

Russell J: A case of hysterical aphonia. *Br Med J* 8:619–621, 1864.

Stemple J: *Clinical voice pathology*, Columbus, Ohio, 1984, Merrill.

Stemple J, Holcomb B: *Effective voice and articulation*, Columbus, Ohio, 1989, Merrill.

Titze I: The role of computational simulation in evaluation of physical problems of the vocal folds. In Stevens K, Hirano M, editors: *Vocal fold physiology*, Tokyo, 1981, University of Tokyo Press.

Van Riper C: *Speech correction principles and methods*, Englewood Cliffs, N.J., 1939, Prentice-Hall.

Ward W: Hysterical aphonia. *Chicago Med J Examiner* 34:495–505, 1877.

West R, Kennedy L, Carr A: *The rehabilitation of speech*, New York, 1937, Harper and Brothers.

CHAPTER 2

Voice Evaluation

Perhaps the most significant change in the treatment of voice disorders has been in the evaluation techniques utilized to describe and diagnose the disorder objectively. Traditional components of the voice evaluation have included medical examination to diagnose the disorder, systematic interviewing of the patient to determine causes, and subjective voice evaluation to describe the vocal symptoms. Now, added to these components is the ability to measure various aspects of voice production objectively and to describe in detail the actual vibratory pattern of the vocal folds. The usefulness of objective descriptions of voice production cannot be denied. To date, objective measures cannot provide a diagnosis and should not be utilized for this purpose. However, acoustic and aerodynamic measures of voice production along with observation of vocal fold vibration through laryngeal videostroboscopy will provide

1. Understanding of the perceptual symptoms
2. A means of systematically describing the vocal condition
3. Pretreatment and posttreatment measures utilized to describe the efficacy of treatment
4. Patient education and feedback.

Many of the case studies presented in this text utilize objective measures of voice production. Indeed, new standards for treatment of voice disorders which are currently being debated will most likely include objective measures for evaluation.

While objective measures are an important adjunct to the traditional components of voice evaluation, these measures are not meant to replace any other component. The physician's eye and clinician's ear cannot be replaced. The most important aspect of the diagnostic voice evaluation is the ability to talk to one's patients: to conduct a patient interview that will yield the necessary diagnostic information. If only one evaluation component were available to me, the patient interview would be my choice.

The primary objective of the diagnostic voice evaluation is to discover etiologic factors specific to the development of the voice disorder. Voice pathologists will use all of their artistic and scientific skills in a systematic evaluation to determine these specific causes. In addition, a detailed analysis of the vocal symptoms, both subjective and objective, will be completed. A systematic management approach will then be devised.

Secondary objectives of the diagnostic evaluation include education and motivation of the patient and the establishment of credibility and trust in the voice pathologist. Most patients have very little knowledge or understanding of the normal voice, to say nothing of their own voice disorders. During the voice evaluation, the voice pathologist will find it useful to explain, in simple terms, normal voicing and how it relates to the patient's current problem. Videostroboscopy, when available, is invaluable as a patient educator and often encourages the patient to become a partner in his or her own care. The more patients understand their voice disorders, the more helpful they will be in answering questions designed to discover the causes of their voice disorders. The well-informed patient will also generally be more highly motivated to follow a regimen to resolve the disorder.

It is also essential that the credibility of the voice pathologist be established early during the evaluation. Many probing questions regarding the patient's personal life must be asked in seeking etiologic factors. It is essential that patients trust the voice pathologist's intent to utilize this information appropriately. Credibility and trust may be developed at the initial patient contact by the voice pathologist who projects a casual yet confident and professional demeanor. This type of relaxed demeanor will reduce anxieties and will establish an atmosphere for easy discussion.

Once the primary etiologic factors are discovered, the vocal symptoms are subjectively and objectively described, the patient has been educated, and the clinician has established credibility, the management plan may then be outlined. When patients understand the causes of the problem and are presented with a systematic management approach, along with a reasonable estimated time for completion, a positive therapeutic attitude is usually developed.

MANAGEMENT TEAM

Evaluation and management of patients with voice disorders have increasingly been accomplished through the teamwork of several professionals. These include the laryngologist and voice pathologist as well as the vocal and/ or singing teacher or coach when required. The laryngologist is trained to examine the laryngeal mechanism and to determine the need for medical, surgical, or referral intervention. The voice pathologist is trained to identify the causes of voice disorders, evaluate the vocal symptoms, and establish improved vocal function through various therapeutic methods. The vocal coach or singing instructor evaluates the efficacy and correctness of performance technique and suggests modifications as deemed necessary. This complementary professional relationship has significantly improved the care of the voice-disordered population.

MEDICAL EVALUATION

A laryngologic examination involves examination of the entire head and neck region as well as a detailed medical history. The examination includes ostoscopic examination of the ears; examination of the oral and nasal cavities; palpation of the salivary glands, lymph nodes, and thyroid gland; and a visual examination of the larynx. The visual examination of the larynx may be performed in the office utilizing indirect mirror observation, a fiber-optic nasal endoscope, or a rigid oral endoscope. The fiber-optic or rigid scopes may be attached to a video camera, permitting the vocal folds to be viewed on a video screen. A laryngeal stroboscope may also be utilized with the video equipment and endoscopes to provide a simulated, slow-motion view of vocal fold vibration.

The vocal folds may also be viewed directly through direct laryngoscopy. During this surgical procedure, the patient receives general anesthesia and a magnifying laryngoscope is placed into the oral cavity and pharynx, yielding a direct view of the larynx. Biopsies and surgical excisions may also be performed through the laryngoscope.

The medical examination may also include special radiographs of the head and neck as well as blood and swallow studies. The final result of the medical examination is a diagnosis of the problem and recommendations for treatment including medical, surgical, voice evaluation and therapy, or any combination thereof.

VOICE PATHOLOGY EVALUATION

When referral is made for a diagnostic voice evaluation, the three major objectives of the voice pathologist are to (1) identify the causes of the disorder, (2) describe the present vocal components, and (3) develop an individualized management plan. Various methods have been utilized to identify the causes of voice disorders. These methods include the formal interview with the patient and a predeveloped case history form to be completed either by the patient or by the patient and clinician. This author finds prepared forms to be restrictive and prefers to use the patient interview format.

Beginning clinicians, however, may find prepared questionnaires useful.

The following interview procedure (as described in Stemple, 1984) describes specific goals for each component of the patient interview as well as pertinent areas of investigation.

Referral

The goal is to establish the referral source, because the referral source should be clearly understood at the beginning of the evaluation. The major referral source will be the otolaryngologist. Referrals may also come from other speech pathologists, or the patient's relatives and friends, or the patient may be self-referred.

Reason for the Referral

The goals are to (1) establish the exact reasons for patient referral, (2) establish patient understanding of the referral, (3) develop the patient's knowledge of his or her voice disorder, and (4) establish the credibility of examiner.

It is important to have adequate information regarding the exact reason the patient was referred. When the patient is referred by a physician, the specific medical diagnosis should be reported along with the physician's expectations. There are many reasons for patient referrals. These may include simply preoperative objective measures of voice, evaluation without management, baseline description of present voice, preoperative trial therapy, postoperative follow-up therapy, or a complete diagnostic voice evaluation with appropriate vocal management. Understanding the physician's expectations will avoid confusion and will help to maintain the necessary working relationships.

It is also desirable at this time to establish the patient's understanding of the referral for "speech therapy." A typical dialogue between a patient (PT) and voice pathologist (VP) might be:

> **VP:** "Do you understand why the doctor referred you here?"
> **PT:** "Not really. The doctor just said I needed speech therapy, but I really don't understand what it is all

about. My speech is OK; I'm just hoarse."

This is an excellent opportunity for the voice pathologist to explain in some detail the three major goals he or she intends to accomplish during the evaluation. The more that patients understand the procedures, the more reliable they will be in communicating pertinent information to the clinician throughout the evaluation.

It is also helpful to establish and develop the patient's knowledge of the voice disorder before proceeding. This may be accomplished by explaining briefly how the normal laryngeal mechanism works and how it is affected by the disorder. With this information, patients will better understand where certain questions are leading and may be able to give more reliable information. Some patients even volunteer pertinent information following this discussion and before questions are asked. For example:

> **VP:** "Do you understand what vocal nodules are?"
> **PT:** "They're some kind of growths on my vocal cords, aren't they?"
> **VP:** "Something like that. Do you know what your vocal cords look like?"
> **PT:** "No not really."
> **VP:** "Well, when the doctor looked down your throat with his mirror, he was essentially looking at two solid shelves of muscle tissue, one on each side. (Draw a diagram or show pictures, or use a video.) Those shelves are the vocal folds, or cords, and we're looking down on top of them. The point here where they meet is your Adam's apple. Can you feel yours? (Gives patient spatial orientation.) Now, the space between the vocal folds is the airway when air travels to the lungs as we breathe.
>
> "Attached to the back of each vocal fold we have two cartilages: one here, and one here. The reason we have these cartilages is so that other muscles that work the vocal folds may have a place

on which to attach. Some muscles separate the folds while other muscles draw them together. This is certainly a simplified explanation, but I think it will give you the basic idea of how the system works.

"To move the vocal folds together we have one muscle attached to each cartilage pulling in opposite directions. These pull the vocal folds to the middle where they vibrate, giving us our voices.

"If these muscles pull too hard, such as when we shout, talk loudly for a long time, or clear our throats, this excessive pull will cause the vocal folds to rub and bang together. (Demonstrate with clapping hands.) If this rubbing and banging is done too much, it will eventually cause some swelling of the tissues that will usually cause a temporary hoarseness. The hoarseness may go away after a day or so, but if whatever caused the swelling persists, the folds will remain swollen and will eventually begin to try to protect themselves from further damage. In your case, they've done this by developing, layer by layer, small callous-like structures, which are called vocal nodules.

"As you've experienced, the nodules cause a change in your voice. Because of the swelling and the nodules, your voice is deeper in pitch; and because the nodules are holding your folds apart when you try to vibrate them, your voice is breathy. You've also probably noticed that when you do a lot of talking your voice weakens, and it becomes quite an effort just to talk. Sometimes by the end of the day, you may be worn out from the effort, and you simply don't feel like talking anymore.

"One final point. Vocal nodules are not cancer, are not related to cancer, and do not lead to cancer. Many people do not understand this, and I think it's important to mention. So you now understand basically what the vocal folds are like and what vocal nodules are?"

PT: "Yes, now I do. I'm glad you mentioned cancer. I was worried about that. But, what do you think caused the nodules? I don't raise my voice very much."

VP: "That's what we're here today to try and find out. I'm going to ask you many questions. I need to get to know who you are and how you use your voice. From that information we will try to determine specifically what has caused your nodules. Any questions?"

It should also be noted that this type of discussion goes far in developing your credibility as an "expert" in this area. You usually will have managed to develop a high level of trust before you begin questions regarding the history of the problem.

History of the Problem

The goals are to (1) establish the chronological history of the problem, (2) seek etiologic factors associated with the history, and (3) determine patient motivation.

This section of the evaluation is designed to yield a chronological history of the voice disorder from the onset of vocal difficulties, through the development of the problem over time, and ending with the patient's present vocal experiences. All questions are designed to yield information regarding the causes for vocal difficulties. Finally, the patient's motivation for seeking vocal improvement is determined. A list of appropriate questions may include the following:

1. When did you first notice you were having some difficulties with your voice?
2. What was the first time you ever experienced vocal difficulties?

3. How did the problem progress from there?
4. What finally made you decide to see your doctor about it?
5. How did the doctor treat the problem?
6. Did your family doctor refer you to the otolaryngologist?
7. Has anyone else in your family ever had voice problems?
8. Is your voice now better in the morning than in the evening or vice versa?
9. Have you ever lost your voice totally?
10. Do you have any occasion at all to raise your voice to shout, or to talk loudly over noise?
11. Do you often talk to anyone who is hard of hearing?
12. Do you have a pet?
13. Not knowing you prior to your vocal difficulties, I don't know what your normal voice is like. If I have a scale of 1 to 5, how hoarse are you right now if 1 is normal and 5 is very hoarse?
14. How much does this problem actually bother you?
15. Are you really interested in doing something about it?

Medical History

The goals are to (1) seek medically related etiologic factors, and (2) help establish awareness of patient's basic personality.

Taking the medical history is the process of seeking out any medically related etiologic factors regarding the presenting disorder. Questions are asked regarding past surgeries and hospitalizations. Chronic disorders are probed, along with the use of medications. Smoking, alcohol, and drug use are explored. The patient's hydration habits are also discussed. The medical history also helps to establish in the clinician's mind how patients view themselves in terms of how they "feel" about their physical well-being. This may be accomplished by asking patients whether, on a day-to-day basis, they feel "excellent, good, fair, or poor." The response to this question will provide the voice pathologist with insight into how patients feel about themselves. Some patients report lengthy medical histories with many chronic disorders, but they indicate that they feel "good" on a day-to-day basis. Other patients with unremarkable medical histories may report feeling "fair" or "poor." This information is helpful in learning the basic personalities of the patients.

Social History

The goals are to (1) know the patient's work, home, and recreational environments; (2) discover emotional, social, and family difficulties; and (3) seek more etiologic factors for the disorder.

The social history finalizes in your mind who the patient is. It yields information regarding work, home, recreational and social lifestyles, and whether these lifestyles contributed to the development of laryngeal disorders. All questions probe for answers to possible etiologic factors. For example,

1. Are you married?
2. How long have you been married?
3. Do you have children? What are their ages? How many are still at home?
4. Does anyone else live in your home? Parents? Aunts? Others?
5. Do you work? Where? How long?
6. Specifically, what do you do in your work?
7. How much talking is required?
8. Does your husband/wife work? Where? How long? What shift?
9. When you're not working, what do you enjoy doing? (Include clubs, groups, hobbies, organizations, and so forth.)
10. Sometimes voice problems arise out of upsetting events. Has anything occurred that has been particularly upsetting to you recently or has caused you to have an increased amount of anxiety?

As you begin the social history questions, it is often helpful to explain to patients that you need to get to know who they are and what they do in order to find the causes for their vocal difficulties. You want the patient to "excuse" you if some of the questions seem personal. This questioning is necessary in order for you to discover all possible causes. Do not be surprised when patients open up to you with many personal, family, social, marital, or work problems. If you have developed your credibility and gained their trust, you will often be given this important information.

Oral-Peripheral Examination

The goals are to (1) determine the physical condition of oral mechanisms, (2) observe laryngeal area tension, (3) check for swallowing difficulties, and (4) check for laryngeal sensations.

A routine oral-peripheral examination should also be conducted to determine the condition of the oral mechanism in its relation to the patient's speech and voice production. Also included is observation of the patient's laryngeal area tension, utilizing visual observation of posture and neck muscle tension as well as digital manipulation of the thyroid cartilage. The patient should also be asked whether any swallowing difficulties are present to determine whether this function has been affected by or is affecting vocal production. Finally, the patient should be asked whether any laryngeal sensations are present. The laryngeal sensations most often associated with voice disorders including aching, dryness, tickling, burning, and a feeling of a "lump in the throat."

Voice Evaluation

The goals are to (1) describe the present vocal components, and (2) examine inappropriate use of the vocal components.

Following the patient interview, the subjective and objective voice evaluations are conducted. Several attempts have been made to standardize the subjective evaluation of voice (Wilson, 1987; Hirano, 1981; Laver, 1980). However, the immense variety of vocal qualities makes this task formidable.

The subjective evaluation of the voice is conducted to describe the present condition of voice production and to determine whether any vocal components such as pitch, loudness, breathiness, and so on are being utilized in a habitual inappropriate manner to the degree of contributing to the development or maintenance of the disorder. Each vocal component is examined separately following a general subjective description of voice quality.

At this point in the evaluation, the examiner has had an adequate sample of conversational speech in which to make a subjective description of the patient's voice quality. Most physicians to whom speech pathologists report patient information are not familiar with formal voice scales; thus, it is adequate for the examiner to report the degree of baseline dysphonia as mild, moderate, or severe. This description is followed, for the future reference of the examiner, by a characterization of the voice, including descriptive terms such as breathiness, glottal fry, and low pitch. The vocal components are then individually examined including:

Respiration. This includes a description of conversational breathing patterns including supportive or nonsupportive clavicular, thoracic, or diaphragmatic breathing patterns. Use of residual air is determined through observation. The s/z ratio is formally tested. Eckel and Boone (1981) demonstrated the reliability of this simple test. When no laryngeal growths are present, the ratio should be near equal. The presence of growths yields a longer voiceless /s/ than the voiced /z/ because of the inability of the folds to approximate adequately.

Phonation. Subjective observations regarding the actual opening and closing of the vocal folds are made through critical listening. These include the presence of hard glottal attacks, glottal fry, and breathiness. These may be observed conversationally throughout the evaluation. You may also recheck simply by having the patient say the ABC's slowly, while listening for specific phonatory behaviors.

Resonation. Observation regarding the type of resonance quality is made. These include normal, hypernasality, hyponasality, and cul-de-sac nasality.

Pitch. The patient's present pitch range is tested either by having the patient sing up a scale from the lowest note to the highest note or by having the patient sigh from high to low. We should remember, if such a thing as an optimum pitch existed, it could not be found in the pathologically disturbed voice. Conversational inflection and pitch variability are more important to describe.

Loudness. The appropriateness of the patient's speaking intensity level during the evaluation is described. It is also important to test the patient's ability to increase subglottic air pressure. This may be done by simply asking the patient to shout "hey." The ability to produce a more solid phonation during a shout is a good indicator of the severity of the problem. If the patient is able to override the dysphonia with increased intensity (which is determined by the ability of the folds to approximate tightly to increase subglottic air pressure), the disorder is perhaps not as severe as when the patient cannot easily increase intensity.

Rate. The rate of a patient's speech may contribute to the development of laryngeal disorder. This is especially true for the individual who speaks exceptionally quickly. During the diagnostic work-up, the rate of conversational speech is described as normal, fast, or slow.

OBJECTIVE VOICE ANALYSIS

Objective measures of voice function, sometimes called phonatory function tests or laryngeal function studies, are then conducted if the appropriate instrumentation is available. Acoustic, aerodynamic, and laryngeal videostroboscopic analyses are utilized to objectively describe vocal function. (Hirano, 1980, provides an excellent reference for these measures.) Common acoustic measures include

- Fundamental frequency
- Frequency range
- Frequency perturbation (jitter)
- Habitual intensity
- Intensity range (maximum/minimum)
- Intensity perturbation (shimmer)
- Signal-to-noise ratio.

Useful aerodynamic measures include

- Airflow volume
- Airflow rate
- Phonation time
- Subglottic air pressure
- Glottal resistance.

Laryngeal stroboscopy demonstrates a simulated, slow-motion view of the vocal fold vibration. This view provides much additional diagnostic information, including

- Configuration of glottic closure
- Amount of supraglottic activity
- Vertical level approximation of the vocal folds
- Condition of the vocal fold edge
- Amplitude of vibration
- Integrity of the mucosal wave
- Nonvibrating areas of the folds
- Symmetry of the vibratory pattern.

Impressions

The goal is to summarize the etiologic factors associated with the development and maintenance of the individual's voice disorder.

The impression section of the diagnostic procedure is utilized as a summary for the causes of the voice disorder discovered throughout the evaluation. These causes are listed in order of perceived importance as they relate first to the initiation of the problem and second to the maintenance of the problem. Remember, the precipitating factor may not be the maintenance factor.

Prognosis

The goal is to analyze the probability of improvement through voice therapy.

The prognosis for improving many voice disorders through voice therapy is generally good. However, many factors influence prognosis (see Chapter 8), including the motivation, interest, and time of the patient; ability of the patient to follow instructions; the physical and emotional conditions of the patient; and the general condition of the vocal folds. The prognosis section permits the voice pathologist to give a subjective opinion regarding the chances for successful remediation based on the diagnostic information. A reasonable time frame for expected completion of the management program should also be stated.

Recommendations

The goal is to outline the management plan. This management plan is then briefly outlined based on the etiologic factors discovered during the evaluation. The plan includes the therapy approaches to be utilized and additional referrals to be made.

ADDITIONAL CONSIDERATIONS

The evaluation format presented here may be classified as semistructured. The basic questions remain the same from patient to patient, but the answers given by individual patients dictate the direction in which the questioning will proceed and the order in which each diagnostic section is reviewed. This format favors the more experienced voice pathologist. The beginning clinician may feel the need for a more structured format. As experience is gained, the structured formats may prove limiting, and the semistructured method is often the method of choice.

Some voice pathologists also feel most comfortable tape recording the entire diagnostic session for later review. This may help in determining the exact vocal components produced during the evaluation and serves as a record of the baseline voice quality. Even if the entire diagnostic session is not recorded, recording of a standard speech sample is necessary for later comparison. It is not unusual for the voice pathologist and the patient to forget the actual severity of the baseline quality. Tape recordings serve as an objective reminder and should be used liberally.

Finally, the American Speech-Language-Hearing Association mandates that patients who undergo speech, voice, and language evaluations must have had a current hearing screening. Audiometric evaluation is important for the patient with a voice disorder. The inability to monitor voice well may result in the use of inappropriate vocal properties. Severe voice disorders are often observed in the hard-of-hearing and deaf populations.

SUMMARY

Successful voice therapy is totally dependent on an in-depth and accurate diagnostic evaluation. Indeed, this author views the voice evaluation as a primary **therapy** tool. The evaluation determines the causes for the disorder, teaches the patient about the disorder, and describes the symptoms that must be modified for vocal improvement to occur.

The remainder of this text is devoted to management techniques for voice disorders. You will realize in studying the many case presentations that selecting the appropriate treatments was dependent on the multidisciplinary evaluations of management team members. For organization purposes voice disorders are classified here as hyperfunctional, hypofunctional, resonance, functional, spasmodic dysphonia, and professional voice disorders. Much cross-over in management approaches is evident and useful for the various disorders. All successful voice therapy, however, begins with accurate diagnosis and planning through the medical examination and voice evaluation.

REFERENCES

Eckel F, Boone D: The s/z ratio as an indicator of laryngeal pathology, *J Speech Hear Disord* 46:147–149, 1981.

Hirano M: *Clinical examination of voice,* Vienna, 1981, Springer-Verlag.

Laver J: *The phonetic description of voice quality,* Cambridge, U.K., 1980, Cambridge University Press.

Stemple J: *Clinical voice pathology,* Columbus, Ohio, 1984, Merrill.

Wilson DK: *Voice problems of children,* ed 3, Baltimore, 1987, Williams & Wilkins.

CHAPTER 3

Management of Vocal Hyperfunction

MANAGEMENT APPROACHES FOR

- Vocal nodules
- Contact ulcer
- Vocal polyp
- Vocal fold edema/erythema
- Vocal abuse/misuse
- Pitch modification
- Loudness modification
- Glottal fry phonation
- Poor breath support
- Low tone focus
- Chronic throat clearing
- Vocal psychodynamics
- Laryngeal tension.

MANAGEMENT STRATEGIES, INCLUDING

- Vocal hygiene counseling
- Environmental manipulation
- Changing pitch
- Changing loudness
- Vocal function exercises
- Reduction of caffeine
- Hydration program
- Esophageal reflux treatment
- Elimination of chronic throat clearing and coughing
- Patient/parent education
- Elimination/modification of children's vocal noises
- Ear training
- Charting for behavior modification
- Teaching "how" to shout

- New psychosocial communication strategies
- Respiratory training
- Tension reduction and relaxation
- Easy phonation onset
- Frontal focus exercises
- Inflection training
- Increasing articulatory precision
- Negative practice
- Yawn/sigh approach
- Humming and chanting
- Voice time-out or recovery time
- Voice use journal
- Listening skill enhancement
- Breathy phonation
- Soft whisper
- Accent method
- Instrumental biofeedback

As described in Chapter 1, knowledge of the common causes of voice disorders is essential when planning appropriate management programs. Many voice disorders and associated laryngeal pathologic conditions are caused by hyperfunction of the laryngeal mechanism. At times, this hyperfunction is simply behavioral, causing harmful mechanical impact to the tissue lining of the vocal folds; examples include shouting, loud talking, screaming, vocal noises, coughing, throat clearing, and inappropriate singing technique. Inappropriate use of the components of voice production such as respiration, phonation, resonation, pitch, loudness, and rate may also lead to a hyperfunctional voice disorder. The direct condition of the tissue lining and underlying muscular strength of the vocal folds may also be implicated in the hyperfunctioning of the vocal mechanism. For example, a dehydrated mucous membrane lining caused by lack of adequate liquid intake, drying medications, smoking, and so on may create mild edema. The additional mass caused by the edema requires greater effort to produce voice. This increased effort may lead to vocal hyperfunction, causing laryngeal muscle strain and subsequent weakness. Indeed, most hyperfunctional voice disorders have multiple causes and therefore multifaceted management approaches.

Vocal hyperfunction will often lead to the development of laryngeal disorders. Some of the more common conditions include

- Chronic laryngitis
- Vocal nodules
- Vocal polyps
- Contact/ulcers/granulomas
- Leukoplakia/hyperkeratosis.

Chronic laryngitis is characterized by long-term inflammation of the laryngeal mucosa. Voice quality may range from a mild to a severe dysphonia depending on the severity of edema. The cause is normally associated with voice abuse/misuse and chemical (smoke, drug, alcohol) insults to the tissue lining.

Vocal nodules are one of the more common hyperfunctional laryngeal disorders caused by direct vocal misuse/abuse. The lesion may begin as a tiny hemorrhage on the medial edge at the junction of the anterior one-third and posterior two-thirds of the vocal folds. This is the point of greatest amplitude and therefore greatest impact of the folds during phonation. As the misuse continues, fibrous tissue forms the nodules, which almost always occur bilaterally. Nodules are most common in male and female children and adult women. They seldom occur in adult men.

Vocal polyps are fluid-filled sacs of tissue. They may occur anywhere along the length of the vocal folds. Usually caused by misuse or tissue abuse, they may be unilateral, pedunculated sacs attached to a stalk, or fluid may collect in Reinke's space and cause expansion or ballooning of the superficial layer of the vocal folds. The latter is often called Reinke's

edema or polypoid degeneration. Smoking is highly implicated in the development of vocal polyps.

Contact ulcers typically develop on the mucosa covering of the vocal processes of the arytenoid cartilages. Causes for these ulcerations—which typically granulate, forming granulomas—are acid reflux, surgical or medical intubation, and occasionally mechanical trauma from voice abuse/misuse such as harsh coughing or throat clearing. Utilization of an inappropriate low pitch has been suggested as a probable cause.

Leukoplakia and hyperkeratosis are classified as premalignant lesions. Leukoplakia appears as a patchy white membrane and is usually located on the anterior third of the true vocal folds. Hyperkeratosis is a layered buildup of keratinized cell tissue. The causes of both disorders include chronic irritations of the chemicals in tobacco smoke, the irritation of alcohol, incessant coughing, throat clearing, and general voice abuse.

COMPLEMENTARY RELATIONSHIP OF SPEECH PATHOLOGIST AND OTOLARYNGOLOGIST

As with most voice disorders, the treatment of vocal hyperfunction-induced voice problems is multidisciplinary and multifaceted. The following case study illustrates the complementary relationship of the speech pathologist and the otolaryngologist. The study demonstrates the utilization of medical/surgical treatment along with voice therapy. Voice therapy focuses on vocal hygiene counseling, environmental manipulation, direct symptom modification, and physiologic exercises used in combination to remediate a chronic voice problem.

CASE STUDY: PATIENT B

Patient B, a 26-year-old, second-grade teacher, was referred by a laryngologist to The Professional Voice Center of Greater Cincinnati for a complete diagnostic voice evaluation, with the diagnosis of large bilateral vocal fold nodules and a left contact ulcer. Patient B first became symptomatic in the fall of 1987, her first year of teaching. In October of that year she became dysphonic. When the hoarseness persisted she sought the opinion of the referring physician, whose examination revealed mild bilateral vocal fold edema. The physician instructed her to reduce caffeine intake and to increase intake of water, and briefly counseled her regarding voice abuse. The patient followed these instructions, and her voice quality improved.

Between the fall of 1987 and late winter of 1991, the patient experienced intermittent periods of hoarseness. She thought the mild hoarseness was fairly normal considering her level of voice use in the school setting. However, in late February of 1991, she became moderately hoarse during an upper respiratory infection. Like most teachers, she continued to work her normal schedule during this illness. She began to notice not only hoarseness but also voice fatigue and a burning sensation on the left side of her "throat." When the upper respiratory infection resolved and her vocal symptoms persisted, she sought the opinion of the laryngologist.

Upon seeing the vocal nodules and the ulcerated tissue located on the vocal process of the left arytenoid, the laryngologist prescribed an antacid and referred patient B for voice testing and therapy. The antacid was prescribed as a precaution due to the implication of esophageal reflux on the development of contact ulcers and granulomas.

The information gathered during the voice evaluation confirmed the nature of the voice abuse which had significantly increased her symptoms in February. Patient B had indeed experienced a mild hoarseness since school began in the fall of 1990. She reported that her voice quality was typically better on Monday and much worse by Friday, but always had some level of hoarseness. On a daily basis, she was more symptomatic, with hoarseness during the early morning. The hoarseness would clear somewhat by mid-morning and then worsen again by mid-afternoon.

With the onset of the respiratory infection Patient B began coughing and throat clearing. These abuses were most likely the causes of the contact ulcer. By the time of the voice evaluation the coughing had decreased, but chronic throat clearing was noted. Her voice use was typical for a second-grade teacher. Students of this age require much instruction. Non-speech times in the classroom were reported to be minimal. In addition, the patient was assigned playground and school-bus duty, which required occasional shouting and raising the voice above noise for conversation.

There was no evidence that patient B misused her voice away from her work environment. Though married and having a 2-year-old daughter, she denied any direct voice abuse or environmental abuse. She reported that her voice improved on weekends and had always returned to normal during the summer months. Her remaining social history was unremarkable as related to this problem.

The patient's medical history was also unremarkable. She was free of any chronic illnesses or disorders; took only the antacid, although she was not symptomatic with "heart burn"; and was a nonsmoker, living and working in a nonsmoking environment. Her liquid intake was not adequate; she drank two cans of caffeinated soda, and two glasses of iced tea per day. She reported that she "loved" teaching and felt "great" on a daily basis.

During the voice evaluation, patient B presented with a moderate dysphonia characterized by a breathy, dry hoarseness. The laryngeal videostroboscopic examination revealed large bilateral vocal fold nodules, worse on the right than the left; bilateral edema and erythema; and an apparent resolving left contact ulcer. The nodules caused glottic closure to demonstrate an hourglass configuration with a slight ventricular fold compression. Both the amplitude of vibration and the mucosal wave were severely decreased bilaterally. The open phase of the vibratory cycle was dominant, while the symmetry of vibration was generally irregular. In other words, she presented with significant tissue changes that would present a challenge to functional voice therapy.

Acoustic measures demonstrated a limited frequency range of 147 to 562 Hz. Her fundamental frequency remained appropriate at 211 Hz. While her jitter measures for sustained vowels were normal, conversational jitter was above normal limits at 2.60%.

Aerodynamic measures yielded significantly high airflow rates for high pitches averaging 305 mL H_2O. Comfort and low pitches were borderline high at 180 and 189 mL H₂0, respectively. The patient was required to push more air through her vocal system to support the vibration due to increased mass and the hourglass glottal chinks. Her subsequent phonation times at all pitch levels were only 11 seconds or less.

Following the voice evaluation and testing a treatment plan was proposed. The plan included:

1. Temporary reassignment from playground and school-bus duties
2. Site visit to determine environment and teaching style
3. Elimination of throat clearing
4. Oral hydration program
5. Symptom modification
6. Vocal Function Exercises

Temporary Reassignment

It was decided to first immediately eliminate the potential for the most obvious voice abuse. The patient therefore requested to be assigned to other duties away from the playground and school buses where voice would not be a factor and she would not be required to raise her voice. If therapy proved successful, reassignment would be temporary; otherwise, it would continue until the end of the school year.

Site Visit

Site visits are time consuming and not always practical. But the value of seeing the patient in the implicated environment cannot be overemphasized. Other useful options to site visits are video or audio tape recordings of the patient in the environment that can be reviewed during therapy.

Patient B's school was convenient to the voice center, so a 1-hour site visit was arranged. Observations made during the visit included:

1. Large room
2. Unusually high (16 to 18 ft) acoustical tile ceilings
3. Sound lost in space
4. Only twenty-four students spread

throughout large room at different "stations"
5. All sounds such as scooting chairs, dropped books, and so forth, were magnified by glass and plastic, but speech was hard to discriminate

It was obvious that patient B indeed "loved" her work. She was very enthusiastic and had complete control of the classroom. Observations made regarding her teaching style included

1. Vocally enthusiastic, but does not shout
2. Room requires that she speak loudly and precisely, not to be heard but to be understood
3. Spends a good deal of time "directing" children when not actually teaching
4. Uses high pitch, limited inflection, and back focus; constantly strains voice.

A tape recording was made during the visit, which was reviewed in therapy.

The opportunity to visit the patient's classroom led to several suggestions. These included:

1. Decrease the physical space by rearranging seating to utilize approximately two thirds of the classroom. With a class size of only twenty-four students, this was easy to accomplish. The patient herself suggested a further change. She physically decreased the room size by utilizing large, free-standing display boards (which were normally in school storage).

2. Soften the acoustics of the room by utilizing the window blinds, pulled halfway down. Utilize fabric in a work display area by hanging a sheet on the wall to display student papers, pictures, tests, and similar exhibits. The large display boards also functioned well as an acoustic barrier.

3. Build into the schedule a vocal "time-out" for both the teacher and the students. Learn to respect and appreciate this silent time as a chance to rest the voice and as a reminder to talk only as loudly as necessary in the newly configured classroom.

4. Develop a sign system for common instructions and requests. It was noted during

the site visit that the patient was constantly correcting and directing students' actions while instructing. When this was brought to her attention she decided to implement an interesting sign/symbol system that would preclude voice commands. She listed the names of the students on a large magnetic board she had in the corner of the classroom. Signs were then made with picture symbols depicting the most common corrections/directions that she found herself making. They included symbols representing such directions as the following: be quiet, don't tilt your chair, slow down, stop talking, talk softer, and pay attention. These symbol pictures were attached to magnets. When the need arose, the patient would place the symbol next to the name of the offending child, all the while continuing her teaching. A list of consequences for receiving more than one symbol correction was established by the teacher and well understood by the children.

Elimination of Throat Clearing

The changes in the previous paragraph proved successful in immediately decreasing the daily laryngeal fatigue and voice struggle. The patient, of course, remained dysphonic. The therapy plan then introduced a behavior modification approach for eliminating the abusive behavior of throat clearing. Until brought to her attention by the therapist, the patient was not aware of her frequency of throat clearing. Throat clearing may be extremely abusive to the tissue lining of the vocal folds and arytenoid cartilages. Once brought to her attention, the patient was surprised by the number of times she cleared her throat during the session. To modify this behavior she was told the following.

"Throat clearing is one of the most abusive things you can do to your vocal folds. When you clear your throat like this (demonstrate), you create an extreme amount of movement of your vocal folds, causing them to slam and rub together (demonstrate using your hands). You should understand that it is not unusual for you to have developed this habit. The vast majority of patients we see with your type of voice problem also have this habit. Sometimes people do not even know that they are doing it. But often they say that they feel something in their throat, like a lump or mucous. The majority of the time, however, when you clear your throat, there is simply nothing there. You are often only feeling a muscle thickness from chronic strain. The only thing you have accomplished is to create more vocal fold abuse.

"We have demonstrated to you with the tape recording from your class that most of the time you clear your throat right before you begin to speak. Also, you are clearing many more times than you realized. This is a sign that throat clearing is very much a habit. Like all habits, it is difficult to break. We are, therefore, going to try to make it easier by giving you a substitute habit that will (1) take the place of throat clearing, (2) accomplish the same thing as throat clearing, and (3) is not abusive. This substitute, nonabusive habit is a hard swallow.

"If you do, in fact, occasionally have an increased amount of mucous on your vocal folds, a hard swallow will accomplish the same thing as throat clearing—minus the abuse. The only difference is that throat clearing feels good. It psychologically gives you more relief than the hard swallow, even though it physically accomplishes no more. It is your goal to overcome this psychological dependence. Understand that this habit is harmful and that it must be broken.

"To break this habit, you need to tell everyone in your family and any friends who are around you often (and whom you feel comfortable in telling) that you are not permitted to clear your throat anymore. When these 'helpers' hear you clear your throat, and they will, they are to immediately point it out to you. You may even consider using your students as helpers. Your task then is to 'swallow hard.' Obviously, it will not be necessary to swallow, since you just cleared your throat. However, this is your first step in substituting the hard swallow for the throat clearing.

"After your family and friends have pointed out your throat clearing to you several times, you will begin to catch yourself. You will clear your throat and almost immediately think, "Oops! I am not supposed to do that." Your response again should be to swallow hard.

"When you have caught yourself clearing your throat several times, you will begin to halt yourself just prior to clearing. Once again, you will substitute the hard swallow, but this time the throat clearing was stopped. By the time you have reached this point, you will be very close to breaking the habit totally. The final goal will be met when you realize that you are swallowing many fewer times than the number of times you used to clear your throat.

"I want you to work very hard on this problem. I think you will be very surprised just how quickly you are able to break this habit. As a matter of fact, the majority of our patients have significantly reduced the habit within 1 to 2 weeks. Most patients, though, cannot do it alone. So please, find other people to help you by having them point out when you are doing it. Any questions?"

Following this explanation, the patient will typically clear his or her throat more times than usual. This is immediately pointed out by the voice pathologist, and the hard swallow substitution is initiated. Often, great gains in habit modification are made during this initial session.

Patient B received help from her husband, mother, and a friend, and was able to totally eliminate the habit of throat clearing within 2 weeks.

Oral Hydration Program

The superficial layer of the vocal folds must be well lubricated to decrease the heat and friction of vibration. A thin, slippery mucous secreted on to the vocal folds serves the same purpose as oil is to the engine of a car. It was explained to Patient B that what she swallows does not touch her vocal folds, but rather is diverted around them. (Video-laryngoscopy is an excellent means of demonstrating anatomic functions.) Therefore, the amount and type of liquid intake will either permit or inhibit the normal mucous flow to the vocal folds. Caffeine, alcohol, and many medications are drying agents. Many times when patients feel as if they have too much mucous on the vocal folds the fact is that they have too little and the consistency is drier, thicker, and stickier than is desirable.

The patient's liquid intake was minimal and caffeinated. She was therefore placed on a hydration program which required a minimum intake of six 8-ounce glasses of water or fruit juices per day. In addition she was asked to decrease her caffeine intake but was not required to totally eliminate caffeine from her diet.

Symptom Modification and Vocal Function Exercises

Direct vocal function tasks were also introduced. These tasks combined a symptom modification approach with physiologic exercises. The tasks included the following:

1. Enhancing awareness of appropriate pitch and loudness during teaching. The initial tape recording was used to demonstrate problems with pitch, loudness, and focus. Direct practice utilizing feedback from a Visi-Pitch instrument was helpful in introducing more appropriate pitch and loudness. The patient was instructed to talk only as loudly as was absolutely necessary in the classroom. The combination of these approaches returned her teaching style to a more conversational mode. Reconfiguring the classroom and improving the acoustics was also a factor in making positive changes in voice production.

2. Vocal function exercises for improvement of muscle function and to balance airflow to laryngeal muscle effort were introduced. Vocal function exercises, as described in Chapter 1, proved helpful in improving the overall condition of the vocal folds and helped to retrain frontal focus. The patient's baseline mean phonation time for sustaining the appropriate notes was 8.5 seconds. This measure improved to a mean of 18 seconds during 6 weeks of therapy.

Significant improvement was noted during 6 weeks of therapy for both subjective observations and objective measures. The patient was experiencing much less vocal fatigue and laryngeal discomfort. Tape recordings made while teaching demonstrated stabilization of new voicing habits and only very occasional throat clearing. She did, however, remain mildly dysphonic, characterized by a slight breathy hoarseness.

Objective measures demonstrated a fundamental frequency of 196 Hz and an expanded frequency range of 165 to 720 Hz. All jitter measures, including conversation, were within normal limits. Airflow rates for comfort and low-pitched voices had decreased to 136 and 150 mL H_2O/sec, respectively. Airflow rate for high-pitched voice also decreased to 240 mL H_2O/sec, but was still above the normal limit of 200 mL H_2O/sec.

Videostroboscopy also demonstrated improvement. The edema and erythema were resolved, and there was no evidence of the contact ulcer. A slight thickness was noted where the left nodule had been. The right nodule was still present but appeared much more cystlike. The glottic closure retained an hourglass shape; however, the glottal chinks were much smaller. The amplitude of vibration was only slightly decreased left and moderately decreased right. The mucosal wave was normal on the left and moderately decreased around the right lesion. The open phase of the vibratory cycle was slightly dominant, while the symmetry of vibration remained irregular.

The results of the therapy program were discussed with Patient B's physician. Considering the cystlike nature and stiffness of the right vocal fold lesion it seemed unlikely that the lesion would resolve with therapy. It was decided to extend therapy for an additional month to be certain that this was the case. When the remaining lesion did not resolve, surgery was scheduled for the 2nd week in June.

The pathologist's report confirmed the lesion to be a cyst. Following surgery, the patient continued vocal function exercises for 1 month and then began a maintenance exercise program for the remainder of the summer. Mean phonation times improved and stabilized at an average of 32 seconds. The voice quality improved to normal. Changes in objective measures included a higher frequency range ($+900$ Hz) and a normal airflow rate at high pitch (160 mL H_2O/sec). Videostroboscopic examination performed just prior to the fall opening of school revealed all observations to be within normal limits except for the symmetry of vibration, which remained irregular at higher pitches.

Patient B was followed monthly until the time of this writing (November, 1991) to confirm her symptom-free status. To date, her voice has remained normal, and she will soon be discharged altogether. The combination of medical/surgical treatment and voice therapy proved successful in remediating a long-term voice disturbance in this patient.

VOCAL HYPERFUNCTION IN CHILDREN

Vocal hyperfunction will occur among all ages and is the most common cause of voice disorders in children. Children with hyper-

functional voice problems pose quite a challenge because, frankly, many children abuse their voice in some way. These abuses may include, but are not limited to shouting, loud talking, screaming, vocal noises, and throat clearing. The following cases will illustrate some important issues when dealing with vocal hyperfunction in children.

CASE STUDY: PATIENT C

In discussing the treatment of children's voice disorders with public school speech pathologists, one of the primary problems is the lack of interaction/cooperation with parents. Because most parents work outside the home, interactions with the school are often limited and difficult to schedule. Because of the reality of limited parental interaction, behavior modification in voice therapy may prove difficult. This was the case with patient C, a 9-year-old fourth-grade child who was identified as being hoarse during the fall speech screening period. A form letter was sent to his home describing the voice problem and suggesting the problem be checked medically either with his family physician or an ear, nose, and throat physician.

Patient C's parents did not respond to the letter, and as school progressed he became more dysphonic. His classroom teacher became concerned and invited the school's speech pathologist to discuss the problem with the parents during a parent/teacher conference. The patient's mother confirmed receiving the form letter, but indicated that her son had "always had a husky voice." She and his father were neither alarmed nor overly concerned. The patient's teacher indicated that her concern focused on how it was affecting the child in the classroom. He had to talk loudly to be heard, because he could not seem to talk softly. This was somewhat embarrassing to him, and he had become reticent to participate in class. In addition, his chronic throat clearing was annoying, and on occasion he had been disruptive during "quiet periods."

The speech pathologist explained the common causes of hoarseness and the possibilities of edema and nodules, the common childhood laryngeal disorders. Patient C's mother left the conference promising to discuss the matter with her child's pediatrician.

Patient C's mother followed through with her promise. The pediatrician placed the boy on an antibiotic for 10 days, which did not modify his symptoms. A referral was made to a laryngologist in December. Indirect laryngoscopy revealed the presence of bilateral vocal fold nodules. Voice therapy was recommended and was scheduled to begin in January. Thus, between identification of the problem in September to referral for therapy, half of the school year had been lost.

Public school speech pathologists often ask if they must wait for a laryngological examination and therapy recommendation. My answer is always, "Yes." From a medical/legal standpoint, we need to know what we are treating. My examples of this rule include the 10-year-old child who was indeed treated for "hoarseness" without improvement for 3 years in the school. When an indirect laryngoscopic examination was finally performed, a congenital web was found to be the cause of her voice problem. Thirty years of therapy would have been of little use. In another case, persistent hoarseness was identified in a 9-year-old girl. An immediate laryngological examination and subsequent direct laryngoscopy with biopsy revealed a squamous cell carcinoma, a shocking and highly unusual diagnosis in a child. Imagine the implications had medical management not been implemented. As it was, this child required total laryngectomy.

In January, Patient C's speech pathologist evaluated his voice production. She described his voice as moderately dysphonic, characterized by breathy, husky, hoarseness and loud volume. He had a pitch range of less than one octave and could sustain the /a/ sound for only 5 seconds. The s/z ratio was 11 seconds to 4 seconds. His phonation was characterized by hard glottal attacks.

Many vocal abuses were also identified. They included

1. Shouting at/with his 6- and 11-year-old brothers (arguing, playing, fighting)
2. Shouting during sporting events (the patient played soccer, baseball, and basketball on organized teams)
3. Chronic, habitual throat clearing

4. Production of vocal noise while pretending to be a professional wrestler; engine noises while playing with cars, trucks, cycles; various vocal sounds while playing with "He-Man" toys, and so on
5. Shouting with extreme high pitch
6. Habitual loud talking.

It was determined to focus therapy on those issues which could be best addressed in school. Parental support would be sought, but realistically was not expected or subsequently received. Patient C's speech pathologist developed a program which consisted of four components.

1. **Education.** Photographs and line drawings were utilized with the patient to describe his vocal folds and to describe how vocal nodules are developed. The boy's inability to talk softly was discussed as related to the inability of the vocal folds to totally approximate. With the nodules holding his vocal folds apart, Patient C was required to force a greater amount of air between the folds to set them and hold them in vibration. This increased effort made him talk louder and caused constant voice strain.

Tape recordings of clear voices, hoarse voices, and his own voice were utilized to demonstrate the voice qualities being discussed. Finally, vocally abusive behaviors such as shouting, loud talking, vocal noises, throat clearing, and so on were discussed and related to the causes of hoarseness. Substitutions for various vocal noises were described, as well as suggestions for eliminating the most abusive noises. Shouting for "play" was contrasted with shouting in nonplay activities. Nonplay shouting—such as calling for another family member from one part of the house to another, yelling for the dog, arguing with his brothers, and so on—were discussed, and appeals made to "think before you shout." Again, without parental cooperation, modifying nonplay shouting may be difficult.

2. **Behavior modification.** Utilizing his classroom teacher, a best friend, and the speech pathologist, Patient C was taught the "hard swallow" method for eliminating throat clearing. A method of charting throat clearing

during school was devised, with the occurrences decreasing significantly within 3 weeks.

Charting was also utilized for shouting activities in school. These included shouting on the playground, during gym class, in the hallway and cafeteria. Appropriate reward systems were developed.

3. **Direct voice therapy.** The patient's increased loudness level, breathiness, and hard glottal attacks were all symptoms of his vocal nodules and not causes of the problem. Direct therapy using Vocal Function Exercises (see Chapter 1) was initiated as a means of indirectly teaching easy onset and frontal focus while restrengthening the laryngeal musculature and balancing air flow to muscle effort.

4. **Teach appropriate method of shouting.** Patient C was a very active, vocally enthusiastic child. He was encouraged to shout during organized sporting events. In addition, it was evident that he lived in a loud, active household. It was therefore determined that it was not practical to expect elimination of shouting behaviors. The speech pathologist decided to teach him "how" to shout.

As the boy's voice quality began to improve with the previous three methods, he was taught a less abusive manner of shouting. As you recall, when the patient shouted, his pitch level went to an unusually high frequency. This would require the vocal folds to be stretched and tensed during this loud phonation. He was, therefore, taught to shout using a low pitch, with improved breathing and breath support. It is felt that the vocal folds will be less abused when absorbing the impact of shouting when the vocal folds are thicker and less tense at lower pitch.

Integrating education, behavior modification, direct voice manipulation, and instructions for less abusive shouting, patient C was able to improve his voice quality and stabilize the voice by the end of the school year to a mild dysphonia characterized by a slight dry hoarseness. More important was his increased participation in the classroom. The speech pathologist did not have the opportunity of a follow-up laryngological examination. However, even without the parents' active participation, patient C's voice therapy could be judged successful.

PSYCHOSOCIAL ASPECTS OF CHILDREN'S BEHAVIOR

Contributed by Moya Andrews, Ph.D.

In the next case study, Moya Andrews, Ph.D., explores the psychosocial aspects of a child's behavior and introduces the facilitating techniques of yawn-sigh, chanting, and humming.

CASE STUDY: PATIENT D

Patient D, aged 4 years, 6 months, was referred by her teacher at the Montessori Preschool because of "hoarseness, loud talking, and frequent attention-getting behaviors in class." She was brought to the speech and hearing clinic by her mother, who had taken the patient from school in time for their 11 A.M. appointment. The mother apologized for the fact that the child insisted she needed to bring a large, "fast-food" milkshake into the diagnostic room with her. "She always has to have a shake," said the mother with a shrug, while the little girl smiled complacently and toyed with her straw. When the speech pathologist suggested that the patient could sit in the waiting room until she had finished her shake, the mother looked distressed and said, "Oh no, she wouldn't like that at all." The patient's smile widened, she tossed her head, did a little dance around the room, and spilled some of the shake on the floor. "Oh dear," said the mother helplessly, "she's just so full of energy."

During the interview, the mother reported that patient D was the youngest of three children. Her two older brothers, aged 14 and 16 years, attended the local high school. The mother, a homemaker, said that the patient had been born in Germany during the time that her husband had been in the U.S. military service. The father was currently employed at a local hospital. "My husband always wanted a daughter, so I suppose we spoil her," said her mother.

Patient D demonstrated many of the classic behaviors associated with vocal abuse: inefficient respiratory pattern; tension in the shoulder, neck, and jaw; phonation breaks; hard glottal attacks; loud conversational level; hoarse vocal quality; weak resonance; limited vocal variety; and frequent throat clearing. She could prolong a vowel for 3 seconds and exhibited hearing sensitivity within normal limits bilaterally. The results of an examination of her peripheral speech mechanism were unremarkable. The otolaryngological report noted small bilateral vocal nodules and redness of laryngeal structures but no evidence of allergies or infections. The school psychologist's report noted above-average intelligence, frequent temper tantrums and episodes of crying, and use of manipulative interpersonal strategies. The child was involved in after-school programs such as ballet, swimming, an art class, and a neighborhood play group. The mother characterized her daughter's behavior in the following way. "She is quite a handful at times, but she's intelligent and has had more opportunities than other children her age because we lived abroad. Also, she has had to be assertive or her brothers ignore her. She is a live-wire and can be difficult, but she is so cute and talented that we can never stay angry with her for long." It appeared that the psychodynamics in the patient's family merited further attention. Further questions resulted in the information that when the patient's vocal behavior was loud and forceful, she usually got what she wanted at home. However, the patient's teacher reported that the child's interpersonal strategies did not help her succeed in her school environment. Rather, she needed to develop more effective interpersonal and vocal strategies in order to establish satisfying relationships with her peers and teachers. Therefore, the therapy program was designed to include work on relevant psychosocial issues as well as modification of abusive vocal behaviors.

General Awareness Phase

Voice therapy programs for children usually begin with a general awareness phase. During this phase the child is oriented to the general area of voice and taught basic concepts and the background information that is necessary before the clinician targets specific symptoms. For example, patient D needed a general awareness of respiration, because that was an area of her behavior that needed to be modified. The clinician used a "science project"

format to teach the girl general information about breathing. Activities were designed to achieve two sets of goals.

I. I can talk about breathing.
   A. I can describe some different ways people and animals breathe.
   B. I can describe how air is used (for example, to sustain life, to make sound, to pant, and so forth).
   C. I can label the body parts used during breathing (such as lungs and windpipe).
   D. I can tell my teacher how to breathe in without tensing her shoulders and neck.
   E. I can time the number of seconds it takes for my teacher to breathe out air.

Another general awareness goal for patient D was for her to develop an understanding of psychosocial factors relevant to vocal communication. The clinician used a "story format" to teach the patient some general principles of communication. Activities were designed for the following goals:

II. I can talk about what happened in stories my teacher reads to me.
   A. I can guess what might happen when storybook characters act in certain ways (utilization of cause/effect).
   B. I can make up different endings to some stories (analysis of choices).
   C. I can explain why some things go wrong for some children in our stories (identification of unproductive strategies).
   D. I can suggest some other ways the characters may handle situations (problem solving).

Sample Stories

1. Jennifer and Mary were both doing puzzles at preschool. Mary finished her puzzle and started to watch Jennifer, who was having trouble with hers. Mary picked up two of the pieces of Jennifer's puzzle, shrieked loudly, and ran across the room. Jennifer ran after Mary and tried to grab the pieces from her, but

Mary quickly threw them under a storage cabinet. It took Jennifer a long time to crawl under the low cabinet and find them.

Answer these questions.

1. How did Mary feel?
2. How did Jennifer feel?
3. Why do you think Mary threw the pieces away?
4. What would you suggest Mary should do next?
5. Does Mary like Jennifer? Explain why or why not?
6. What would you do if you were the teacher?

2. Ann told Cathy that she was mean and no one wanted to play with her any more. Cathy felt very badly, but she didn't want Ann to know, so she knocked over the glue and then screamed loudly that Ann had knocked the glue over on purpose and ruined Cathy's work. Cathy screamed so much she got red in the face and the teacher had to tell her to have a drink of water to calm down. The teacher also told Ann to go and work on the other side of the room. So Cathy felt she'd paid Ann back.

Answer these questions.

1. What do you think the other children in the class were thinking during the uproar?
2. Why do you think Ann said Cathy was mean?
3. How do you think Cathy could have solved the problem differently?
4. What would Cathy wish Ann had said instead?

3. During recess, Emily was playing by herself. A new girl named Lindy stood nearby. Emily asked Lindy if she wanted to play with her in the sandbox. Lindy was pleased when Emily quietly asked her about her family and where she lived. Lindy thought Emily was a really friendly girl.

Answer these questions.

1. Why did Lindy think Emily was friendly to her?
2. Why didn't Emily talk more about herself?
3. Describe how it feels on the first day at a new school.
4. What advice would you give to someone who wanted to make friends?

4. Mrs. Brown's class was having a discussion about different ways to talk. They had two boxes. One box was labeled "loud talking," and one box was labeled "soft talking." The children had to think of times when they talked in loud or soft voices. The teacher wrote their ideas on pieces of paper and they put them in the correct box. Here are some of their ideas. You decide which box they go in! In the library; at a ball game; telling secrets; visiting a sick relative; calling the dog; saying goodnight; fighting with my brother; making friends; calling for help; calming a frightened animal; when I'm not getting my fair share; when my mom has a headache.

Specific Awareness Phase

During the specific awareness phase of therapy, the child is taught to focus on specific behaviors, discriminate between behaviors, and describe pertinent behavioral characteristics. This creates a perceptual and linguistic framework that prepares the child to modify critical behaviors during the subsequent production phase of therapy.

The goals for patient D included

1. Identification of abusive vocal behaviors exhibited by others
2. Description of the salient characteristics of vocal behaviors
3. Discrimination of differences between appropriate and inappropriate behaviors
4. Explanation of ways inappropriate behaviors can be avoided or changed

Targets

Respiration
- Use lower chest breathing
- Use more replenishing breaths

- Eliminate unnecessary upper torso tension

Phonation
- Use easy onsets
- Use easy breathy quality*
- Decrease tension
- Decrease loudness level in conversational speech
- Employ vocal variety (not only increased loudness)

Interpersonal
- Increase question asking
- Improve listening/talking ratio
- Use "other" referenced statements in addition to "self" referenced ones

Resonance
- Improve resonance
- Increase articulatory precision

Because patient D needed to modify a number of different behaviors subsumed under four different areas, it was decided to present the behaviors as a set or a gestalt. Consequently, the appropriate behaviors were associated with one storybook character and the inappropriate behaviors with another. The "beautiful ballerina's" voice was relaxed and "airy," and her lips danced when she used them. She made music by humming on the front of her face and the music was carried over into the voice as she chanted words. The ballerina voice was characterized by appropriate breathing patterns, easy onsets, resonance, and lack of laryngeal tension. The voice was light and musical and easy to listen to. Listeners felt relaxed and pleased when they heard it. In contrast, "tense Tessie's" voice was characterized by laryngeal effort, hard glottal attacks, excessive loudness, and inefficient breathing patterns. Patient D was given ample opportunity to identify the two patterns and their effects on listeners, during discussion of stories.

---

*A clear quality is not realistic until the nodules have subsided.

Sample Stories

1. The beautiful ballerina came onto the stage wearing a frothy white tutu. She breathed deeply and her lower chest swelled with air. She stood with her lovely head, neck, and shoulders relaxed and poised. The audience admired her graceful posture and relaxed expression. As she began to dance she hummed to the music and the bones of her face vibrated. "Hmmmm" she hummed as she glided smoothly across the flower-strewn stage under the glittering chandelier.

Answer these questions.

1. Describe how the ballerina breathes.
2. How does she hum?
3. Explain how she keeps her body relaxed.

2. Tense Tessie tightens her jaw and neck and raises her shoulders when she breathes in. She pushed hard with her throat and makes a little click or grunt on words such as:

1. I'm always eager.
2. But everywhere I go.
3. I jerk instead of glide.
4. (I feel all stiff, you know!)

Answer these questions.

1. Can you tell Tessie what she must do to breathe more efficiently?
2. How can she relax her neck?
3. Can you tell which words Tessie makes with a hard start?

Sample Activity
When your teacher tells you an action, do it first the way tense Tessie would do it and then do it the way the beautiful ballerina does it. Explain the difference.

Production Phase

During the production phase of therapy patient D learned to produce and monitor target vocal behaviors in structured and controlled situations. Initially, cues and monitoring were provided by the clinician. Gradually, however, the patient learned to assume more and more of this responsibility. For this patient, the production goals were sequenced as follows:

I. Produce each target behavior correctly (in isolation).
   A. With instructions, cues, and presentation of the model.
   B. With instructions and cues.
   C. With instructions.
   D. Spontaneously.

II. Prolong-repeat the target behavior.
III. Stop and start the target behavior at will.
IV. Demonstrate both the appropriate and inappropriate forms of the behavior (negative practice).
V. Produce the target behavior, varying length of utterance.
   A. Isolated sounds.
   B. Syllables.
   C. Words.
   D. Phrases.
   E. Sentences.

VI. Produce the target behavior, varying the complexity of processing.
   A. Imitation.
   B. Automatic responses.
   C. Limited repertoire of responses.
   D. Simple self-generated responses.
   E. Complex self-generated responses.

VII. Produce the target behavior, varying the timing of the response.
   A. Predictable response time.
   B. Unpredictable response time.

VIII. Describe the characteristics of one's own production in terms of the following.
   A. Preparatory set.
   B. Strategies used.
   C. Reactions of self.
   D. Reactions of others.

IX. Monitor one's own production.
   A. When cued verbally.
   B. When cued nonverbally.
   C. After practicing aloud.
   D. After thinking about it first.
   E. Spontaneously.

Sample Materials

Facilitating Techniques
- Yawn/sigh
- Humming
- Chanting.

Facilitating Contexts

1. Minimal pairs to teach breathy onset. "Think" the [h] in the second word of the following pairs:

whose	ooze
hear	ear
hair	air
has	as
his	is
how	ow
ha	ah
hoe	oh
heel	eel
high	eye
hobo	oboe

2. Words and phrases containing only vowels and voiced continuant consonants for continuity of tone and maximum vibration of facial structures:

[z]	[l]	[m]	[v]	[th]
zulus	lovely	Maisie	Vivian	them
zoo	lazy	Molly	violin	those
Zoro	long	mowing	vision	these
Zelma	lions	money	Vera	there
zero	lying	Moses	Volvo	then

Sentences

1. Mow the lawn.
2. Move the Volvo.
3. Vivian is lazy.
4. The lions were lying in the zoo.
5. Molly loves violins.
6. My mom never loses money.
7. Noses are nozzles.
8. I was living in Germany then.
9. Zionsville is near there.
10. Nellie is never nosy.

3. Words, phrases, and sentences loaded with "front" sounds to promote articulatory movement and forward tone focus:

Words

1. Whirl
2. Bounce
3. Jump
4. Wobble
5. Tap
6. Tumble
7. Topple
8. Toddle
9. Pretty
10. Dainty.

Sentences

1. Pop goes the weasel.
2. Pitter patter water splatters.
3. Fit as a fiddle.
4. Tap with your toes.
5. Pearl buttons to button up.
6. Touch Tilly's white tulle tutu.
7. Leap up and down.
8. Tiptoe through the tulips.
9. Puppies snap and yip and yap.
10. You yell at little lizards.

Sample Activities

1. Be the dancing teacher and "sing" as you count for ballerinas to practice at the bar: "One and two and three and four."

2. Play "singing Simon says," and sing the instructions for dance movements.

3. Look at this stack of cards with the names of foods (for example, eggs, apples, onions). Use the carrier phrase "I eat" and make a sentence with each card in the stack. You get a point for each word you say with an easy onset. Try lengthening the vowel sound.

4. Find the sounds that will help you vibrate your voice on the front of your face. ("I'll say some words, and you tell me which sounds helped you when you repeated the words.")

The Carry-Over Phase

The clinician arranged with the teacher for patient D to present some of her "science projects" in her school classroom. Patient D enjoyed the opportunities for attention as she explained and demonstrated some of the information she had learned about respiration. The teacher also implemented a unit on "voice pictures" into her classroom curriculum and provided opportunities for patient D to be the "expert" on how to make pictures with her voice without talking loudly or in a tense manner. The patient demonstrated "high jumps" and "broad jumps" and "long worms" and "soft fur" using vocal variety, and she served as the judge when the teacher organized a "voice-picture" competition. The patient also starred in another classroom activity where picture cards were used. For example, two cards—one with a bird (blue jay) and one with a letter (blue J)—were held up. The listeners had to identify which card patient D was referring to.

The patient's mother routinely observed therapy sessions and observed the ways in which the clinician insisted on mature, direct interpersonal interactions. The mother also met for several sessions alone with the clinician and the school psychologist so that she could talk about ways to help the patient at home. The teacher and the parents agreed to give the patient lots of attention and praise when she used mature, nonabusive vocal strategies.

Patient D's father agreed to read stories with his daughter each evening before bedtime and to reinforce appropriate voice use. For example, he used phrases such as "I really like these times when we talk quietly together. You make me see the pictures in my head, and the stories come alive for me," and "you have the prettiest 'quiet voice' I know." The parents set up rules during meal times to ensure that everyone had a turn to talk and that loud interruptions and shouting down other siblings was not reinforced. When patient D lapsed into her immature, manipulative patterns of interacting, the parents calmly said, "Let's replay that in a more grown-up way."

Fortunately, patient D's parents understood the importance of addressing the psycho-social issues underlying their daughter's vocal behavior. Their commitment to change and, not coincidentally, patient D's progress were remarkable. From the outset, their interest in their daughter's well-being was reinforced, and the clinician served as a facilitator encouraging them to expand their range of parenting skills.

Patient D attended therapy for 2 years, twice weekly for 45-minute sessions. After she was dismissed from therapy she was followed for a year to ensure that gains were maintained.

USE OF PATIENT/FAMILY EDUCATION AND BEHAVIOR MODIFICATION

Contributed by Leslie Glaze, Ph.D.

In her treatment of a 7-year-old child, described in the following case study, Leslie Glaze, Ph.D., uses specific patient/family education, behavior modification, "recovery time," and the development of a picture journal.

CASE STUDY: PATIENT E

Patient E, a 7-year-old girl, was referred to the voice pathologist by the otolaryngologist, who had diagnosed bilateral vocal fold nodules. She was described by her mother as active, energetic, and frequently "difficult," based on "temper tantrums" and episodes of yelling and screaming with her mother and 5-year-old brother. Her second-grade schoolwork was average, and she did not pose behavior problems at school. Her parents had divorced 2 years previously, and custody has been split jointly, with her primary residence at the mother's home, and extended summer vacations spent at her father's home. Patient E, her mother, and her brother were being seen in joint family counseling sessions weekly to resolve problems with discipline and communication at home. The patient reported that her favorite activities were watching videos, playing outside with neighbor friends, riding her bicycle, and gymnastics.

Patient E's medical history showed no serious disease. She had been in good health since birth, with very infrequent middle ear infections during the first 4 years of life. She had no history of allergies, postnasal drip,

chronic colds, sinus infections, or other upper respiratory infections. She had not had injury to the throat, nose, or neck, and had no evidence of hearing loss. She had never been hospitalized, had no chronic medical problems, and was not on any medication. The patient reported that she drank approximately three cans of caffeinated soda per day and drank milk with meals. Little or no water was consumed on a regular basis.

History of the Problem

Patient E was referred to the otolaryngologist by her school nurse following a (at minimum) 2-year history of chronic hoarseness and occasional episodes of losing her voice. Her first- and second-grade teachers noticed the problem and brought it to the attention of her mother and the school nurse. The patient had no evidence of other speech or language problems.

The otolaryngologist visualized the larynx during an indirect mirror examination, and observed "soft-appearing, moderate-sized bilateral vocal fold nodules." The remainder of the head and neck examination was negative, including normal appearing ears, nose, mouth, pharynx, and neck.

The patient's mother reported that she believes her daughter's voice had worsened gradually over about a 3-year period, during the period when the parents were separating and there was an escalation in vocal arguments, crying, and tantrum behavior by both the patient and her brother. Her mother reported that in two consecutive summers, her daughter's voice had improved following vacations with her father. The mother believed this improvement was attributable to the fact that the patient's father is a psychologist who manages the children's behavior differently, such that fewer tantrum and/or vocally abusive episodes occur. The principal goal of the current family counseling sessions is to learn to adopt some of these behavior management styles at home.

Evaluation Procedures

Patient E received a standard battery of vocal function testing in the voice laboratory, including videostroboscopic examination of the larynx to assess the vibratory pattern of the vocal folds and the size of the vocal fold nodules; acoustic analysis of sustained vowels and sentence productions to assess frequency, loudness, and perturbation in habitual and range tasks; and aerodynamic measures of airflow rate, volume, and intraoral air pressure estimates. Following is a summary of relevant pretreatment measures.

1. **Visual-perceptual.** Patient E's stroboscopic examination was conducted by means of a rigid endoscope without the need for topical anesthesia. The recording revealed moderate-sized, bilateral vocal fold nodules at the anterior two-thirds junction of the vocal folds, with no evidence of edema or hemorrhage. Mucus stranding between the vocal nodules was persistent. The nodules appeared to vibrate with the vocal folds, although mucosal wave and amplitude were reduced at the midline bilaterally, presumably as a result of stiffness posed by the lesions. Phase symmetry and periodicity were always irregular. Supraglottic hyperfunction was evident throughout sustained vowel productions because of a mild, but consistent, medial compression and "bulging" of the ventricular folds.

2. **Acoustic analysis.** The patient's mean fundamental frequency was 237 Hz, with a low and high range from 157 to 314 Hz. Sustained /i/ vowel produced mean jitter of .09 msec, shimmer of 6.7%, and a signal-to-noise ratio of 14 dB, as measured by the C-Speech software program (Milenkovic, 1987). All of these measures represent subnormal performance based on the expected acoustic measures for the patient's age and sex (Glaze, et al., 1988). Intensity measures of the patient's minimum (62 dB SPL), habitual (70 dB SPL), and maximum (87 dB SPL) loudness productions were all within the expected range for her age and sex (Glaze, 1990).

3. **Aerodynamic measures.** Airflow measures were taken during sustained vowel productions; intraoral pressure measures were estimated from repeated productions of /pi/. Mean airflow rate was 270 cc/sec, which is considered excessive, suggesting "air leak" through the laryngeal valving mechanism. Intraoral pressure was measured at 8.3 cm

H_2O, which is also greater than the expected norm of approximately 5 cm H_2O.

Voice Description

Audio-Perceptual. — Patient E's voice quality was judged perceptually by the voice pathologist during informal conversation and sentence productions, using the four-point GRBAS scale (normal, mild, moderate, or severe impairment), measuring overall (general) voice performance (G), roughness (R), breathiness (B), weakness or aesthesia (A), and strain (S). Patient E exhibited moderate amounts of roughness and strain, a mild amount of breathiness, and no evidence of weakness, as judged from the initial evaluation. The patient also sang the song "Happy Birthday to you," to assess pitch-changing ability during a familiar singing task, and demonstrated five pitch breaks. In conversation, the patient was intermittently aphonic for one-two syllables' duration on an average of once each sentence. Her habitual loudness level was not excessive, nor did she exhibit signs of hard glottal attack during casual conversation.

Description and Rationale for Therapy Approach

Based on the patient's history and the evaluative findings, it seemed that the causes and maintaining factors for the patient's hyperfunctional voice problem were found in two factors:

1. Acute vocally abusive behaviors
2. Chronic, ongoing stress in the family setting.

Consequently, the treatment goals targeted reduction of specific vocally abusive behaviors and, in conjunction with the family counselor, support for continuing development of alternative behavioral management techniques that may reduce overall household tension and opportunities for vocal abuse. Four treatment goals were established for the patient, organized within a therapy regimen focusing on patient and family education, elimination of vocal abuse, and increased self-awareness and self-determination of voice productions by the patient.

Goal 1. — Patient E, her mother, and her brother learn about the origin and resolution of vocal nodules, the risks of additional vocal deterioration, and the effects of vocally abusive behaviors on vocal fold structure and function.

Rationale. — Especially with children, patient education and knowledge of pathologic processes can lead to motivation, a sense of responsibility, and "ownership" toward the voice problem and the rehabilitative process. For patient E, viewing the videostroboscopy recordings of her larynx were particularly illustrative. Another example of vocal fold injury was simulated by having the patient and her brother clap their hands together for a 3-minute period, so that they could feel how tired and hot their hands were after clapping hard together for that time. From session to session, patient E was "quizzed" by the voice pathologist to ascertain her level of understanding of the disorder and the cause-effect relationship between voice behaviors and rehabilitation. The patient appeared to enjoy displaying her new breadth of knowledge each week.

Goal 2. — Patient E and her mother participate in a home program designed to reduce vocal abuse and to provide "recovery" time for each instance. The patient and her mother monitor and record on a chart all instances of vocally abusive behaviors at home, including, screaming, yelling, excessive crying, and "tantrum" behavior. For each instance of vocal abuse incurred at home, patient E will conduct a 10-minute period of silent "recovery" time, to be spent in a relaxed, quiet activity of the patient's choosing. Each week, the patient and the voice pathologist will predetermine a target maximum of vocally abusive episodes. If, at the end of the week, the patient and her mother determine that the target goal has been met, a specific reward (selected by the patient and her mother) will be granted.

Rationale. — Home programming for systematic reduction of vocal abuse allows the

greatest potential for success of therapy and generalization of the therapeutic goals. In my experience, without home compliance, the prognosis for improvement with therapy is limited. A token system of charting vocal behaviors provides opportunities for increased awareness and recognition of abusive behaviors; motivation for reducing those instances (target maximum, reward); and, most importantly, a defined alternative response immediately following an abusive incident (recovery time). This recovery time is not meant to be punitive, but neutral; it serves as an extended reminder (10 **silent** minutes) of the incident, and stands as a signal that "damage" to the vocal folds must be met with a period of "recovery." In the case of patient E, it was especially important that the family was able to separate distinctly the patient's voice program responsibilities from other general household chores and disciplinary events. During the course of therapy, the patient displayed increasing adherence to the program, with successive reductions of vocal abuse incidents in five out of seven regular treatment sessions.

Goal 3. — Patient E will eliminate all colas and caffeinated beverages from her diet, and drink a minimum of five 8-oz glasses of water per day.

Rationale. — Evidence of mucus stranding and reports of patient E's typical caffeine consumption raise questions about possible insufficient hydration of the vocal fold tissues. By increasing water intake and avoiding caffeine, she may be assured adequate hydration for voice production.

Goal 4. — In conjunction with her family therapy, patient E will keep a daily journal of pictures, drawings, or written material describing her voice use that day, based on feelings and events that created opportunities for positive or negative voice use.

The family counselor began this journal project earlier with the patient and her brother to encourage greater self-awareness regarding their feelings. With the counselor's permission, a voice use component was added for the patient to allow her to relate everyday stress responses to her vocally abusive behaviors. She made schematic drawings of the nodules in her throat, drew pictures for her room to remind her not to yell (such as a drawing of a lion "roaring" with a big X over the mouth), and wrote large signs to use instead of yelling (for example, "LEAVE ME ALONE").

Results of Therapy

Patient E received seven sessions of voice therapy over the course of 3 months, and attended two follow-up sessions, at 1 and 3 months following treatment. At the final session (approximately 6 months from initial diagnosis), post-therapy measures and judgements were obtained.

Visual-Perceptual

Patient E's vocal fold nodules resolved, as judged by the patient and her voice pathologist from visual records of her pre-treatment and post-treatment stroboscopic recordings, and confirmed by the otolaryngologist based on repeated indirect mirror examinations. At the last follow-up examination, no midline vocal fold lesion was evident under either method of inspection. Under stroboscopic light, vibratory movement exhibited normal phase closure, with normal mucosal wave and amplitude, and no evidence of supraglottic hyperfunction. Phase symmetry and periodicity were still irregular.

Acoustic Analysis

The patient reduced jitter and shimmer, and increased signal-to-noise ratio and semitone range based on sustained vowel tasks, as measured previously. Post-test acoustic measures were grossly within expected norms for the patient's age and sex. Habitual pitch and loudness tasks did not change.

Aerodynamic Measures

Mean airflow rate decreased 120 cc/sec from initial measures, for a final mean rate of 150 cc/sec, which was within expected normal limits for this patient. Mean intraoral pressure was measured at 5.7 cm H_2O, which is also decreased from initial measures, and within expected limits.

Audio-Perceptual

Patient E's voice quality improved markedly, as judged perceptually by the patient, her mother, and the voice pathologist. She eliminated pitch breaks and intermittent aphonia, and reduced parameters of breathiness, strain, and roughness from her voice as measured perceptually by the GRBAS scale. The patient and therapist rated conversational voice productions as normal overall (G), mildly rough (R), with no evidence of breathiness (B), weakness (A), or strain (S). During singing of the song "Happy Birthday to you," the patient had no pitch breaks.

The positive outcome of this treatment plan is attributable to the patient and family compliance with the home programming effort. During the course of treatment, it seemed apparent that patient E developed a sense of self-awareness and responsibility toward her voice problem. Thus, her decisions about good voice use were motivated by her own sense of self-determination and satisfaction.

VOCAL HYPERFUNCTION IN ADULTS

Contributed by Gordon Blood, Ph.D.

Whether occurring in adults or children, the histories of vocal dysfunction have many similarities. The details of the causes and courses of treatment are extremely variable and unique to each individual. This variability is what taxes the knowledge and creativity of the voice pathologist.

Gordon Blood, Ph.D., describes his therapy approach in terms of a strict research paradigm in the following case study.

CASE STUDY: PATIENT F

The patient was a self-referred 19-year-old woman who indicated that her voice problem had existed for approximately 6 months, with the onset coinciding with excessive cheering during the football season. She also remarked that she had been treated for two upper respiratory tract infections during the same time period and had an allergic history to penicillin. She complained of hoarseness, intermittent dysphonia, and tender laryngeal and neck muscles. She reported that speaking was at times a "real effort, and hurt." She stated that she often found it necessary to shout and talk over other people. She thought that the problem continued to change, although it was worse now than a month ago. She reported no family history of laryngeal misuse or abuse, and rated her present voice as a 8 on a 1 (normal for her) to 10 (very different from normal) scale. She had recently entered a period of stress in her life because of "constant roommate problems" and a self-reported "minor eating disorder." She had never been in voice therapy or participated in any type of relaxation training.

She was seen by the otolaryngologist at our clinic and medically diagnosed through indirect laryngoscopy as having bilateral vocal nodules. The patient indicated that she occasionally suffered from excessive nasal drainage and took over-the-counter medication. She was not taking any prescription medications and was healthy "except for the two 1-week long upper respiratory infections."

The patient was an active student taking a full academic course load and a self-proclaimed "party person on weekends, which began on Thursday." Her socializing consisted of at least 3 ounces of alcohol each day during the weekend, usually in loud clubs or bars, accompanied by her friends. She spent an average of 15 hours a week working as a waitress. During her free time, she "talked a lot" to her friends on the telephone and reported that much of her library time was consumed by "talking with people she hadn't seen for a while."

Voice Assessment

The results of voice evaluation revealed a moderate dysphonia characterized by breathy-tense components and use of glottal fry. She was able to sustain the /s/ for 16 seconds, the /z/ for 11 seconds, and the /a/ for 10 seconds. She demonstrated numerous interruptions and pitch breaks while phonating from a low to high /o/ and /i/. She was able to count vigorously to 100 and produce a sharp glottal attack and cough. Musculoskeletal tension testing revealed pain in response to kneading the larynx, resistance to movement, self-reported occasional pain radiation to the ear,

and minor improvement in the voice upon palpation and downward movement of the larynx. The patient recanted "typical voice usage for a day" and revealed that she shouted, talked over others, and spoke a minimum of 8 hours a day. Her defense was that waitressing demanded talking, and that keeping her social contacts was very important to her. It appeared that she had very little quiet time, and that weekends were more vocally abusive than weekdays.

I use two instruments to evaluate pitch, perturbation, breathing patterns, and easy onset of phonation. The Visi-Pitch (Kay Elemetrics) revealed that her fundamental frequency averaged 165 Hz for 3 days (taken at different times) during baseline data collection. Her perturbation factor percentages averaged 1.54% for the same baseline period. Variations in loudness were also obtained from the Visi-Pitch and revealed higher intensity levels when using higher frequency levels. The computer-aided fluency establishment trainer, the Cafet, (Goebels, 1988) was also used to evaluate breathing and easy onset. This consists of a microcomputer, circuit board, respiratory sensor and clip-type microphone. The respiratory sensor (chest bellows) is used as a noninvasive measure of airflow worn at the level of the solar plexus. The microphone is worn on the collar and is battery dependent. The computer screen provides color, visual feedback of measures of maximum and minimum bellow expansion. The image is plotted on the computer screen as a purple line following the contour of a breathing cycle. The patient controls the breath curve on the screen and can use the visual feedback to establish a smooth breath curve, using a supportive breathing style. If there is no movement, the purple breath line remains horizontal. Results revealed that the patient had a normal amount (22) of breathgroups per minute, a low percentage (18%) of error-free breathgroup trials, a moderate percentage (36%) of breathgroups with breath holding, and a high percentage (79%) of breathgroups with fast airflow. The other measure that the Cafet provides is a measure of slow rise of volume, also labeled easy onset. The patient must extend onset for 0.3 second without having her volume rise more than 70% during any 0.1 second. She must also reach full volume within 1.2 seconds. Seventy-two percent of all breathgroups had early onsets, 15% showed late onsets, while 0% of easy onsets were recorded.

Selection and Course of Treatment

The treatment selected for this patient was based on the goal of restoring normal voice. The approach is a combination of vocal re-education about abuses and misuses, respiratory training, easy onset of phonation, and relaxation training. In order to maintain the research/clinical orientation, I prefer to set up therapy using a multiple baseline on a number of dependent measures. These measures change for each patient. Results of the assessment indicated that the number of abuses, musculoskeletal tension, overall stress, low pitch, and a low percentage of error-free breathing patterns contributed to and/or maintained the voice problem. The dependent measures evaluated for this patient included number of abuses identified and eliminated, fundamental frequency, perturbation factor, relaxation measures, maximum phonation time, measurements of error-free breathgroups, and easy onsets. I also use social validation measures by having patients rate their own voice improvement, and 20 impartial, nontechnical listeners rate the improvement in the overall quality of the voice from baseline and follow-up sessions.

The clinical/research design included (1) baseline probes (A phase); (2) an overall treatment component phase, including education, abuse reduction, breathing, and easy onset components (B phase); and (3) overall treatment, with a relaxation component phase including education, abuse reduction, breathing, easy onset, and relaxation components (B + C phase). The clinical treatment is an interactional design A–B–BC–B–BC with follow-up, which permits examination of the effectiveness of the overall treatment (B) and the specific effect of the treatment with the relaxation component (BC).

Three 15-minute baseline sessions (A phase) were conducted, during which data on all the dependent variables were collected. Spontaneous speech samples were recorded for later analyses. The first session (B phase)

was conducted at the beginning of the week for 2 hours and began by taking measurements on the Visi-Pitch, three 61-second spontaneous speech samples on the Cafet, and maximum phonation time and relaxation ratings. A review of anatomy and physiology of laryngeal musculature and video tapes of fiberoptic and stroboscopic views of normal and pathologic vocal folds were used for voice production and education. Also during this session, identification of vocal misuses and abuses were discussed. It was discovered that amount of talking time, shouting, irritants (caffeine and alcohol), use of glottal fry, loud talking in noisy bars, and environmental stress were the primary vocal abuses. The patient was directed to set up a chart to isolate the behaviors and reduce talking time to at least 5 hours a day. Strategies for elimination of the abuses included walking over to talk to friends, speaking to small groups of one or two people instead of six to eight people, using a low-pitch shout with deeper breath support to call orders at the restaurant and cheer at football games, being a better listener, and using a digital massage of the laryngeal mechanism for muscle tension. She was able to demonstrate these target strategies and was informed that we would begin working on breathing and easy onset of phonation in the next session. She indicated that she could accomplish these goals, and the next therapy session was scheduled. The second therapy session began with collection of data on the Visi-Pitch and Cafet, as well as relaxation ratings and maximum phonation time, and then reviewed the assignments to determine involvement and compliance. We also listened to a therapy audio tape and agreed that her voice sounded "improved from the last session." The remainder of the session was spent on explaining the Cafet unit and the relationship between breathing and good voice. The emphasis of ongoing respiration as a continuous event characterized by the inspiration and expiration was reinforced by establishing a breathing curve visually on the computer screen. The patient then progressed from articulating vowels, single-syllables, bi-syllables, words, short phrases, and conversation to reach the criteria of 20 consecutive correct productions during the next 11 sessions. The patient was also required to use easy onset of phonation by monitoring the slow rise of volume used in an easy onset. The therapist's modeling, supplemented with the computer graphics, allows patients to adjust their onset of phonation with minimal instruction and confusion. All remaining sessions (sessions 3 to 13) began with the collection of data from Visi-Pitch, Cafet, relaxation ratings, and maximum phonation time. Sessions 3 and 4 (B phase) paralleled session 2 and included Cafet and Visi-Pitch data collection, 15 minutes of review of the modification of abuses, and 30 minutes of Cafet training. Sessions 5, 6, and 7 (BC phase), included, in the following order, 15 minutes for reinforcing the new strategies for modification of vocal abuse, 15 minutes for Cafet training, and 15 minutes to introduce the relaxation phase of therapy through progressive relaxation. The patient was given a relaxation tape and asked to use the tape for 30 minutes each evening. Sessions 8, 9, and 10 (B phase) eliminated the relaxation component to determine its effectiveness on the sessions 2, 3, and 4 and continued to review modification of vocal abuses and Cafet training. Sessions 11, 12, and 13 (BC phase) reintroduced the relaxation component and completed the therapy.

Results of Intervention

The results are summarized in Tables 3–1 and 3–2. Table 3–1 shows the positive effects of the treatment program (B phase) and the treatment program plus relaxation phase (BC) on the percentage of easy onsets, fundamental frequency, and maximum phonation time. The target behaviors progressively increased as a result of the treatment package (B phase) and the treatment package plus relaxation (BC phase). Intervention with the Cafet produced impressive results for easy onsets as seen during the second B phase. There appeared to be no direct changes in three of the dependent measures as a result of the relaxation component. It should be noted that these positive increases in fundamental frequency, use of easy onset, and maximum phonation time were not significantly changed as a result of relaxation, nor were there any reversals in the trends of the data. It may be that relaxation may not effect these parameters. A reciprocal trend was found for percentage of breathgroup errors, perturbation factor, and ratings of relaxation (Table 3–2). A progressive decrease in perturbation numbers and breathgroup

TABLE 3–1.

Positive Increasing Trends in Three Target Behaviors as a Function of Treatment Phases for a Hyperfunctional Voice Patient

	Treatment Design Sessions*					
Target Behaviors	A (Baseline)	B (1–4)	BC (5–7)	B (8–10)	BC (11–13)	F-U (1–2)
Fundamental frequency (cycles/sec)	165	182	194	207	213	210
Maximum phonation time (sec)	10	13	15.5	17	17.2	16.8
Use of easy onsets (%)	0	15	26	78	92	86

*A = baseline; B = treatment; C = treatment plus relaxation; F-U = follow-up

TABLE 3–2.

Negative Decreasing Trends in Three Target Behaviors as a Function of Treatment Phases for a Hyperfunctional Voice Patient

	Treatment Design Sessions*					
Target Behaviors	A (Baseline)	B (1–4)	BC (5–7)	B (8–10)	BC (11–13)	F-U (1–2)
Breathgroup errors (%)	82	68	42	21	6	8
Perturbation factor (%)	1.5	0.67	0.36	0.22	0.22	0.49
Relaxation rating (scale of 1 to 7)	6.5	5.8	2.0	3.5	1.3	1.8

*A = baseline; B = treatment; C = treatment plus relaxation; F-U = follow-up

errors can be seen for both the treatment and the treatment plus relaxation. Examination of the patient's ratings of relaxation shows her to be more relaxed during the training phase and less relaxed without the relaxation component. It appears that the patient perceived herself in a more positive fashion and "more relaxed and in control" during the relaxation component. For patients with environmental and emotional stressors, simply providing basic relaxation training may serve to alleviate some of the stress and compliment the overall treatment package. Although the relaxation component has significant effect on the other dependent measures, it also did not reverse the trends of the results. It may serve to complement a voice therapy regimen with patients demonstrating excessive daily stress or specific laryngeal tension.

Overall, the results suggest that this was an effective treatment for this patient. She rated her overall voice quality as 2.0 on a rating scale from 1 (abnormal voice) to 7 (normal voice) at the baseline sessions compared to a rating of 6.5 at the follow-up sessions. Analyses of 20 nontechnical listeners rating her overall voice quality on a rating scale from 1 (abnormal voice) to 7 (normal voice) revealed a change from a baseline mean average of 2.7 to the first follow-up session mean average of 6.1. This provides social validation of the results presented.

Follow-up and Dismissal

The patient was scheduled for a second laryngeal examination and presented no abnormalities. She was dismissed from therapy and told to contact the clinic within 1 month for a follow-up, personal appointment. At that time data were collected on all the dependent measures, and the client was counseled on her progress. To reinforce continuity of care, the patient was encouraged to call if there were any problems and was scheduled for a final visit approximately 3 months later, at the beginning of the new semester. Tables 3–1 and 3–2 provide evidence that the patient maintained her clinical success in all areas during the follow-up sessions. It appeared that the treatment approach was effective. The patient expressed appreciation, and casual observation

suggested that she appeared more relaxed and relieved about her voice problem. Other areas of her life also were self-reported to be "more in control."

OBJECTIVE METHODS FOR EVALUATION OF VOCAL FUNCTION

Contributed by Janina Casper, Ph.D.

In the next case study, Janina Casper, Ph.D., describes many of the objective methods utilized to evaluate vocal function as well as a management approach utilizing breathy phonation.

CASE STUDY: PATIENT G

The treatment approach, actually a group of therapy techniques, to be described in this case report has been found to be very effective in the treatment of patients who present with benign vocal fold lesions and/or hyperfunctional use of the vocal mechanism. The approach will be described as it was used in the case of patient G.

Patient History

Patient G, an attractive 40-year-old woman, presented with a 2-year history of voice difficulty and a great deal of emotionality and anxiety about the problem. (In my experience, it is not at all unusual for patients to be highly emotional about a voice problem, often seemingly out of proportion to its severity.) Her symptoms, that is, the complaints she described, included constant hoarseness with occasional loss of voice and pain lateral to the larynx bilaterally and extending downward into the upper chest.

Patient G is an elementary school art teacher who teaches five to six class sessions per day in an old school building. She enjoys teaching and puts much energy into preparation and presentation of her classes. She lives with her husband and three children, ages 14, 10, and 8 years, in a close and compatible family unit. She is an outgoing, friendly person who enjoys social interactions with family and friends, likes to talk, but does not characterize herself as a loud person. She is a nonsmoker, has no medical complaints with the exception of some allergies, and takes no medicines on a regular basis.

History of the Problem

Patient G initially sought medical attention for her persistent hoarseness from a family physician, who prescribed a course of antibiotic treatment. When this failed to relieve the symptoms, she was referred to a local otolaryngologist, whose diagnosis was irritation of the vocal folds. She was advised to "rest her voice." She attempted to follow that broad advice, particularly over two summers when she was free from her teaching responsibilities. Her emotional description of these periods revealed her attempts to isolate herself from others and from social interactions, actually fearful of times when she might have to talk. Her family was aware of the problem and reduced their communicative demands on her. Despite these attempts, her voice remained somewhat hoarse, and when she resumed teaching, the symptoms quickly recurred. Additional medical attention included another laryngological examination, with a diagnosis of chronic rhinitis and chronic laryngitis. The treatment recommendation included use of a nasal douche solution three to four times daily and, once again, vocal rest. An allergy work-up was done which showed marked sensitivity to molds, cats, and a number of pollens, and mild reactivity to milk products. She eliminated milk products from her diet for a period of time without positive results. She also made some environmental adjustments but has not had desensitization treatment. At about this time, the patient had a short, unsuccessful course of voice therapy at a facility close to her home community.

The report of her first laryngological examination at our facility makes no mention of allergic mucosal changes, but she was found to have a unilateral mid-fold vocal polyp. Surgical excision of this lesion was recommended and carried out using microdirect laryngoscopic technique. Following surgery she is reported to have had improved voice and was allowed to return to her teaching duties after a brief period of recovery.

Two-and-one-half months later, patient G returned with recurrent hoarseness. At this time she was evaluated by the entire voice clinic team (two otolaryngologists, a voice scientist, and a speech pathologist) and was found to have bilateral vocal fold nodules with thickening in the mid-cord area. The team recommended a 6- to 8-session course of voice therapy.

Pretreatment Evaluation

Patient G had a complete laryngological and voice evaluation. The results of that evaluation will be presented through a discussion of the signs: that is, the observable and measurable characteristics of the problem.

Perceptual Signs

The clinician's judgement of voice quality was that it was moderately hoarse with moderately severe breathiness. Pitch range seemed to be restricted. The patient demonstrated mild to moderate overall tension and strain in speaking. Using a 5-point rating scale of overall voice acceptability, where 5 is most acceptable, the team rating for patient G was 3 (Casper et al., 1990).

Stroboscopic/Laryngoscopic Signs

Vocal fold edge was described as mild/moderately irregular bilaterally. Figure 3–1, the stroboscopic image during phonation, demonstrates the presence of the nodules, the irregularity of the vocal fold edge, and the hourglass configuration of incomplete glottic closure. Phase closure was judged to be more open than closed. Vertical level of the folds was equal; amplitude was slightly decreased on the right and moderately reduced on the left. Normal mucosal wave was noted on the right fold, with a slightly decreased wave on the left side. This was consistent with a finding of partial absence of vibratory behavior, or an adynamic segment, on the left vocal fold. Phase shift and periodicity were sometimes irregular. Hyperfunction, as exhibited by squeezing of the larynx anteroposteriorly and increased ventricular fold adduction, was not observed.

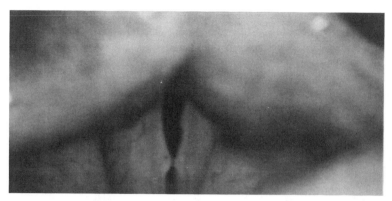

FIG 3–1.
Pretreatment stroboscopic image during phonation.

TABLE 3–3.

Pretreatment Acoustic and Physiologic Signs

Acoustic Signs	Physiologic Signs
Average fundamental frequency = 201.01	Abduction quotient = 0.74
Phonational range = 18.22 semitones	Closing slope = −464.57
Average sound pressure level = 68.66 dB	Mean flow = 167.45 mL/sec
Dynamic range = 31.6 dB	Peak flow = 299.86 mL/sec
Signal-to-noise ratio = 12.46 dB	Leak flow = 36.75 mL/sec
s/z ratio = 1.6	Open quotient = 55.37
Maximum phonation time = 19 sec	
Shimmer = 5.91	
Jitter = 0.03	

Acoustic Signs and Physiological Signs

The C-Speech software program was used to compute the acoustic measures reported here, with the exception of noninstrumental measurement of the s/z ratio and maximum phonation time. Acoustic measures are summarized in Table 3–3, together with physiologic measures. Measures of the physiological signs—airflow and the opening and closing of the vocal folds—were obtained using the techniques of inverse filtered airflow and electroglottography, respectively.

Therapy techniques are simply means by which we attempt to elicit changes in phonatory physiology through a behavioral approach. There is no magic in the technique itself. Its effectiveness lies in its ability to elicit the desired behavior from a given individual. It is probably the case that a number of techniques may produce the same result, and that a given technique is not equally effective with all patients.

In instances of benign vocal fold lesions or of hyperfunction, the goals of therapy are to eliminate those abusive behaviors that we believe had a role in the development of the problem and a continued role in its maintenance; to restore the vocal fold mucosa to a healthy condition and phonatory physiology to normal, thereby restoring improved voice production; and to prevent recurrence. Producing voice is a semi-involuntary, holistic type of activity that most individuals perform quite unconsciously and without thought. Of course, we monitor the sound of our voices through the auditory feedback loop, but we are not conscious at each moment of loudness, pitch, degree of tension, and similar vocal features as isolated phenomena. Because this is so, it seems that a therapy technique that accomplishes its desired result in a holistic manner may be easiest for patients to learn and may be most beneficial. That core technique for this group of patients is the use of breathy phonation.

Breathy phonation can also be described as a confidential voice quality, talking so as not to be overheard by others. It differs from whispering in that some voicing is present. We have examined laryngeal behavior fiberoptically in a number of subjects with and without vocal disease as they produced voice (Casper et al, 1989; Casper et al, 1990). Although some variability was observed in the glottal configuration, there was some degree of incomplete glottal closure in all cases. Aerodynamic measurements revealed increased mean and leakage flows consistent with the incomplete glottal closure. These observations confirmed that breathy phonation usually elicits the desired behavior.

Why is incomplete glottal closure a desired behavior? Indeed, breathy speech is often considered poor voicing. That may well be true if a breathy voice quality is used habitually by an individual. As a therapy technique, however, it is used for a specified time period and with a specific purpose and must not be confused with the desired end product of therapy. It has been my experience that breathy phonation accomplishes the following.

1. Because the vocal folds do not make contact or make it very gently, the amount and force of the contact is reduced, thereby reducing the constant irritation of the vocal folds.

2. Breathy phonation automatically reduces intensity, often a factor in both the cause and maintenance of the problem, and thus, it effectively eliminates talking in noisy surroundings or above ambient noise because it is inaudible in such situations.

3. Because airflow is increased when using breathy phonation, the patient must also renew air supply more frequently, thereby automatically reducing rate of speech and the tendency of some speakers to push voice out on the last remnant of available air.

4. Breathy phonation cannot be produced in a tense or strained manner, and thus, its use helps to eliminate patterns of increased musculoskeletal strain in voice production. (Patients with laryngeal lesions or edema need to work harder to produce voice and tend to adopt such habits unwittingly. They will tell you that unless they "push" they make no sound, and it is that "push" that must be eliminated.)

5. The emphasis on using a lot of air and allowing that air to keep flowing freely while speaking also eliminates strain without direct attention to the strain, but rather focusing on a positive behavior that can be identified by feel and sound.

Patients must often be taught how to produce breathy phonation. The presentation of a model and the instruction to talk in a confidential voice may be sufficient in some instances, or may at least elicit a close enough approximation of the desired quality so that additional trials and instruction will suffice. However, it may be necessary with some patients to start at a more basic task, such as the sigh and the yawn/sigh to teach easy, unimpeded airflow and unstressed voicing. All patients need to practice breathy phonation so that they can become adept at producing it at will and become accustomed to its sound.

When teaching breathy phonation, it is important for the clinician to be aware of some pitfalls. The term breathy must be taken literally. It is not enough for the voice just to be lowered in intensity. The breathiness must be very soft and without any evidence of pushing or forcing air out. The phonation produced must remain well focused, be at the patient's comfortable pitch level, and must not be monotonic. Patients often have a tendency to lower the pitch and the focus of the voice when using breathy phonation. (Be wary of perceptual judgments of pitch, as they are often incorrect. Measure it to verify perception.) Instruct patients to increase water intake because of the drying effect of increased airflow over the vocal folds. Always progress gradually from step to step, allowing enough time for the patient to learn a task and acquire a level of comfort and experience with it. As therapy progresses, increase the amount of voicing used without increasing strain.

Course of Therapy

Therapy began with a simplified explanation of the process of phonation, using pictures, diagrams, and other aids. The effect on this process of the existing disorder or abusive behaviors was also explained. This was followed by an exhaustive exploration of the patient's voice use—at home, work, recreation, and other situations. Patient G was instructed to keep a log for the first week indicating where she used her voice, with whom, the level of ambient environmental noise, the length of talking time, and so forth. (Patients are almost always surprised by what they learn from this activity and have a rewarding sense of having made important and personally meaningful discoveries.)

During the first session, patient G was also instructed in some rules of vocal hygiene and provided with an overview of what the therapy protocol would involve. She was instructed to (1) reduce overall amount of talking to those times when it is necessary, (2) refrain from any loud talking, (3) eliminate all throat clearing, (4) drink much water, and (5) practice assigned exercises as many times as possible, but at least four to five times per day for short periods of time.

Because the problem was of such long standing, and because she had developed habitually strained and tense phonatory behavior, therapy began with the sigh. She was instructed to sit in a relaxed upright posture, to "take a nice and easy breath," and to allow that breath to leave the body in a sigh. Whether or not sound accompanies the sigh at first should not be an issue. She was further instructed in allowing her body to determine when it needed the next breath, and in keeping the inhalation and exhalation as a gentle, unbroken cycle. It is important to make sure that patients do not hold the breath prior to releasing it. In future sessions, the sigh is expanded to include production of slightly more voicing, to voicing as a soft hum, to voicing that begins gently at a higher pitch and glides down and out.

Patient G was also instructed in producing the yawn/sigh by opening the mouth wide, retracting the tongue, breathing in deeply through the open mouth and then releasing the sound as a combined yawn and sigh. She was told to place her fingers lightly on her larynx so that she could feel its descent as the mouth is opened wide and the tongue retracts. The larynx is to remain in that lowered posture until the completion of the sigh.

After 1 week of voice therapy, patient G reported the absence of all pain. Her throat felt relaxed; and she was using fairly breathy

phonation about 90% of the time. Practice on increasing the breathiness of phonation was tied to practicing "talking on the sigh" and on the yawn/sigh. This was begun with a single word per sigh and progressed to short sentences in which all the words began with vowels. During therapy sessions the Visi-Pitch was used to monitor fundamental frequency, frequency variability in speech, intensity level, and other aspects of phonation.

As voice quality improved and patient G became more proficient in phonatory tasks and manipulation of phonatory behavior, some therapy time was devoted to placement or focus of the voice, but always flowing. Although the amount of breathiness was in reality being gradually reduced, the concept of maintaining a flow of air helps patients to avoid strain and tension at the laryngeal level. It is a concept that is incompatible with tension, which tends to shut off air supply. The final two therapy sessions were devoted to helping the patient become comfortable in using full voicing without strain, and even increasing loudness.

Post-treatment Evaluation

At the conclusion of eight sessions of voice therapy, which took place over a 9-week period of time, patient G returned for complete post-treatment assessment at which time all the measures obtained initially were repeated with the following results.

Perceptual Signs

The voice acceptability rating made by the Voice Team was 4.5 (with 5 being normal). Voice quality was perceptually judged to be clear, with very slight breathiness. Tension or strain during phonation were not observable. The patient described an absence of pain and believed her voice was back to its "normal" quality.

Stroboscopic/Laryngoscopic Signs

Vocal fold edge in the patient's larynx was found to be smooth bilaterally, although there was still a slight tendency toward an hourglass appearance during phonation. Figure 3–2 shows the comparison between the pretreatment appearance of the patient's vocal folds

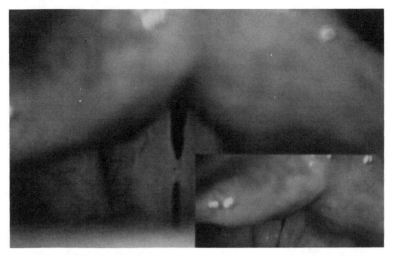

FIG 3–2.
Comparison of pretreatment stroboscopic image during phonation and post-treatment image *(inset)*.

TABLE 3–4.

Post-treatment Acoustic and Physiologic Signs

Acoustic Signs	Physiologic Signs
Average fundamental frequency = 217.76	Abduction quotient = 0.3
Phonational range = 34.39 semitones	Closing slope = −1549.65
Average sound pressure level = 71.85 dB	Mean flow = 102.83 mL/sec
Dynamic range = 42.82 dB	Peak flow = 295.74 mL/sec
Signal-to-noise ratio = 22.49 dB	Leak flow = 11.90 mL/sec
s/z ratio = 1.1	Open quotient = 56.12
Maximum phonation time = 25 sec	
Shimmer = 1.50	
Jitter = 0.01	

and their post-treatment appearance. Phase closure was described as being just slightly more open than normal. Amplitude, mucosal wave, vibratory behavior, periodicity, and phase symmetry were all judged to be normal and regular.

Acoustic Signs and Physiological Signs

The values for these signs are shown in Table 3–4. Of more clinical impact however, are Figures 3–3 and 3–4, which demonstrate the percent change following treatment. All of the values changed in the hoped for directions, being consistent with improved vocal function. The dramatic change in the abduction quotient is objective evidence for the reduction in breathiness, while marked change in the closing slope measure attests to the increased efficiency of voice production.

The laryngologist's post-therapy examination summary included the following statement: "Patient G has had an excellent voice result with speech therapy. She is now back to her premorbid condition. Stroboscopic examination shows excellent return of function with a slight nodular diathesis with mucus collection at the nodal point." The patient was examined again 3 months after termination of treatment, during which time she had resumed teaching. The findings at that follow-up visit were essentially identical to those reported following treatment. It was recommended that patient G pursue further treatment of her allergy condition.

Case Summary

This case demonstrates the use of a group of treatment techniques designed to eliminate

Acoustic Measurements

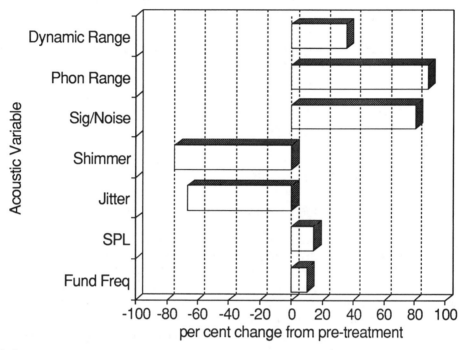

FIG 3–3.
Percent change in acoustic measures following treatment.

Aerodynamic Measurements

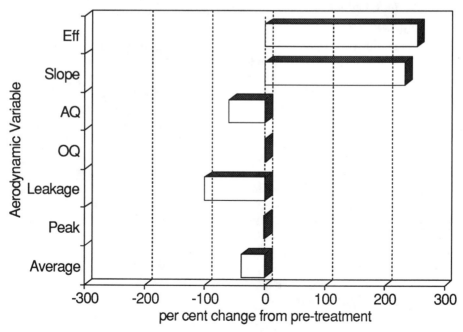

FIG 3–4.
Percent change in aerodynamic measures following treatment.

vocally abusive behaviors, restore the vocal folds to a healthy condition, and teach/retrain appropriate voice use behaviors. However, there are some caveats to bear in mind. Although we have found these techniques to be effective with many individuals, they are not being presented as "the sole" method for consideration. They must be applied sensibly, and the emphasis placed on any one of the techniques must be guided by the patient's needs and responses to therapy. There is still much we do not know about benign vocal fold lesions, their cause, the selectivity factors that allow them to occur in one patient and not in another person who may be equally vocally abusive, or the role of allergy in their development, maintenance, and recurrence. In the case of patient G we have concern about her continued nodal diathesis, the prenodular sign of mucous piling up at the nodal point. We are continuing to monitor her in the hope that we can prevent recurrence of the condition. The therapy time spent on discussion of techniques of vocal hygiene, a constant thread throughout, should also prove to be helpful in avoiding recurrence.

"SOFT WHISPER" TECHNIQUE

Contributed by John Hufnagle, Ph.D.

Next, Jon Hufnagle, Ph.D., presents a case study demonstrating his technique utilizing a "soft whisper" as a facilitating approach to improved voice.

CASE STUDY: PATIENT H

When patient H was first seen she was a 20-year-old healthy female college student who developed a dysphonic voice during her sophomore year. She reported that she never had difficulty with her voice until that time. The difficulty started in September, at the beginning of the school year. At that time she was elected "rush" chairperson of her sorority. She started to use her voice in a strenuous fashion soon after the election. She reported that in the initial stages the voice would be better in the morning and during the weekdays. However, on weekends the voice deteriorated. After 2 months of having problems, she came to the university clinic. During the initial evaluation she reported that she was having difficulty maintaining voice during the day, particularly at night when she was participating in sorority activities. The situation was worse during the weekends. By Sunday nights she reported she was almost aphonic.

Voice Evaluation

Samples of the patient's voice were obtained by having her read the "Rainbow Passage" (Fairbanks, 1960), saying the vowels /i/, /a/, and /u/ for 5 seconds, and engaging her in conversation. The passage, vowels, and 1 minute of conversation were recorded on a reel-to-reel tape recorder, using appropriate recording techniques (Izdebski, 1981). Perceptually, her voice was rated 5 on a scale of 1 to 7, with 1 being normal and 7 being severe. She was judged to have moderate breathiness, a moderate to severe degree of constriction, a slightly low pitch, and a low focus of the voice.

During the evaluation patient H did not exhibit any grossly obvious breathing anomalies. Her vital capacity was 3.5 liters. Maximum phonation times for the vowels /i/, /a/, and /u/ were 15, 12, and 13 seconds, respectively. The s/z ratio was 1.67, with the /s/ being 20 seconds and the /z/ being 12 seconds. The phonation quotient (using the /a/) was calculated to be 291, which should be considered high and out of the range of normal.

Jitter and signal-to-noise ratio (SNR) were obtained using commercially available software. A 1,000-ms section of the /a/ was isolated. Ten tokens of 100-ms each were measured and averaged together to obtain a mean jitter (ms) and SNR (dB). The mean values for jitter and SNR were .033 and 18.64, respectively. (Normal adult values obtained using similar analysis and software are jitter $< .04$ ms, and SNR > 20 dB (Milenkovic, 1987). Fundamental frequency for the vowel was 175.45 Hz. Average fundamental frequency for the second sentence of the "Rainbow Passage" was 180.23 Hz.

Patient H was referred to a local otolaryngologist, who found small to moderate size bilateral vocal cord nodules by examination with a flexible nasoendoscope. Voice therapy was recommended.

During the initial therapy session, patient H was placed on a week of soft whisper to facilitate a target voice (Boone and McFarlane, 1988).

Rationale for Using Soft Whisper

Whisper has been criticized as a form of vocal rest in vocal rehabilitation programs because it is believed harmful to the vocal mechanism, aggravating an existing dysphonia (Boone, 1977; Brodnitz, 1958). However, recent investigations appear to be in conflict with these historical views of whisper (Solomon et al., 1989; Monoson and Zemlin, 1984; Hufnagle and Hufnagle, 1983).

Whisper has been defined as an aperiodic noise caused by rapidly flowing air passing through the glottis (Daniloff, Schuckers, and Feth, 1980). Two types of whisper have been identified and discussed in the literature: soft whisper and stage whisper. Recent investigations have focused on identifying differences and similarities between the two. The variables investigated were glottal configuration, vibratory patterns, aerodynamics, and supraglottal involvement.

A difference in glottal configuration has been found to be dependent on the type of whisper being used. During low-energy whisper (soft whisper), Monoson and Zemlin (1984) observed an inverted "V" or a bow-shaped glottis. Solomon et al. (1989) found that the vocal folds were either straight or parallel to each other or the vocal processes were "toed in" slightly. A summary of the literature appears to indicate that during soft whisper the vocal folds are straight in configuration, creating an inverted "V" glottal shape, or they are slightly bowed. As the effort of the whisper increases, the vocal processes begin to "toe in". As effort continues to increase, the classical "Y" shape with a posterior chink becomes more prominent, with a long triangle initially and a short triangle at the extreme of stage whisper. In all situations the vocal folds were apart, more pronounced in soft whisper than in stage whisper (Solomon et al., 1989; Monoson and Zemlin, 1984; Pressman and Kelemen, 1955).

Very little disagreement can be found about vocal fold vibration during whisper. An overwhelming majority of researchers agree that no vibration is present during whisper, either low effort or high effort (Monoson and Zemlin, 1984; Solomon et al., 1989; Sawashima and Hirose, 1983; Vilkman et al., 1987; Pressman and Keleman, 1970; Daniloff, Schuckers, and Feth, 1980).

Airflow during whisper has been generally shown to be significantly greater than during voiced speech. Monoson and Zemlin (1984) and Lehiste (1962) demonstrated that soft whisper has airflow rates twice that of normal phonation. Supraglottal constriction has been observed during whisper. However, the degree of constriction appears to be dependent on the type of whisper produced. Solomon et al. (1989) noted constriction of the supraglottal structures (structures between vocal folds and the rim of the epiglottis) during high-effort whisper much more than during low-effort whisper.

In the only clinical study to date, Hufnagle and Hufnagle (1983) investigated whisper to determine the efficacy of soft whisper as a facilitating procedure for voice therapy. Ten women diagnosed by an otolaryngologist as having vocal fold nodules participated in the study. The subjects were instructed in the use of soft whisper and then instructed to use soft whisper for 7 days. Prewhisper and postwhisper audio recordings were made. Listeners were instructed to choose the recording (prewhisper or postwhisper) which had the better vocal quality. The results showed a significant preference for the vocal quality following a week of soft whisper, indicating that soft whisper did not have a deteriorating effect on vocal quality. Therefore, this study suggests that soft whisper is not harmful.

The above review of the literature suggests that soft whisper may provide an efficient, rapid, and easily understood method of eliminating vocal abuse and restoring a more normal voice. It appears that soft whisper is nonabusive and can be used in the initial stage of therapy to facilitate a target voice. The clinician then can reinforce and habituate the target voice, train phonatory efficiency and help the patient identify potentially abusive behaviors.

Description of the Procedure

Soft whisper is used in the beginning of therapy to obtain or facilitate a model or target voice. The patient has only to follow the directions for a period of time and the voice will improve. As with all facilitating techniques, patient compliance is necessary. The clinician should be the judge as to the appropriateness of the procedure with a particular patient. As with all facilitating techniques, those that may work for one patient may not work for another patient with the same kind of voice problem. The type of problems that seem to benefit most from soft whisper are problems associated with muscular tension dysphonia (Kaufmann and Blalock, in press).

Implementing soft whisper with patient H, the following points were adhered to.

1. An audio recording of the voice should be obtained for baselining purposes. The recording should consist of a 1-minute sample of the voice during conversation, recitation of the "Rainbow Passage," and recitation of the vowels /i/ and /a/. These samples should be obtained using appropriate recording procedures. A high-quality recording is very important because it will be used to judge change. The recording is usually obtained during the initial voice evaluation.

2. During the first therapy session, a thorough explanation of the procedure and the necessity of the patient to follow the directions should be emphasized. With children it is necessary that a parent be present during this time. Also, if the child is in school, the teacher needs to be informed that the child will be using soft whisper for a short period of time. During this time the teacher should be instructed not to require the child to do activities that require full voice, such as oral reading or a class presentation.

3. The patient should be instructed to use soft whisper in a one-to-one situation only. He or she should not attempt to communicate to a group of people in a large room or to people in an outdoors situation. Telephone use should be limited.

4. The patient should not mouth a word, which requires holding a breath (closing the vocal folds).

5. The patient should be instructed to not say more than three or four words on a breath stream. To do more puts a strain on the respiratory system which can be reflected in the laryngeal system. In other words, the whisper will progress more towards a stage whisper.

6. The clinician should practice soft whisper with the patient for an extensive period of time during the first session. Many people do not know how to whisper softly. Many will use a breathy voice.

7. If the patient is a child, the family must become involved. For example, when the family is together, perhaps at night, all members of the family could use soft whisper. A reward system could be established.

8. The patient should use soft whisper for 5 to 7 days, the time period being dependent on the schedule of the patient. If the patient has a previously scheduled activity over the weekend, then the time period should be adjusted appropriately. The clinician should try to see the patient once or twice during the soft whisper period. During these short sessions, the clinician can answer any questions and reinforce the patient.

9. Following the period of soft whisper the patient should be recorded again using the same material previously used. The pretreatment and post-treatment recordings should be evaluated by the clinician and patient. The improved voice can then be used as a basis of explaining how and why the voice problem started and what is needed to improve the voice permanently.

Following 1 week of soft whisper, patient H's voice improved. Quality was judged to be a 4. Breathiness and focus improved slightly. Pitch was judged not to have changed. However, a significant change in constriction was noted. Acoustic analysis found jitter to be 0.017 and SNR 23.33. Prewhisper data was 0.033 for jitter and 18.64 for the SNR. However, because of her old habits, her voice deteriorated through the session. But, goals were set and the patient was able to hear her more normal voice. For the patient, it was very motivational being able to hear her improved voice.

During the next six therapy sessions, the clinician reinforced the more normal voice productions, developed phonatory efficiency, helped the patient identify periods of vocal abuse, and created an awareness of potentially abusive behaviors. After seven sessions it was determined the patient's voice was within normal limits, and therapy was discontinued. Post-therapy laryngeal examination revealed no vocal cord nodules.

Because of either habit, the presence of edema or mass lesions, or laryngeal muscle strain, many persons with voice disorders produce voice with a strained "back-focus" of the laryngeal tone. These patients are essentially muscling the tone at the level of the folds, thus restricting full pharnygeal/oral/nasal resonation. Backward focus leads to laryngeal fatigue and vocal hyperfunction.

REFOCUSING LARYNGEAL TONE

Contributed by Linda Lee, Ph.D.

In the following case study, Linda Lee, Ph.D., describes the history of refocusing laryngeal tone along with a management technique for facilitating a more appropriate frontal focus.

CASE STUDY: PATIENT I

Patient I, a 21-year-old female college senior, came to the University of Cincinnati Speech and Hearing Clinic because of vocal fatigue and periodic loss of voice. She reported that her voice had always been what she described as "rough" and would "give out" after long periods of talking, but daily fatigue had coincided with the start of student teaching in her major area of elementary education. Her voice production became increasingly effortful as the day of teaching progressed and improved on weekends.

The patient was a nonsmoker in good health, with the exception of allergies, which caused sinus congestion in the spring. She used an antihistamine (Seldane) during this period and took no other medication. Her daily fluid intake included caffeinated tea and orange juice at breakfast, iced tea during the day, and diet cola at dinner. Water intake was limited to occasional sips at the school water fountain or following exercise.

Patient I's teaching schedule consisted of 5 hours in the classroom. She had a 1-hour preparation break late in the morning, half an hour for lunch (shared with a group of teachers in a lounge), and two breaks in the afternoon (6 minutes each). The patient lived with two other nonsmoking roommates and described herself as socially outgoing. Her interests included dining out, biking, and traveling. Singing activities had been eliminated several years previously.

Laryngeal Examination

Patient I was examined by an otolaryngologist, who found edema of the vocal folds. An expectorant (Humibid) was prescribed on an as-needed basis.

Voice Evaluation

Subjective Observations

Patient I's voice production during conversation consisted of 60% to 75% glottal fry. Phonation at the initial portion of most sentences was at the lower end of her frequency range but had good tonal quality. Mild laryngeal and jaw tension were noted during conversation. The focus of the voice was low and back. Respiration was characterized by shallow breathing during conversational speech.

Objective Analysis

Fundamental frequency was determined with a Visi-Pitch (Kay Elemetrics). During production of sustained vowels /i,a,u/, the fundamental frequencies averaged 192 Hz for comfortable pitch, 405 for high pitch, and 182 for low pitch. The total frequency range was 168 to 475 Hz during reading; the average fundamental frequency was 185 Hz.

Maximum phonation times for vowels averaged 11 seconds at comfortable pitch, 7.5 seconds at high pitch, and 9 seconds at low pitch. She sustained the /s/ for 20 seconds and the /z/ for 14.

Impressions

Patient I had a voice disorder characterized by the frequent use of glottal fry phonation and a low, back-focus. The disorder was further complicated by a lack of hydration of the system, poor breath support, and a vocally demanding schedule.

Prognosis

The prognosis for eliminating the voice disorder was considered good, based on the patient's recognition of the problem, motivation, and willingness to assume the responsibility for change.

Recommendations

Patient I was enrolled in voice therapy twice weekly. Her goals consisted of the following.

1. Learn physiologic exercises for improving vocal function, as described in Stemple (1984). These exercises will be performed twice daily.
2. Improve vocal hygiene by increasing hydration and reducing laryngeal tension.
3. Improve respiratory support for speech.
4. Use a forward, frontal focus for her voice.
5. Eliminate the use of glottal fry phonation.

Management Program

Following initial counseling and introduction to therapy, patient I was trained in the use of the vocal function exercises. These exercises were reviewed at the initial part of each therapy session. The patient immediately switched from caffeinated to noncaffeinated beverages and increased her intake of water to eight glasses per day by carrying a thermos of ice water to school with her. She also substituted fruit juice for some of her colas. A final immediate change was in the arrangement of her room at school, so that the environment was as free of competing background noise as possible.

The mechanics of speech breathing and importance of respiratory support for speech were explained. The patient learned to inspire to a higher lung volume by placing one hand on her chest and one on her abdomen during speech. This tactile cue was enough to remind her to take a deeper breath at the beginning of sentences and at phrase boundaries. Occasion-

ally, the tactile cue was supplemented by marking breathing places on her reading passages. The tactile cue was dropped as soon as the pattern began to habituate.

The majority of the therapy sessions were aimed at changing the focus of the voice. Therefore, this aspect of management will be described in detail.

Philosophy of Treatment for Altering Tone Focus

Focus refers to the resonation of the voice in the airways. Forward focus allows the voice to resonate fully throughout the pharyngeal cavities. When an obstruction such as the presence of laryngeal or upper airway tension impedes resonance, the focus of the voice is shifted away from its ideal placement. The result is a voice that tires easily and lacks flexibility and vibrancy.

The concept of altering focus has been addressed in two bodies of literature: voice disorder and singing. Techniques for altering focus in both bodies are similar, although terminology varies and some authors rely more heavily on imagery than information. Singers most often refer to "placing the voice" in their attempts to control focus. Lamperti (1931) is probably the most poetic in his address of the subject:

"Noise is a naked skeleton. Tone is fleshed in its own harmonics, and clothed in the overtones of surrounding space." (p. 40)

"When the top and bottom of the lungs are equally full of compressed air, the voice will focus in the head, and awake all the resonance in the head, mouth, and chest. Diction then is master over all." (p. 43)

Constriction at any point alters focus. Christy (1961) talks about moving focus away from the larynx by releasing it of tension. He states that the voice places itself if resonance is free and balanced. A common technique of singing teachers is to ask the student to place the voice "into the mask" behind the eyes, out in front, behind the teeth, and so forth. Although this imagery will work for some, Christy believes that the voice should not be "put" anywhere. He feels that this concept leads to fixing or setting of the muscles of phonation or articulation, thereby moving the constriction from one part of the airway to another. The resonance tends to be "imprisoned" and the individual pushes the voice, leading to even tighter muscles and a more deteriorated tone (Emil-Behnke, 1945; Fawcus, 1986).

Improper focus is rarely an isolated problem. However, when focus is moved forward, improvements may be seen in other aspects of phonation. Tetrazzini (1975) stated that if breathing is correct and the focus of the tone is correct, other problems will probably resolve. This was the philosophy applied to the present case. Therapy was aimed at altering patient I's focus rather than the glottal fry production, believing that tone would improve as a secondary effect.

Orientation to the Management Approach

The concept of resonance is not an easy one to communicate to the client. I rely more on sensation than the ear when teaching focus. Every client I have helped with focus has had an "ah-ha!" experience, in which the idea suddenly became meaningful. Always searching for new and better ways to explain this concept, I ask them to describe the difference between the back-focus and the more forward placement. Each has said it "feels different"; that the energy is now experienced anywhere from the alveolar ridge to the front of the mouth. They also typically say that phonation is easier or more comfortable to produce. When a patient hears his or her voice on a tape recorder, most recognize that it sounds brighter and louder. One client said, "Oh, that's my bedroom voice!" When we managed to stop laughing and her face returned to its normal color, she explained that she uses that voice when she and her husband are talking in bed and they do not want to wake the children in the next room. What she did not realize is that her properly focused "bedroom voice" probably carried farther than the disordered one!

The importance of providing a model for each stage of treatment cannot be overemphasized. Patients required some time to learn to change focus at will without altering fundamental frequency, but the change truly has

been worth a thousand words. Adding a bit of tension in the laryngeal and lower tongue area does the trick for me. Tape recording is also a part of every session and is used often as a form of feedback. Finally, I am a firm believer in homework. In addition to the vocal function exercises, patient I was given drills to complete at home. Sometimes I asked her to tape record these drills; always I made sure she did not need my cues or feedback in order to complete them.

Treatment Stages

A number of resources were used when developing a plan for the treatment stages, especially Colton and Casper (1990) Fawcus (1986) and Boone (1983).

Step 1. — I began by asking patient I to read a passage while concentrating on where she felt the most sensations; where she felt the "energy" of her speech. Invariably, clients with low, back-focus point to the throat. I then talked about the need to pull that energy forward, stating that when it is confined in the laryngeal area, sound is restricted. I explained that the voice receives its quality or character by resonating through the passages above the throat, and that she needed to open these cavities to take advantage of them.

Following this orientation to the treatment approach, patient I was instructed to hum at a comfortable pitch. She was encouraged to relax, enjoy the process, and phonate without pushing. I checked to be sure her jaw was dropped and relaxed, the tongue was limp, and there was no laryngeal tension. With some clients, relaxation exercises are needed prior to this activity.

We then produced the nasal consonants /m/ and /n/ with vowels in consonant-vowel (CV) combinations. These were repeated on a comfortable pitch so that one sound dissolved into the next and the nasal was emphasized. Patient I was encouraged to feel the vibration created at the sides of her nose and on the facial bones.

Other clues which may help bring focus forward at this stage include the following:

1. Pretend you have a comb with a tissue over it. Put the comb in front of your lips and

make a vibrating noise on it. Pretend you are moving the place of sound vibration from your vocal folds to the front of your lips.

2. Make a "motorcycle noise" by vibrating your lips together. Extend phonation and change vowels (for example, bbbrrrr /i/, bbbrrr /o/).

3. Trill your tongue on the top of the alveolar ridge. Move your lips to shape different sounds. With all three of these techniques, extend the forward placement of vibration by moving into CV combinations with front placement.

4. Finally, produce a rather loud, well-supported sigh on the vowel /o/ or /a/, beginning at the higher end of the frequency range and phonating without break into lower midrange. This technique should extend the more forward focus usually produced at the higher pitches into the comfortable frequency range.

Step 2. — Using the humming procedure, patient I produced CVCV combinations. Initially, the consonants were all nasals (such as /mona/). Later, one /z/ (*not* /s/) was added, such as /mozo/ or /mizi/.

Step 3. — Patient I read short sentences which were loaded with nasal and other voiced consonants. The sentences were chanted slowly on a comfortable pitch, connecting the sounds together to make the sentence very "legato." She was reminded to take an adequate breath at the beginning, relax, and concentrate on the feelings of vibration. Examples of the sentences used are

1. My mother makes much money.
2. Nana made lemon jam.
3. Many mice munch on melons.
4. Mary meets me at the market.
5. Monogamy is monotonous.
6. Many moonrocks are mined on Mars.
7. Mudpies are made in mud.

Although some sources recommend using shorter phrases first, I have discovered that the sentence gives the client time to develop the feeling of resonation.

Step 4. — This stage usually proves to be the most difficult, because it is the transition from

chanting to speaking. Using the same sentences as in step three, patient I first chanted the whole sentence. Next, following my model at her comfortable pitch, she chanted the first word and spoke the sentences **as a question with rising intonation.** At first, as soon as she ended the chanted word, she dropped into back-focus. She was reminded to emphasize the nasal sounds just as she had during the chanting and take her time producing the sentence. Occasionally, she needed reminders to take an adequate breath or to relax her jaw. Patient I spent 1 week at this stage. When she could produce the questions without first chanting the entire sentence and with 90% success, she followed the same procedure but used falling intonation. It was at this stage that the patient had her "ah-ha!" experience and began to show consistency.

Step 5. — Patient I was ready to move into longer utterances, but she needed the nasal context to keep the focus forward. We used the following paragraph, initially marking breath groups.

Minnie mariner loved the water. Many members of her family had been in the Navy. Her uncle was a fisherman. He remembered many moments netting tuna in the pouring rain. When Minnie was a little girl, she dangled slimy worms to catch sunfish. Nothing was more fun than watching the sunfish nibble the worms. When she was seventeen, Minnie learned to sail. She named her boat Minerva. Sometimes, her best friend, Nancy Noman, went with her. Their mothers never minded their sailing. When the dinner bell rang, Nancy and Minnie always came home.

Step 6. — Patient I was now 4 weeks into therapy. Her maximum phonation times on the vocal function exercises had increased to an average of 20 seconds at all pitch levels. Inspiring to higher lung volumes was more automatic, and signs of tension were gone during practice. Exercise sentences were free of glottal fry, although it still entered into conversational speech.

Nonnasal sentences with many forward consonants were introduced (for example, "Ted bought a baby bed"). A light articulatory contact was encouraged. If this patient had experienced difficulty with this step, questions containing nasals in the initial word only would have been used, followed by statements.

Step 7. — As patient I became accustomed to sentences and paragraphs which were not controlled for phonetic context, short segments of conversation were added. Whenever she slipped into old patterns, she was reminded to take a better breath, hum for a moment to regain focus, drop her jaw, and so forth, as she repeated the phrase. Short periods of conversation were extended outside the therapy room by establishing specific times, places, and conversation partners.

Step 8. — When the patient could converse without losing focus the majority of the time, background noise was added with a radio in the therapy room. We also left the therapy room to converse in other environments and with different people.

Step 9. — Finally, patient I role-played some of her teaching activities in a large classroom. Here, she sometimes needed reminders about breath support. She also tape recorded parts of her lessons at school so that we could evaluate them together.

Results of Therapy

Patient I improved the quality of her voice production by creating a more forward focus, increasing breath support, and releasing tension. These changes resulted in an elimination of glottal fry. She was dismissed after 7 weeks of therapy, with the advice that she continue the vocal function exercises at least once a day and maintain her present level of fluid intake. She no longer experienced laryngeal fatigue and was very happy with her new manner of speaking.

ACCENT METHOD
Contributed by Danna Koschkee, M.A.

Vocal hyperfunction may also be a symptom of many other medical disorders and disabilities. In the next case study, Danna Koschkee, M.A., discusses a voice therapy technique known as the Accent Method (Smith and Thyme, 1976, 1978), which enhances improvement not only in phonation but also in the interplay of phonation among respiration, resonation, and articulation.

CASE STUDY: PATIENT J

Therapy efficacy studies, using the Accent Method for treatment of functional voice disorders, have been reported by several European investigators (Smith and Thyme, 1976, 1978). Their results have documented increases in vocal intensity, frequency range, and general intelligibility. Earlier use of the Accent technique with stutterers and clutterers demonstrated the method's applicability in improving timing, fluency, and prosody of speech. Despite the apparent effectiveness of this approach in improving the "control aspects" of speech production, no case studies utilizing Accent therapy in the treatment of dysarthria have been reported previously.

The purpose of this case presentation is to describe use of the Accent methodology in treating a closed head injury patient, 13 years following the head trauma. The discussion includes a rationale for the treatment approach and provides specific information regarding procedures and effectiveness of the intervention method in this case.

Rationale

Selection of the Accent Method for treatment of a patient with a closed head injury was based in part on the technique's holistic or whole-system approach toward phonatory improvement. Deficits in pulmonary support, voice initiation, underarticulation, and coordination of resonation with speech are emphasized in this method. Because of the interplay among the various subsystems (respiration, phonation, resonation, and articulation) necessary to produce the Accent rhythms, the goal is not to isolate but rather integrate these functions so that the result is automatic regulation.

Furthermore, other whole-system approaches such as Melodic Intonation Therapy (MIT) have proved effective in improving total communication skills across populations (aphasics, apraxics, dysarthrics, and Down's syndrome individuals). Like MIT, the Accent Method utilizes intoned rhythms, distinct/accentuated stress patterns, and slowed tempo to facilitate productions.

Physiologically, the Accent method purports to: (1) increase pulmonary output, (2) reduce glottic waste, (3) reduce excessive muscular tension, and (4) normalize the vibratory pattern produced during phonation. According to the technique's originators (Smith and Thyme-Frokjaer), the technique rests on the myoelastic and aerodynamic therapy of voice production. They state that because voice production is created by subglottal air pressure and transglottal airflow, stronger air pressures below the vocal folds (that is, the abdominal expiratory activity) results in an increased amplitude of vibration and a more normalized closed phase in the glottal cycle. The filtering process of the vocal tract is improved, presumably as a result of a longer duration of the vocal fold contact within one single period and a higher flow through the glottis in the opening phase, which together counteract the damping effect of the resonances in the vocal tract. The reported acoustic effects of treatment are (1) increased energy of the fundamental frequency, (2) increased energy in the F2 to F3 region, (3) reduced irregular pitch perturbations, (4) optimal fundamental frequency, 5) increased fundamental frequency range, nd (6) increased dynamic range.

Patient History

Patient J, a 30-year-old woman, was involved in an automobile accident in October 1979 and sustained severe closed head injury, which resulted in significant cognitive deficits, spastic left hemiplegia, and severe dysarthria. She remained in a coma for approximately 6 months and then received extensive rehabilitation during the next 7 years, including speech therapy. Her major areas of deficit were respiratory, laryngeal, and velopharyngeal dysfunction. Medical evaluation resulted in a diagnosis of a mixed level paresis involving the recurrent laryngeal nerve, superior laryngeal nerve, and pharyngeal components, with greater involvement on the left side. Surgical interventions undertaken to improve glottic closure included two collagen injections (1984) and an Ishsiki (type I) thyroplasty (1990). A pharyngeal flap procedure was performed in 1980 to reduce velopharyngeal incompetence.

Pretreatment Status

Prior to initiation of Accent Therapy and 13 years following her trauma, the patient was evaluated with a comprehensive battery of vocal function tests. At the time of testing, her intellectual functioning was reported to be within the average range, as were her receptive and expressive language skills. She stated that she was highly motivated to improve her voice further. Previous phonosurgery had resulted in reduced problems with swallowing and choking but minimal improvements in voice. She continued to present a mild degree of velopharyngeal dysfunction, most prevalent during the production of plosives, fricatives, and affricates, although her speaking voice was not perceived as excessively nasal.

Examinations

The test battery included perceptual, aerodynamic, acoustic, and videostroboscopic examinations. All tests were administered three times within a 1-week period in order to monitor baseline performance. Baseline stability fell within a 10% range of the overall mean response for all measures except mean airflow rate and habitual fundamental frequency. The baseline instability demonstrated on these two measures was considered characteristic of the patient's performance since high variability was observed across tasks over time. A summary of overall baseline mean responses (average of B1, B2, and B3) is reported below.

Perceptual Judgments

On the GRBAS scale, a 4-point, equal-appearing-interval scale where 1 represents normal and 4 represents severe (Hirano, 1981), overall grade or severity was rated 4, roughness 2, aesthenic 4, breathy 4, and strain 4.

Aerodynamics

Air flow measures, obtained using the Nagashim PS-77 Phonatory function Analyzer, showed a high degree of variability within tasks although the mean airflow rate ($\overline{X}$ = 192 cc/sec) fell at the upper end of the normative range. Typically, the patient demonstrated peak airflow (500 cc/sec) during pre-exhalation or voice onset followed by a sloping decline in airflow rate during sustained phonation. Maximum phonation time was significantly reduced ($\overline{X}$ = 1.8 seconds) as was the total phonatory volume ($\overline{X}$ = 260 mL) expended during maximum phonation time. Intraoral pressure measurements fell well below normal ($\overline{X}$ = 1.1 cm H_2O).

Acoustics

Simultaneous recordings of fundamental frequency and intensity were obtained using the Phonatory function Analyzer. Generally, habitual fundamental frequency was aperiodic, although the overall mean value of 223 Hz fell within normal limits for an adult woman speaker. Frequency range was significantly reduced (9 semitones) as was vocal intensity range (13 dB/SPL). Habitual speaking level was lower than expected at 64 dB. Analysis using the C-Speech software program revealed a near-normal value for jitter (.05 msec) while shimmer and SNR fell well outside of the acceptable range.

Videostroboscopy

Videostroboscopic examination with a rigid endoscope was completed during several phonatory and breathing tasks. It was observed that the patient had symmetrical closure, but periodicity was inconsistent, at times both regular and irregular. Glottic closure was complete in the membranous portion of the glottis, but a large posterior glottal chink was present. Although it is typical to see a posterior glottal chink in women, the chink appeared somewhat larger than is typically seen. A slight abduction of the left arytenoid seemed to be a contributing factor. Both amplitude and mucosal wave were small bilaterally. No nonvibrating portions of the larynx were observed. During respiratory tasks, the patient showed inconsistency in her ability to abduct the vocal folds. In between phonatory tasks, abduction was minimal. During maximum inspiratory tasks, the patient inconsistently abducted to what appeared to be a normal level. During phonation, it was noted that there was hyperfunction of the glottal structures, that is, the

vocal folds were closed with extreme force. Unfortunately, there did not appear to be adequate respiratory force to overcome the closure of the vocal folds. Thus, there was airflow escapage from the posterior glottal chink but limited movement and subsequent phonation coming from the vocal folds.

Impression

The patient exhibited voice problems that were due at least in part to inadequate breath support, poor respiratory and laryngeal coordination, and hyperfunctional closure of the membranous portion of the glottis. Although marked improvement in vocal functioning could not be expected, it was felt that the patient would benefit from a voice therapy program directed at improving respiratory support, increasing relaxation, and improving coordination between the respiratory and laryngeal systems. The Accent Method was selected as the behavioral approach to treatment.

Accent Therapy Methodology

The preparatory stage, the steps preceding Accent Therapy, were no different from those used routinely in planning any treatment program, and included (1) establishing baseline stability, (2) probing for stimulability, (3) identifying patterns of vocal dysfunction, and (4) predicting expected outcomes from treatment.

For our closed head injury patient, expected outcomes included (1) an increased phonatory volume elicited during a maximum phonation task, (2) an improved distribution of airflow over time (that is, reduced range of airflow/variability on maximum phonation time), (3) reduced hyperfunction of the glottal structures visualized during videostroboscopy, (4) increased frequency range of phonation, and (5) increased intensity range of phonation.

Accent Therapy Procedures

1. **Facilitate diaphragmal/abdominal breathing.** Since normal respiration at rest is diaphragmal/abdominal, the clinician needs only to elicit or facilitate this breathing pattern to begin Accent Therapy. Generally, a recum-

bent position works well, with gravity helping the patient to achieve a comfortable abdominal breathing pattern. However, in dysarthric individuals such as this patient, increased problems with swallowing and/or choking are likely to occur, so a sitting position was used. Once the patient had established abdominal breathing at rest, she was instructed to place one hand on the stomach to monitor the abdominal movements. The clinician simultaneously demonstrated abdominal breathing and upper body relaxation. A brief description of the action of the diaphragm (a lowering movement against the intestines or soft abdomen) to increase the chest cavity was provided. The patient was asked to gain a feeling of control as air was sent up and out with the contraction of the expiratory abdominal muscles. It was explained that this control is important for achieving changes in loudness and pitch. The patient was asked to "watch me and do what I do" as the clinician demonstrated fricative-like sounds, first sustained and then with a two-beat rhythm consisting of one small (weak) sound and one long (strong) sound. Throughout Accent practice, changes in body positioning (sitting, standing, walking, swinging the arms) were used to encourage automatic regulation of the breathing pattern.

Sample Sequence-Breathing Exercises

Sustained productions:

s — — — sh — — — f — — —

Two-beat rhythms (underlined sounds are stressed):

s–S̲ — —
sh–S̲H̲ — —
f–F̲ — —

2. **Utilize rhythmic vocal play.** Phonation began as soon as the correct breathing pattern was established. Voice was introduced with soft, breathy onsets at a low-intensity level. The clinician demonstrated the rhythm, and the patient imitated the accent pattern. On each main (stressed) beat, there was to be a smooth abdominal contraction. Eventually, the exercises were carried out at three different speeds: largo, andante, and allegro tempos. In implementing the Accent Method, the clinician can utilize arm movements, tapping, or beating on a drum to help establish the rhythms. Beating on a drum was not used in

this case, although it is used routinely by some clinicians.

The largo tempo consisted of one to two main stresses in a three-beat rhythm in which breathy phonation and consonantal resistance were used at the lips and tongue. The clinician alternated between one-beat and two-beat stresses.

Sample Sequence-Largo Tempo

zh–Z̲H̲
zz–Z̲Z̲–Z̲Z̲
yoi–Y̲O̲I̲
vv–V̲V̲–V̲V̲

In the andante tempo, phrases increased in size to three main beats in a four-beat rhythm, and breathiness was eliminated. This step provided variability in pitch, intensity, timbre, and time.

Sample Sequence-Andante Tempo

woo–W̲O̲O̲–W̲O̲O̲
yea–Y̲E̲A̲–Y̲E̲A̲–Y̲E̲A̲
yee–Y̲E̲E̲–Y̲E̲E̲–Y̲E̲E̲

In the allegro tempo, the voice exercises consisted of an unstressed vowel followed by five stressed vowels. The speed was doubled, and the main beats were divided into two faster beats. Phrase length, intensity, and a rich variety of sounds were incorporated into the practice as well as the other tempo patterns. This step gave more variety to the voice and approached the natural prosody used in conversation.

Sample Sequence—Allegro Tempo

yea–Y̲E̲A̲–Y̲E̲A̲–Y̲E̲A̲–Y̲E̲A̲–Y̲E̲A̲–Y̲E̲A̲
da–Y̲A̲–Y̲A̲–Y̲A̲–Y̲A̲–Y̲A̲
ba–B̲A̲–B̲A̲–B̲A̲–B̲A̲–B̲A̲
no–N̲O̲–N̲O̲–N̲O̲–N̲O̲–N̲O̲

3. **Transfer rhythms to articulated speech.** The final stage of Accent therapy involved transferring the rhythms to real speech. The process included (1) repetitions after the clinician, (2) reading aloud, (3) monologue, and (4) conversation. Marking passages for phrasing and stressing was particularly useful in aiding transference.

Effects of Accent Therapy

Throughout treatment, an abbreviated protocol was administered at the beginning of each therapy session to monitor the course of improvement. The protocol consisted of three trials on each of the following tasks: maximum phonation time, frequency range, and intensity range. Measures obtained using the PS-77 Phonatory function Analyzer, were plotted on to a Treatment Response Form (Koschkee, 1991) to generate a vocal behavior profile. Following ten 45-minute treatment sessions, a complete reevaluation of vocal functioning was performed.

The first and most dramatic change observed over time was increased phonatory volume produced on maximum phonation time. Before therapy, the total phonatory volume expended was only 260 mL compared with 2 L of air used after nine treatment sessions. Several other aerodynamic measures showed some degree of improvement, including intraoral pressures, maximum phonation time, and airflow rate variability. Intraoral pressure increased from 1.1 cm H_2O to 2.5 cm H_2O, and maximum phonation time was increased from 1.8 seconds to 4.9 seconds. An overall reduction in range airflow (minimum to maximum values) was evident by session 10. In general, there were fewer instances of peak flow and air wastage occurring during pre-exhalation and voice onset. Mean flow continued to fall at the high end of the normal range during reevaluation (220 cc/sec). During the middle of treatment (sessions 3, 4, and 5), an increase in mean flow was observed, placing those values above normal limits. However, as therapy progressed (sessions 6 through 10), mean flow rate returned to the pretreatment level. This pattern appears to be fairly typical during the phonation exercises, particularly when the largo tempo is being used where breathy voice is encouraged.

Acoustically, no changes were demonstrated in habitual fundamental frequency, habitual intensity, or intensity range of phonation. The patient did report, however, feeling more comfortable producing a louder voice. In less neurologically impaired individuals, an increase in intensity range would likely result based on clinical observation. Frequency range of phonation did increase from 9 semitones to 26 semitones. There was no change in jitter (.05 msc), which was already borderline acceptable, but shimmer and SNR did improve, although they continued to fall well outside of the acceptable range. A follow-up videostro-

boscopic study did not reveal significant changes after ten treatment sessions.

In summary, following a 10-day intensive Accent therapy program, the patient exhibited improvements in respiratory function, voice onset, and frequency range. These changes were considered significant given the patient's anatomic and physiologic capabilities.

To this point several case studies have documented the condition of voice and voice change with acoustic, aerodynamic, and stroboscopic measurements. Many of the instruments used to make these measurements may also be used as therapy training tools. Visual feedback from acoustic instruments of pitch and intensity are often useful when modifying these vocal components. Observation of the stroboscopic image is extremely educational and truly makes the patient a partner in the rehabilitative process. Direct feedback of airflow rates can be monitored and manipulated when teaching focus and glottal onset.

ACCENT METHOD PLUS DIRECT VISUAL FEEDBACK OF ELECTROGLOTTOGRAPHIC SIGNALS

Contributed by Eva Carlson, M.Sc.

In the next case study, Eva Carlson, M.Sc., combines the Accent Method of therapy with direct visual feedback of electroglottographic signals to modify vocal hyperfunction.

LARYNGOGRAPHY

For the past 7 years the Fourcin "laryngo-graph" has been in daily use for routine voice assessment and visual feedback in treatment, in the department of speech and language therapy at St. Thomas' Hospital London (Fourcin and Abberton, 1971; Fourcin, 1974, 1981).

The laryngograph is an electroglottograph (EGG), but Fourcin chose to call his version a "laryngograph," and this particular EGG technique is therefore called electrolaryngography (ELG). The resulting waveform is called "Lx" (larynx excitation) and is customarily shown in a positive-going direction (on y axis) for in-

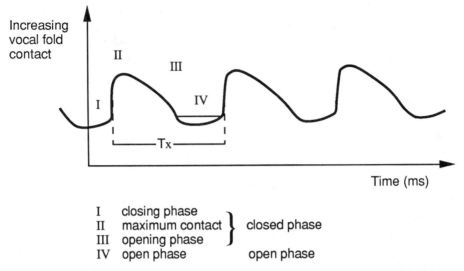

FIG 3–5.
Laryngographic waveform (Lx).

creasing vocal fold closure (Fig 3–5). The opposite tends to be the case in most other reports of EGG data, where the EGG waveform is shown in a negative-going direction for increasing vocal fold closure.

Two surface electrodes are placed either side of the thyroid cartilage at the level where the strongest Lx signal is achieved on phonation. The Lx signal reflects the variation in electrical conductance between the electrodes, as the vocal folds open and close. The amplitude of Lx indicates the amount of vocal fold contact. The greater the tissue contact the greater the current flow between the electrodes and the higher the amplitude (Gilbert et al., 1984). The Lx signal does not differentiate between the degree of vertical or horizontal closure but gives an integrated measure of the total current flow between the electrodes.

Voice therapy is often aimed at teaching patients to improve their breath support to achieve the right balance between subglottal pressure and laryngeal adduction forces, rather than just varying laryngeal resistance for voice production. The resulting aerodynamic changes and laryngeal tension characteristics give rise to increased Lx amplitude and steeper rise in Lx waveform. It is hypothesized to be due to the Bernoulli effect playing a greater part in glottic closure, resulting in increased tissue contact and a faster rate of closure of the vocal folds.

A male patient with an extremely "pressed" voice assessed in February 1988, was helped to produce voice with considerably less effort using Lx for visual feedback. At the end of a period of voice therapy (Fig 3–6, B), he sustained waveforms of higher amplitude and with steeper closing phase gradients, indicating faster closure rate. If anything, he was producing a voice with rather "whispery" quality in his effort to reduce laryngeal tension as evidenced by the long open phase, particularly at "high [i]" (see Fig 3–6, B).

The speed of vocal fold closure is an important factor in determining voice quality (Fourcin, 1981; Kelman, 1981; Sundberg, 1987) and can be monitored by looking at the steepness of the rising portion of the Lx waveform (Fig 3–6). Colton and Conture (1990) measured the "closing time" of the EGG waveform, defined as the time from the start of the closing phase of the EGG signal (Fig 3–5) to the point of maximum closure. They found that lesions on one or both vocal folds often increased the closing time.

The duration of the closed phase is another indicator of the efficiency of the voice source (Fourcin, 1981). During the open phase (Fig 3–5), acoustic energy is lost in the subglottis. However, in "pressed" and hyperkinetic voice, the closed phase occupies an excessive amount of the whole period and gives rise to characteristic Lx waveshapes (Fig

3–6, A). In patients with a lot of subcutaneous fat overlying the thyroid cartilage, common in women, or in older men with short necks, where the larynx has dropped to a point where the thyroid alae are difficult to access, the Lx signal is full of "noise" and is not a reliable source of information of glottal dynamics. Colton and Conture (1990) report that they were unable to get reliable EGG signals from 15% of their patients.

However, in clinical practice a poor signal can sometimes be useful for comparison purposes. Figures 3–7, A and B show the waveforms from a subject who had radiation therapy for glottic carcinoma and later asked for help with his voice, as it was deteriorating despite no evidence of recurrence of the tumor. The Lx waveforms from December 8, 1989 (Fig 3–7, A) show some periodicity but so much noise in the signal that a scientist would no doubt consider

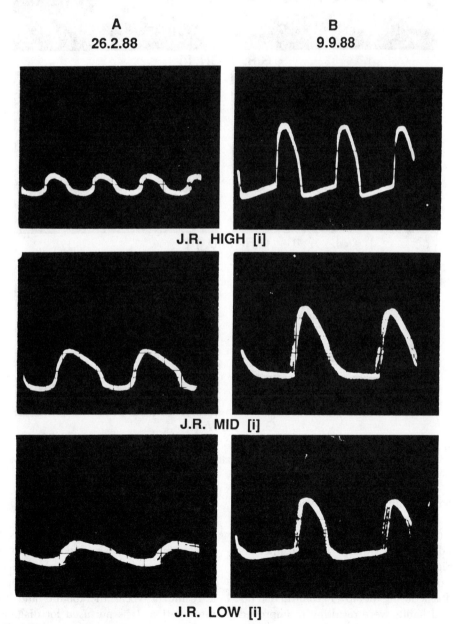

A
26.2.88

B
9.9.88

J.R. HIGH [i]

J.R. MID [i]

J.R. LOW [i]

FIG 3–6.
A, pretherapy pressed or hyperkinetic waveform. B, posttherapy waveform demonstrating reduced laryngeal tension.

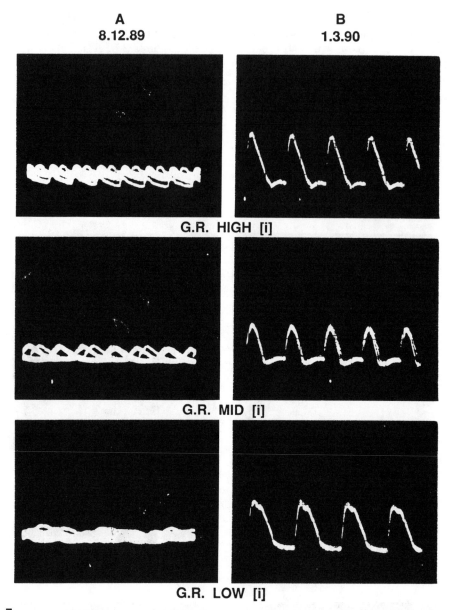

FIG 3–7.
A, Lx waveform demonstrating signal noise in patient after vocal cord radiation therapy. **B,** Lx waveform of same patient after voice therapy.

them worse than useless. However, as a basis for clinical comparison of the patient's later ability to produce and sustain Lx with good amplitude and no evidence of signal interference (Fig 3–7, B), they serve a useful purpose. The amplitude of the Lx waveform was used for feedback during therapy, to confirm that his new vocal habits were resulting in improved glottal dynamics. He used the waveform to monitor this and gain confidence in his ability to vary pitch and volume without effort, in a variety of vocal exercises, conversation, and reading aloud.

This case study aims to describe how the Lx waveform, and fundamental frequency parameters derived from Lx, can be used to give visual feedback of changing glottal dynamics as a result of vocal therapeutic and surgical intervention. It is not used for diagnosis but may, as will be shown later, reflect observed organic vocal fold changes that interfere with vocal fold contact.

Abberton and Fourcin (1984) and Abberton et al. (1989) give a detailed description of the laryngograph and the measurements derived from the Lx signal. Limitations of the technique are well summarized by Baken (1987) and more recently by Colton and Conture (1990) and by Childers et al. (1990). Suggested improvements and development of the technique are described by Rothenberg (1991). Finally, simulation of EGG waveforms from computer modeling of glottal configurations, incidentally with the same orientation in space as Lx and strongly reminiscent of waveforms produced in the clinic, are reported by Titze (1990).

Equipment Used

The Laryngograph Processor, which is a development of the original Laryngograph, is linked to a BBC Master microcomputer, a Cumana dual discdrive, and an Epson FX80 printer. A Telequipment S61 oscilloscope is used to show the Lx waveform in real time. The input from the laryngeal surface electrodes and an RS professional dynamic microphone is recorded on a Sony TC 144CS stereo cassette tape recorder.

Objective Voice Parameters Derived From Lx

The ELG parameters that we use most for voice assessment and visual feedback during treatment are the following:

1. The Lx waveform itself (Fig 3–5), showing a closing phase, a point of maximum contact, an opening phase, and an open phase (Abberton et al. 1989). It is used as a basis for calculation of fundamental frequency, Fx, by measuring the time, Tx, between successive vocal fold closures (Fig 3–5). The Laryngography Processor allows the simultaneous recording and display of Lx and the corresponding speech waveform recorded through a small electrode microphone (see Figs 3–8, 3–10, and 3–12).

2. The recorded Fx data from several minutes of conversation or reading aloud, plotted in a probability histogram, Dx (Distribution of excitation), and giving statistical information

on the recorded data (see Figs 3–9, 3–11, and 3–13). The frequency scale is logarithmic to correspond to pitch perception and divided into 128 equally spaced "bins" between 30.52 Hz and 1,000 Hz (Abberton et al., 1989). Second- and third-order Dx plots give an indication of the amount of regularity in the sample in that they only admit the instances where two and three adjacent Fx samples, respectively, fall into the same frequency "bin." A harsh, "irregular" voice will show a dramatic decrease in the "total sample" carried into second and third-order Dx distributions. An estimate of voice regularity can be expressed as a proportion of the total sample carried into second and third order (% TS).

3. A different way of illustrating first-order Dx data is in the form of a Cx plot (cross plot of FX) or "scatter plot" (Figs 3–9, 3–11, and 3–13). This plots adjacent pairs of Fx values against each other. The frequency scales are divided into 64 logarithmically equally spaced "bins." The density of the markings reflect the number of occurrences of transitions at that position. A smooth, regular voice will show a dense, narrow plot along the diagonal, the length of which reflects the frequency range of the voice. A thick, "cigar"-shaped diagonal and significant scatter away from it, indicate an irregular, rough voice.

The Cx plot gives the visually most striking display of improvement in voice quality, and patients often ask for copies of their "before" and "after" speech or reading Cx plots as souvenirs.

Rationale for Using ELG for Visual Feedback in Voice Therapy

It is the ability to noninvasively and continuously, reflect glottal dynamics during a variety of phonatory tasks, that makes an EGG device an invaluable asset in the voice clinic. As the technique is easily applied, it can be used routinely for assessment of most voice patients, although there are a minority of patients for whom the technique is not suitable (Colton and Conture, 1990).

The use of laryngeal electrodes for recording and analysis of voice fundamental frequency allows the clinician to interact with the patient in a natural conversation, several min-

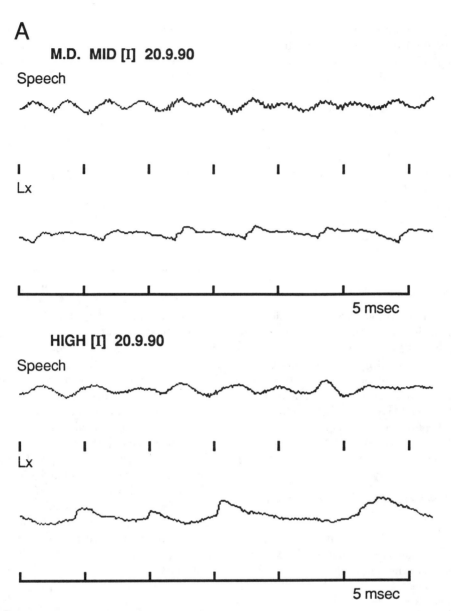

A

M.D. MID [I] 20.9.90

Speech

Lx

5 msec

HIGH [I] 20.9.90

Speech

Lx

5 msec

FIG 3–8.
A, Lx waveforms for /i/, demonstrating massive laryngeal effort. (*Continued.*)

utes in duration. Many of our patients are not confident readers, and a reading sample is not always obtainable, nor does it always give a true impression of the patient's habitual voice production. The electrodes are impervious to extraneous noise, and the recording can be carried out in an ordinary clinic environment, provided certain minimum standards are adhered to regarding sound attenuation. The patient is instructed not move his or her head, and is seated on a swivel chair to allow the person to turn toward the therapist without turning the head. During recording, the therapist can observe patterns of vocal fold contact during conversation and other phonatory tasks, as reflected in the shape of the Lx waveform.

A tendency to excessive laryngeal movement during speech, common in hyperkinetic dysphonias and in vocal fold palsy, gives rise to gross movement of the Lx baseline during speech. This can in itself be used for visual

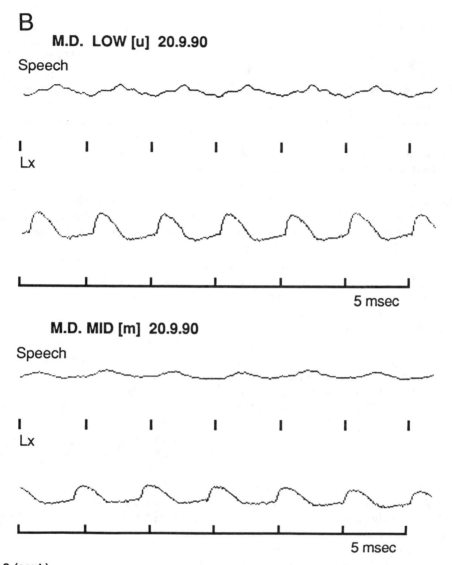

B

M.D. LOW [u] 20.9.90

Speech

Lx

5 msec

M.D. MID [m] 20.9.90

Speech

Lx

5 msec

FIG 3–8 (cont.).
B, Lx waveforms for /u/ and /m/ with reduced laryngeal effort, reduced intensity, and abdominal breath support.

feedback, to heighten the patient's awareness of excessive laryngeal activity. The effect of reduction of this is clearly observable in the cessation of major gross baseline movement.

This feature, and other potential sources of "noise," are obvious problems in the scientific application of EGG and ELG (Childers et al., 1990; Colton and Conture, 1990; Rothenberg, 1991) and are often a reason given for not using the technique. However, the increasing body of quantitative research into EGG waveforms produced by healthy and dysfunctional subjects (Kelman, 1981; Colton and Conture,

1990; Orlikoff, 1991) provide confirmation of the validity of many EGG features that we have found useful in therapeutic application of ELG for visual feedback.

Many of the reservations expressed in the literature about the drawbacks of EGG as a research tool need not be seen as reasons for not using it in a clinical situation. There is less need for scientific stringency in the application of ELG as a therapeutic tool, for comparison of the same patient with himself at different stages in the therapeutic process, and for use as immediate visual feedback of glottal dynamics.

CASE STUDY: PATIENT K

Patient K was a 47-year-old woman who worked as a cashier at a staff restaurant. She started smoking 7 years before presentation and smoked 25 cigarettes a day. She was happily married and had two grown children and two grandchildren. Patient K was referred by her general practitioner to the otolaryngologist in April 1990. She reported progressive hoarseness over a 3-year period which had recently been aggravated by an upper respiratory tract infection. Indirect laryngoscopy showed an irregularity of the anterior end of her right vocal fold, and she was admitted for microlaryngoscopy on July 7, 1990. A hemorrhagic polyp was removed. A small nodule on the left vocal fold, opposite the polyp, was observed but not removed on this occasion. She was sent home on "voice rest" and referred for voice therapy. On October 10, what was described as a large polyp on the anterior end of her left vocal fold was removed. Her progress in voice therapy between Sept 17, 1990, and Nov 19, 1990, is described in the following sections.

Description of Voice

Patient K's voice quality on her first visit for assessment and treatment on September 20, 1990, was extremely "harsh" and "whispery" and produced with massive "laryngeal tension" in the terminology used by Laver et al. She had poor breath control and was continuously clearing her throat of excessive mucus. She was distressed over comments on her extremely low-pitched, rough voice that were continuously made at work.

The Lx waveforms for /i/ recorded on September 20, 1990 (Fig 3–8, A) were produced with massive laryngeal effort. There is some contact periodicity but very limited tissue contact at mid /i/, a gradual closure, and an extremely long closed phase. Each period corresponds to a very damped speech waveform. The attempt at a high pitch /i/ resulted in a extremely irregular pattern of closure.

Instruction, on the same occasion, to reduce laryngeal effort, to reduce intensity, and to use abdominal breath support, immediately resulted in more normal appearing periodic Lx waveforms on production of /u/ and /m/ at mid-pitch (Fig 3–8, B). There was increased tissue contact as evidenced by the increased Lx amplitude, and this time a long open phase indicating a "whispery" quality. This was used as proof of the patient's potential ability to produce a better voice quality with less effort, despite the continuing presence of a left vocal fold polyp. The weak speech waveforms of /u/ and /m/ are due to the rather inexpert therapist not having increased the gain on asking the patient to reduce intensity.

The Dx and Cx plots and fundamental frequency statistics of conversational speech on this occasion (Fig 3–9) show extremely abnormal distribution of Fx values. Central measurements, in this case the mode, is the only usable one, are extremely low for a 47-year-old woman.

There was a lot of "noise" in the signal because of gross laryngeal movement throughout the recording. Continuous need to clear mucus and possibly interference of the polyp on phonation must also account for some of the extreme scatter of Fx values. The second- and third-order Dx plots based on only 8.5% and 2.3% of the original sample (% TS), respectively, indicate an extremely small amount of regularity of vocal fold vibration in the sample, in second order within a 90% range of 104.3 Hz to 201.3 Hz. Another feature of the second-order Dx plot is its marked bimodality. One might hypothesize this reveals a "diplophonia" possibly due to different parts of the vocal folds vibrating at different frequency, which would not be implausible, knowing the presence of the vocal fold polyp. Some of this limited "regularity" of vibration within a similar frequency range is carried into third order. Perceptually the voice did not sound diplophonic, as there was so much other "noise" present.

The Cx plot reveals a very wide scatter along the diagonal throughout the range, illustrating a very limited amount of regularity of vocal fold vibration.

Description of Therapy Approach

The voice therapy offered in our department is preceded by a detailed explanation of the vocal mechanism using a model of the

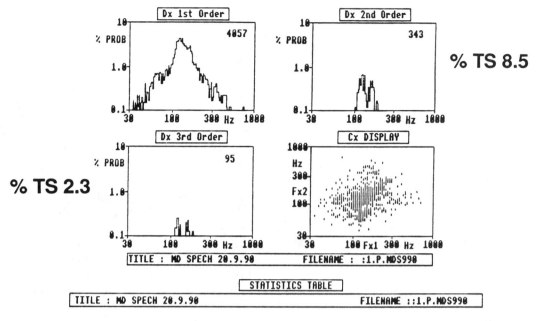

% TS 8.5

% TS 2.3

TITLE : MD SPECH 20.9.90   FILENAME : :1.P.MDS990

DISTRIBUTION TYPE	Dx 1st Order		Dx 2nd Order		Dx 3rd Order	
SAMPLE TOTAL	4057		343		95	
MEAN	133.5	Hz	137.2	Hz	144.9	Hz
MODE	122.9	Hz	126.4	Hz	122.9	Hz
MEDIAN	133.5	Hz	133.5	Hz	141	Hz
STANDARD DEVIATION	0.20	LOG-Hz	0.10	LOG-Hz	0.08	LOG-Hz
80% RANGE	75.1 237.3	Hz	113.2 185.3	Hz	119.6 190.6	Hz
90% RANGE	60.3 329.7	Hz	104.3 201.3	Hz	116.4 201.3	Hz

STATISTICS TABLE

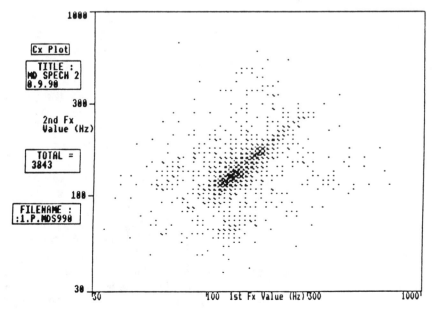

FIG 3–9.
Dx and Cx plots and fundamental frequency of conversational speech.

larynx and xeroradiograms of the vocal tract at rest and during phonation. The aim is to give the patient as much understanding of the mechanism as possible to "demystify" the voice problem. The therapy is loosely based on the "Accent Method" described by Smith and Thyme (1976, 1978). This approach emphasizes the control of subglottal pressure to "drive" the voice source to achieve increased speed and duration of vocal fold closure through the Bernoulli effect. This results in less air wastage and the acoustic effect of increased number and intensity of overtones (Smith and Thyme, 1978). The amplitude of the Lx waveform feeds back this change in glottal aerodynamics during voice exercises, as it responds to increased amount of tissue contact and reduction in force of adduction, as described previously. Accentuated breath pulses, controlled by abdominal muscles, are taught in a progressive series of exercises, which start with control of expiratory airflow during production of voiceless fricatives. The intensity of the sounds is varied by varying the expiratory force in different rhythms. Gradually, vowel sounds are introduced with soft attack and produced in increasing sequences and also in varying rhythmical patterns. The advantage with the method is the emphasis on reduction of laryngeal effort and concentration on the abdominal muscles as the power source for voice production. We also emphasized in this case the use of an open vocal tract. Chewing, humming, "playing on the lips," and "chanting" on a monotone were used to help the patient gain confidence and control over breath support for voice production, before embarking on gradually more speech-like exercises. The aim is to develop the control of a relaxed, comfortable, and flexible voice in speech and reading, appropriate in pitch, quality, and volume to the patient's sex and vocal needs.

Results of Therapy

Patient K was seen for voice therapy twice weekly and practiced recorded exercises at home between visits. The aim of therapy was to reduce volume, reduce laryngeal effort, and increase pitch using the breath control that was taught in clinic. Reassessment on October 3, 1990, shows improved control of vocal fold vibration in well-defined Lx waveforms showing improved tissue contact and steeply rising closing portions of the wave (Fig 3–10, A–C). The open phase occupies still the major portion of the cycle, however, resulting in a poorly differentiated acoustic output.

An interesting feature of the closing portion of the Lx waveform appears at low /i/ (Fig 3–10, C). The high amplitude indicates increased tissue contact, and the closed phase occupies more of the total period than at mid and high pitch. There is, however, a recurring irregularity at the same point in the rising portion of the waveform, which has the effect of delaying complete closure. This illustrates the claim of Colton and Conture (1990) that the closing time is affected by organic changes of the vocal folds and that EGG and ELG sometimes reflect this interference. Because of different modes of vibration of the vocal folds at different pitches and with different types of voice production, the effect of organic lesions on the Lx waveform varies. In this case it would seem that the vocal fold polyp mainly interferes with vibrations at low pitch. Both at mid and low pitch, however, there is also evidence of variability in tissue contact from one cycle to the next as seen in the slight variation in amplitude from one cycle to the next.

The Dx and Cx plots illustrating conversational speech on this occasion (Fig 3–11) show a marked improvement in regularity and range of Fx values. Central measurements are markedly higher than on the previous occasion, although the 90% range is still somewhat low and narrow. There is a marked increase in the % TS carried into second and third order, showing an increased amount of regularity of vocal fold vibration as a result of the changes made by patient K in her vocal habits. The best proof of her improvement was comments on her voice from her manager at work, who told her she was "beginning to sound like a human being." Her husband had commented that she did not "sound like a navvy off a building site any longer." These comments also serve to illustrate what she once sounded like to others, and the understandable distress it caused her.

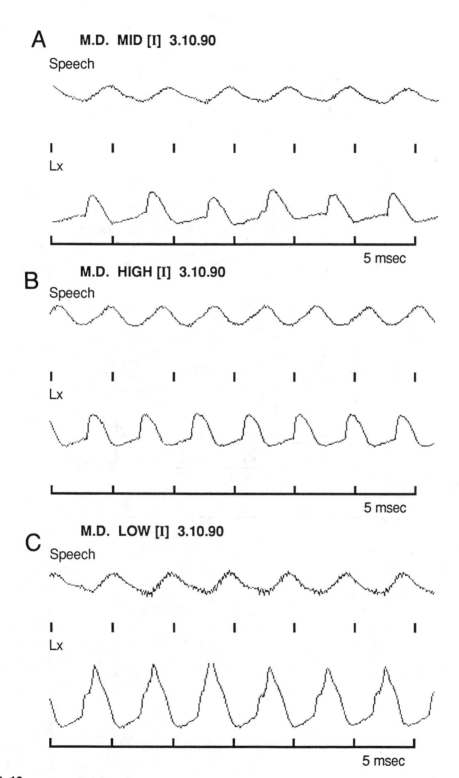

FIG 3–10.
A, Lx waveform for mid /I/ posttherapy. **B,** Lx waveform for high /I/ posttherapy. **C,** Lx waveform for low /I/ posttherapy.

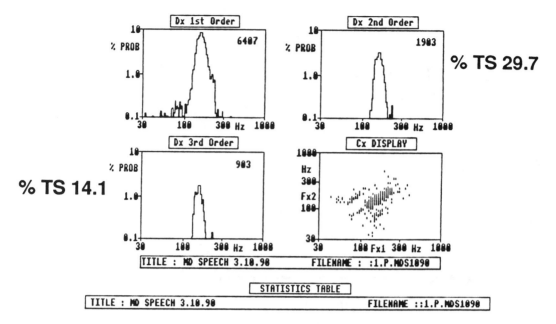

% TS 29.7

% TS 14.1

DISTRIBUTION TYPE	Dx 1st Order		Dx 2nd Order		Dx 3rd Order	
SAMPLE TOTAL	6407		1903		903	
MEAN	157.3	Hz	157.3	Hz	157.3	Hz
MODE	161.7	Hz	157.3	Hz	157.3	Hz
MEDIAN	161.7	Hz	161.7	Hz	161.7	Hz
STANDARD DEVIATION	0.11	LOG-Hz	0.05	LOG-Hz	0.04	LOG-Hz
80% RANGE	133.5 195.8	Hz	141.0 185.3	Hz	141.0 180.3	Hz
90% RANGE	113.2 218.6	Hz	137.2 195.8	Hz	141.0 190.6	Hz

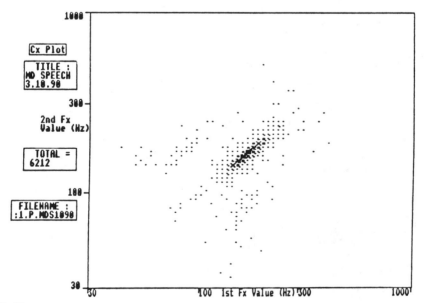

FIG 3–11.
Dx and Cx plots of conversational speech prior to vocal fold surgery for anterior polyp.

Patient K had another microlaryngoscopic treatment on October 10, 1990, for removal of the anterior polyp from her left vocal fold. Both vocal folds were observed to be edematous. Voice therapy continued after an initial postoperative period of voice rest. She stopped smoking at this time, and this was still the case on the last voice assessment, 5 weeks later on November 19, 1990.

On this occasion (Fig 3–12), the Lx plot shows overall, regular periodicity and higher fundamental frequency, well-defined closure, and longer closed phase compared with October 3, 1990 (Fig 3–10, A–C).

Fundamental frequency analysis on this occasion (Fig 3–13) shows a marked increase in central measurements and a higher and wider 90% range. A strong tendency to use hard glottal attacks and glottal stops, characteristic for certain London accents, which tends to lower the range is probably responsible for the bimodality of the Dx distribution.

The therapist remarked in her notes that the patient's voice sounded "lighter and was produced with considerably less laryngeal tension than previously." Her husband now described her as sounding "gentler."

TREATMENT OF SEVERE DYSPHONIA

Contributed by William Kramer, Ph.D.

In the following case study, William Kramer, Ph.D., presents the case of an active 76-year-old woman with severe dysphonia. The case ably demonstrates that a "normal" voice is not always the possible end result.

CASE STUDY: PATIENT L

Patient L, a 76-year-old woman, had severe dysphonia, due in part to bilateral vocal nodules. This diagnosis was made at the Mayo Clinic, Rochester, Minnesota, where she was being seen for a periodic check-up and evaluation of what she described as chronic obstructive pulmonary disease (COPD). She was referred by her local physician (an internist) who is not an otolaryngologist. She is a former registered nurse, having retired from a nursing career over 20 years previously. At the time of her initial evaluation and subsequent therapy in the spring and summer of 1989 she was living in her own home with her husband of over 50 years. During the course of her marriage, she and her husband traveled extensively throughout most of the United States (including Alaska and Hawaii) and Europe. Since her husband's death in the fall of 1990 she continued to live at home by herself. Her two married children live at a great distance from her home in the Midwest, and one of her initial therapy concerns was her intelligibility when making long-distance telephone calls.

Patient L is mentally and physically active. Depending on her schedule, she swims for an hour in the morning, five to six days each week. She attends movies, civic theatre, and symphony concerts on a regular basis; is active in her church; and volunteers to drive some of her "older" friends who are unable to do so. Her ambulatory skills and general coordination are excellent, and she is mentally alert and enthusiastic about life in general. Her visual acuity is quite functional with the aid of eyeglasses (she still makes quilts) and her pure-tone threshold test revealed only a mild-to-moderated loss at 4 and 8 kHz. She has never smoked. Her alcohol consumption is moderate, consisting mainly of an occasional drink before or with meals.

Evaluation

First seen in June of 1989, the patient reported the onset of the voice problem to have occurred approximately 5 years previously, with the actual diagnosis of vocal nodules being made in 1985 while she was at the Mayo Clinic. She attributed the development of her nodules to a chronic cough that had persisted for the previous 16 years. She described her voice as being "awful and hoarse," and described the dysphonia as "severe." She reported no pain upon phonation, but did indicate vocal fatigue after prolonged talking. No deterioration in voice was noted as a function of time of day (A.M. versus P.M.), or the day of the week (Monday versus Friday). She reported allergies to penicillin, most antihistamines, and cough syrups.

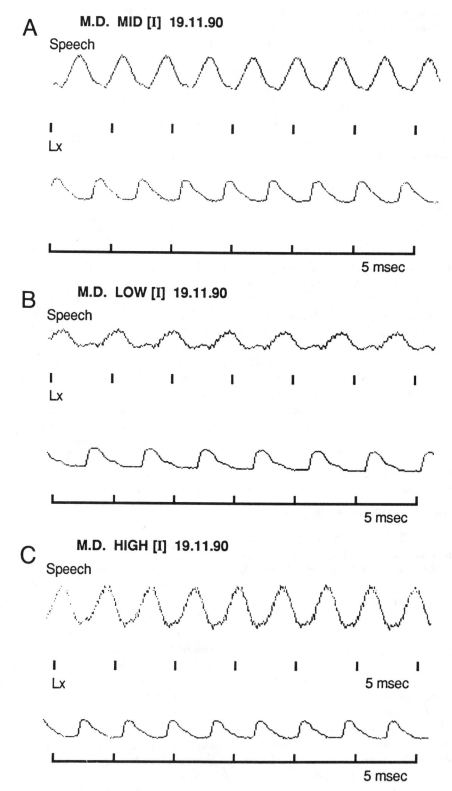

FIG 3–12.
Lx waveforms for mid, low, and high /I/ 5 weeks after surgery.

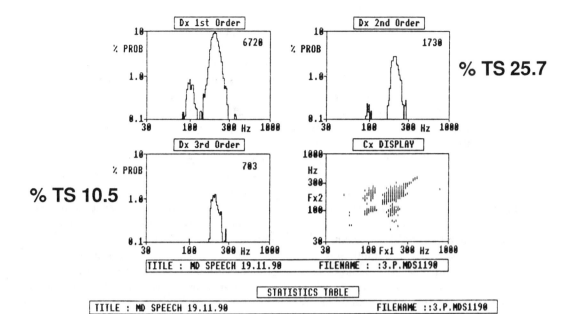

TITLE : MD SPEECH 19.11.90

STATISTICS TABLE

TITLE : MD SPEECH 19.11.90   FILENAME ::3.P.MDS1190

DISTRIBUTION TYPE	Dx 1st Order		Dx 2nd Order		Dx 3rd Order	
SAMPLE TOTAL	6720		1730		703	
MEAN	195.9	Hz	201.3	Hz	206.9	Hz
MODE	206.9	Hz	201.3	Hz	212.7	Hz
MEDIAN	201.3	Hz	206.9	Hz	212.7	Hz
STANDARD DEVIATION	0.11	LOG-Hz	0.08	LOG-Hz	0.07	LOG-Hz
80% RANGE	166.2 237.3	Hz	185.3 243.9	Hz	185.3 250.7	Hz
90% RANGE	104.3 257.6	Hz	161.7 250.7	Hz	180.3 257.6	Hz

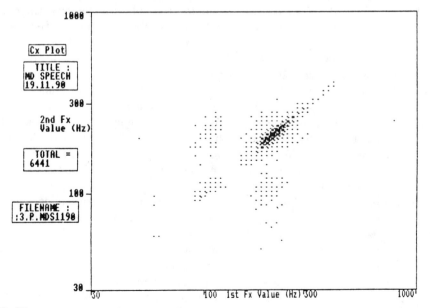

FIG 3–13.
Dx and Cx plots of conversational speech following surgery.

Subjective

During the initial interview, her voice was hoarse and low in pitch. She exhibited both pitch breaks (upward) and phonation breaks. Hard glottal attacks were evident on vowel-initiated words, and general hypertonicity in speech was the norm. The final words in most sentences were spoken in a glottal fry as she attempted to speak using what little expiratory reserve volume she had left.

At nearly 1-minute intervals she exhibited a forceful hacking cough (nonproductive) which lasted for approximately 20 seconds. This persistent hacking cough was apparently so habituated that she was not aware of its severity or frequency until the therapist brought it to her attention.

Objective

Maximum phonation time for the vowel /a/ averaged 6 seconds over three trials, and she was able to sustain /i/ for 6 seconds as well. This short duration was considered symptomatic of both her vocal nodules and her reduced lung capacity due to COPD scarring.

Her prolongation of the /s/ and /z/ phonemes was similarly short, and the seemingly normal s/z ratio of 1.0 was considered an artifact of this short (6-second) duration. Hypertonicity of the strap muscles of the neck and the platysma was evident throughout her conversation and the maximum phonation time and s/z trials. She was unable to sing up or down the musical scale when initially asked to do so using the numbers 1 through 8 (one octave).

Subsequent probes of voice range, using the Visi-Pitch for visual feedback, revealed a frequency range for 98 to 150 Hz, with an average fundamental frequency of 134.8 Hz and a pitch perturbation (jitter) measuring from 8.4 on isolated vowels to as high as 12.8 in conversation speech, with both measures being well above the expected norm. Laryngeal videostroboscopy was not yet available but was utilized for post-therapy testing.

Therapy

Therapy prognosis was initially guarded, based on the patient's age and her 16-year history of pulmonary distress and vocal abuse of persistent coughing. Encouraging signs, however, included her physical activity, mental alertness, and enthusiasm. Correspondingly, a therapy regimen was designed on the premise that improved vocal function would likely result from reduction of two primary abuses: her persistent cough, and her use of an inappropriately low pitch.

The rationale behind this is that the voice is a function of the vibration of mucosal and muscle tissue, and that the health of this mucosal and muscle tissue is best ensured by proper hydration and exercise. Just as muscle tonus of arms and legs responds to increased blood flow and the oxygenation obtained through exercise, the laryngeal musculature should respond in a similar fashion.

The first therapy suggestion, then, was that patient L increase her fluid intake by four large glasses of water daily. It was thought that this would accomplish two things: increase the lubricity of her vocal fold mucosa, and subsequently reduce the tickling sensation resulting in her cough. She agreed to do this and noticed a reduction of her persistent cough within a matter of only a few weeks.

Following this rehydration of her larynx and resultant reduction in her coughing behavior to one cough per hour (as opposed to once per minute), the "physical therapy" approach to her voice rehabilitation began. Her use of an inappropriately low-pitched voice (135 Hz) was targeted as the next abuse to be eliminated.

In the experience of this clinician, a great deal of success in voice therapy has come about by simply obtaining greater sustained phonation on vowels. This sustained phonation of vowels is thought to be enhanced by the use of appropriate pitch and loudness levels and better approximation of the vocal folds. Although improper breath support is often thought to be a factor in short vowel duration (defined here as less than 10 seconds), the majority of patients seen by this clinician exhibit no pulmonary or neurologic disease affecting respiration. The vast majority of patients are far more likely to exhibit short vowel duration as the result of faulty approximation of the vocal folds.

In the case of patient L we were faced with a short vowel duration of only 6 seconds, but it was unclear as to whether this resulted from poor breath support (COPD related) or poor fold approximation attributable to the vocal nodules.

The initial goal was to raise her pitch level on sustained vowels. When asked whether or not she had any familiarity with the musical scale or the piano keyboard, the patient said that she had once sung in the choir at church and had considered a voice major instead of nursing. She also played the dulcimer, and was familiar with the musical scale. A visual handout was then given to her with a likeness of the piano keyboard on it from C2 (65 Hz) to F5 (740 Hz), with the corresponding frequency in Hertz written above each note.

With the aid of the Visi-Pitch and voice modeling of the clinician, she was stimulable and able to raise her own pitch and to sustain the vowel /i/ at 160 Hz. The choice of the vowel /i/ for initial volume attempts is thought to obtain greater success in vocal fold approximation because of the attendant elevation of the larynx by the hypoglossus during this high-front vowel production. Subsequent attempts at sustained /a/ and /u/ production yielded similar increases in fundamental frequency, but these two vowels also exhibited a much greater jitter factor.

Patient L received voice therapy for 50-minute sessions twice weekly for approximately 2 months (9 weeks) following her initial evaluation. During this time she tried various other voice facilitation techniques. Noting that the approximate duration of a single syllable rarely exceeds .25 second, it was pointed out that, even with a limited phonation time of 6 seconds, she could use phrases and sentences of almost twenty-four syllables without resorting to vocal fry.

To aid in her understanding of hard glottal attack, she was asked to contrast the sound and "feel" of vowel-initiated words such as (ice) with those preceded by a voiced continuant (rice). The use of intonation exercises ("I like THAT coat/I like that COAT") and monitoring of her frequency range seemed to help her understand her own vocal dynamics. She became quite adept at reading the Visi-Pitch screen during production of isolated vowels

and in phrases and sentences. The concept of pitch perturbation was explained to her and she became adept at "predicting" whether or not her perturbation would be high (over 1.0) or low (under .9) based on how her voice felt and sounded. Within weeks she was able to replicate isolated vowels at various frequency levels, and was experiencing less vocal fatigue at the end of the day.

Results

Following the 9-week regimen of voice therapy during which patient L increased her intake of fluids, reduced her coughing, and raised her fundamental frequency, patient L's voice was much clearer, and she was quite pleased with the progress she had made. She reported increased positive feedback from her husband and her children, and returned to the Mayo Clinic for some additional evaluation and treatment of her pulmonary distress. A written report of her therapy progress to date was sent with her, along with a request for results of their laryngoscopic findings.

Laryngoscopic findings at this time revealed no nodule on the left vocal cord, and the nodule on the right cord had been reduced to half its original size. In light of this therapeutic success, it was recommended that her therapy continue. Additional therapy obtained a fundamental frequency of 190 Hz on isolated vowels, words, and phrases, and a perturbation of less than 1.0% (r = .40 to .88).

Following her husband's death in September, 1990, the patient's voice became noticeably worse. This was also during a period when her therapy had been reduced to one session per week (for maintenance), and this clinician's injuries in a motorcycle accident precluded him from actively participating in her therapy or its supervision.

At patient L's request, she was re-enrolled in therapy in June, 1991. Her voice at that time was still somewhat hoarse, with some breathiness as well. Her conversational speech at that time had an average fundamental frequency of 184 Hz. Her longest sustained vowel was 7 seconds, some glottal fry was noticed, and an occasional facial grimace and hypertonicity of the strap muscles of the neck were noted.

A videostroboscopic examination of the larynx was performed in June, 1991, at Ball Memorial Hospital, Muncie, Indiana, with the following results:

1. Glottic closure was incomplete. A small anterior and posterior chink were noted adjacent to some cord thickening on the right side.

2. Vibration was typically aperiodic, although some periodicity was observed.

3. Vibration was asymmetrical.

4. Amplitude was normal for the left vocal fold, but there was some stiffness observed in the right fold as the thickened area had less movement.

5. The mucosal wave was normal for the left vocal fold, whereas the right vocal fold had some stiffness involving the posterior two thirds.

Conclusion

Although this elderly patient still presented with some noticeable dysphonia, the results of therapy were considered successful to a limited extent. This judgment of (qualified) success is based on the following:

1. Speaking fundamental frequency increased from 135 Hz to almost 190 Hz, approximating more closely the norm for her age and gender.

2. Frequency range improved to one octave (D3 to D4; 147 Hz to 294 Hz), which allows her to sing "Happy Birthday" to her grandchildren. (The range for "Happy Birthday" is exactly one octave.)

3. Pitch perturbation had decreased from 8.4% on isolated vowels to an average of .29%.

4. Increased hydration appeared to have had measurable effect on reducing her cough from once per minute to once every hour.

5. Subjectively the patient felt that her voice was stronger, fatigued less easily, and was better heard by her friends and relatives.

6. Substantial improvement was achieved in the first 2 months of therapy (bilateral nodules reduced to a unilateral nodule half the original size).

7. Improvement was achieved with a nodule patient who should be considered to be atypical from the standpoint of her age and medical history.

REFERENCES

Abberton E, Howard DM, Fourcin AJ: Laryngographic assessment of normal voice: a tutorial, *Clin Linguistics Phonetics* 3:218–296, 1989.

Abberton E, Fourcin AJ: Electrolaryngography. In Code C, Ball M, editors: *Experimental clinical phonetics*, New Hampshire, England, 1984, Croom Helm.

Andrews ML: *Voice therapy for children*, San Diego, 1991, Singular Publications.

Baken RJ: *Clinical measurement of speech and voice*, London, 1987, Taylor Francis Ltd.

Boone D: *The voice and voice therapy*, ed 3, Englewood Cliffs, N.J., 1983, Prentice-Hall.

Boone D: *The voice and voice therapy*, ed 2, Englewood Cliffs, N.J., 1977, Prentice-Hall.

Boone D, McFarlane SC: *The voice and voice therapy*, ed 4, Englewood Cliffs, N.J., 1988, Prentice-Hall.

Brodnitz F: Vocal rehabilitation in benign lesions of the vocal cords, *J Speech Hear Disord* 23:112–117, 1958.

Casper JK, Colton RH, Woo P, et al: Investigation of selected voice therapy techniques in a patient population, paper presented at 19th Annual Symposium: Care of the Professional Voice, Philadelphia, June 1990.

Casper JK, Colton RH, Brewer DW, et al: *Investigation of selected voice therapy techniques,* paper presented at 18th Annual Symposium: Care of the Professional Voice, Philadelphia, June 1989.

Childers DG, Hicks DM, Moore GP, et al: Electroglottography and vocal fold physiology, *J Speech Hear Res* 33:245–254, 1990.

Christy VA: *Expressive singing*, vol 2, Dubuque, Iowa, 1961, WC Brown.

Colton RH, Casper JK: *Understanding voice problems*, Baltimore, 1990, Williams & Wilkins.

Colton RH, Conture EG: Problems and pitfalls of electroglottography, *J Voice* 4:10–24, 1990.

Daniloff R, Schuckers G, Feth L: *The physiology of speech and hearing: an introduction*, Englewood Cliffs, N.J., 1980, Prentice-Hall.

Emil-Behnke K: *The technique of singing*, London, 1945, Williams and Norgate.

Fairbanks G: *Voice and articulation drillbook*, ed 2, New York, 1960, Harper & Row.

Fawcus M: *Voice disorders and their management*, New Hampshire, England, 1986, Croom Helm.

Flynn P, Andrews M, Cabot B: *Using your voice wisely and well*, Tucson, Ariz, 1990, Communication Skills Builders.

Fourcin AJ: Laryngographic assessment of phonatory function. In Ludlow CL, Hart MO, editors: *Proceedings* of the conference on the assessment of vocal pathology, Bethesda, Md, 1981, National Institute of Health.

Fourcin AJ: Laryngographic examination of vocal fold vibration. In Wyke B, editor: *Ventilatory and phonatory control systems*, Oxford, U.K., 1974, Oxford University Press.

Fourcin AJ, Abberton B: First application of a new laryngograph, *Med Bio Illus* 21:172–182, 1971.

Gilbert HR, Potter CR, Hoodin R: The laryngograph as a measure of vocal fold contact area, *J Speech Hear Res* 27:178–182, 1984.

Glaze L, Bless DM, Susser R: Acoustic analysis of vowel and loudness differences in children's voice, *J Voice* 4:37–44, 1990.

Glaze L, Bless DM, Milenkovic P: Acoustic characteristics of children's voice, *J Voice* 2(4):312–319, 1988.

Goebel M: *CAFET, a computer aided fluency establishment trainer. User's manual for installation and therapy.* Annandale, Va, 1988, Annandale Fluency Clinic.

Hirano M: Clinical examination of voice, New York, 1981, Springer-Verlag.

Hufnagle J, Hufnagle K: Is quiet whisper harmful to the vocal mechanism? A research note, *Percept Mot Skills* 57:735–737, 1983.

Izdebski K: Magnetic sound recording in laryngology, *Am J Otolaryngol* 2:34–40, 1981.

Koufman JA, Blalock PD: Functional voice disorders. In Koufman JA, Isaacson G, editors: *Voice disorders*, Philadelphia, 1991, WB Saunders.

Kelman AW: Vibratory pattern of the vocal folds, *Folia Phoniatr* 33:73–99, 1981.

Koschkee D: Treatment reponse form, presented at Scientific Advances: The Assessment and Treatment of Voice Disorders, Madison, Wisconsin, April 1991.

Lamperti GB: *Vocal wisdom*, New York, 1931, William Earl Brown.

Laver J, et al: A perceptual protocol for the analysis of vocal profiles. In Work in progress, University of Edinburgh Department of Linguistics 14:139–155, 1981.

Lehiste I: Acoustic characteristics of selected English consonants. Part IV: a study of /h/ and whispered speech (Report No. 9, contract AF 49-638-492 AFOSR 2093), Ann Arbor, 1962, University of Michigan.

Milenkovic P: Least mean square measures of voice perturbation, *J Speech Hear Res* 30:529–538, 1987.

Monoson PK, Zemlin WR: Quantitative study of whisper, *Folia Phoniatr* 36:53–65, 1984.

Orlikoff RF: Assessment of the dynamics of vocal fold contact from the electroglottogram; data from normal male subjects, *J Speech Hear Res* 34:1066–1072, 1991.

Pressman JJ, Kelemen G: *Physiology of the larynx*, rev ed, Rochester, N.Y., 1970, American Academy of Ophthalmology and Otolaryngology.

Rothenberg M: A multichannel electroglottograph, *J Voice*, March 1992.

Sawashima M, Hirose H: Laryngeal gestures in speech production. In MacNeilage PF, editor: *The production of speech*, New York, 1983, Springer-Verlag.

Smith S, Thyme K: *Accent metoden: Special paedagogisk Forlag A-S* , Herning, Denmark, 1978.

Smith S, Thyme K: Statistic research on changes in speech due to pedagogic treatment (the Accent Method), *Folia Phoniatr* 28:98–103, 1976.

Solomon NP, McCall GN, Trosset MW, et al: Laryngeal configuration and constriction during two types of whispering, *J Speech Hear Res* 32:161–174, 1989.

Stemple JC: *Clinical voice pathology*, Columbus, Ohio, 1984, Merrill.

Sundberg J: *The science of the singing voice*, De Kalb, 1987, Northern Illinois University Press.

Tetrazzini L: *The art of singing*, New York, 1975, Da Capo Press.

Titze IR: Interpretation of the electroglottograph signal, *J Voice* 4:1–9, 1990.

Vilkman E, Aaltonen O, Raimo I, et al: Stress production in whisper, *J Phonetics* 15:157–168, 1987.

CHAPTER 4

Management of Vocal Hypofunction and Resonation Disorders

MANAGEMENT APPROACHES FOR

- Laryngeal myasthenia
- Bowed vocal folds (senile laryngitis)
- Vocal fold paralysis
- Hypernasality
- Hyponasality
- Cleft palate.

MANAGEMENT STRATEGIES, INCLUDING

- Patient education
- Laryngeal muscle relaxation (tension reduction)
- Respiratory support training
- Frontal focus
- Vocal function exercises
- Modification of telephone voice
- Elimination of throat clearing
- Hydration program
- Optimize auditory acuity
- Steaming and humidification
- Caffeine reduction
- Visual biofeedback
- Auditory feedback
- Sustaining vowels
- Singing
- Emotional/psychological support
- Environmental manipulation
- Glottal attack and pushing exercise
- Teflon injection
- Vocal fold medialization

- Pitch and loudness modification for resonance disorders
- Non-speech phonation
- Articulation therapy
- Negative practice
- Palatal surgery
- Pharyngeal flap surgery
- Auditory, visual, tactile feedback.

While the majority of voice disorders fall into the category of vocal hyperfunction, hypoadduction of the vocal folds for either functional or organic reasons may occur. Normal voicing is dependent on near total closure of the vocal folds. (The larynges of many women and some men will demonstrate a normal posterior glottal gap of the vocal folds upon adduction.) Air pressure from the lungs builds and eventually overcomes the resistance of the adducted folds, and a puff of air escapes. This release of air creates a sudden drop of air pressure between the vocal folds, creating a suction. This drop in pressure, along with the static positioning of the adducted folds, draws the vocal folds back together completing a vibratory cycle.

When the vocal folds do not totally approximate, then a greater amount of air pressure and airflow is required to create and maintain phonation. The speaker, therefore, must work harder to produce voice. The perceptual quality of voice, and effort to produce it will be directly reflected by the size of the glottal gap. The larger the glottal gap, the breathier the voice will be. Voices of hypoadducted vocal folds will range from a mild breathiness to complete whispered aphonia.

Vocal hypofunction may result from both functional and organic reasons. Functional hypoadduction of the vocal folds may be caused by laryngeal myasthenia, emotional dysphonias, or conversion disorders. Laryngeal myasthenia, in this context, is a descriptive term used to describe laryngeal muscle fatigue in an otherwise medically/emotionally healthy individual. This is the patient who reports that his/her voice quality is normal in the morning, but as the day progresses, becomes weak, hoarse, and breathy. The result of this vocal fatigue is hypoadduction of the vocal folds, usually with increased supraglottic tension. The patients complain that the harder they try to produce voice, the worse the quality becomes. One might argue, correctly, that the original cause of laryngeal muscle weakness was hyperfunctional vocal behavior. However, stroboscopic observations of many of these patients made during the fatigued state, demonstrate unusual anterior glottal chinks and occasional spindle-shaped chinks. These chinks create the vocal hypofunction condition.

Breathy voice productions are also evident in many patients who present with both functional emotional dysphonias and conversion aphonias and dysphonias. Discussion of these disorders and management suggestion are included in the following chapter.

Vocal hypofunction may also be the result of organic reasons. Organic causes include neurologic disease, vocal fold paralysis, and bowed vocal folds. Many neurologic diseases cause dysarthric speech patterns. Neurologic voice disorders are components of the dysarthria with breathiness being a common symptom of hypokinetic dysarthrias (Aronson, 1990).

Vocal fold paralysis may also be caused by neurologic disease but is more often caused by peripheral nerve damage or peripheral disease (Willatt and Stell, 1991). Vocal fold paralysis may be unilateral or bilateral. It may be caused by damage or disease to the tenth cranial nerve from the brain stem to the muscle, or to the external branch of the superior laryngeal nerve (cricothyroid muscle) or the recurrent laryngeal nerve branches (all remaining intrinsic laryngeal muscles). Location of the lesion along the nerve pathway will determine the type of paralysis and the resultant voice quality.

MANAGEMENT FOR LARYNGEAL MYASTHENIA

The following case studies describe therapeutic and surgical management approaches for vocal hypofunction. The studies include direct therapy facilitating techniques for improving fold adduction, the use of Teflon injections to decrease glottal chinks, and vocal fold medialization techniques.

CASE STUDY: PATIENT M

Patient M was a 36-year-old systems analyst for a large computer networking company with no previous history of voice difficulty. Eight months prior to the voice evaluation, he had experienced bronchitis with associated harsh coughing and hoarseness. Within 2 weeks, all symptoms had resolved. Since that time, however, the patient had noticed that his voice was not quite as "strong" and that it seemed to get "tired" easily. At first, the voice fatigue occurred only occasionally and was usually associated with a very busy work day or a normal social gathering. In the previous 2 to 3 months, however, the "tired" voice had become a daily occurrence and, according to the patient, was getting worse.

On a daily basis, the patient's voice quality was slightly hoarse when he awakened at 6 A.M., cleared to nearly normal by 8 A.M., but then began fatiguing, often by 11 A.M. The fatigue was accelerated if he was required to talk on the telephone or make a presentation to a small group. The patient described his voice quality, when the voice was fatigued, as being "breathy and muffled, almost like talking out of a barrel." He described an increased effort to talk and complained that the harder he tried to talk, the worse the quality became.

Except for persistent throat clearing, patient M was not a voice abuser. By his own admission he was a "couch-potato." When not working at his computer at work, he was working on his home computer, watching television, or reading. Social activities were limited to family gatherings, movies, and quiet dinners with friends. He had been married for 10 years and had no children. His wife was an accountant.

The patient's medical history was unremarkable; no surgeries, other hospitalizations or chronic disorders were reported. The patient took no medications; had never smoked, though he grew up in a smoking environment; and drank alcohol only occasionally. His liquid intake was not adequate, consisting mostly of morning coffee and evening iced tea, both caffeinated. The bronchitis, experienced 8 months ago, was an unusual occurrence for this normally healthy man.

Laryngeal videostroboscopic examination revealed grossly normal-appearing vocal folds bilaterally. Glottic closure demonstrated a moderate-sized anterior glottal gap with a slight ventricular fold compression. The bilateral amplitude of vibration and mucosal wave were moderately and slightly decreased, respectively. The open phase of the vibratory cycle was slightly dominant, while the symmetry of vibration was irregular during extremes of pitch and loudness. No mass lesions, paresis, or paralysis were evident.

This vocal fold condition left patient M with a mild dysphonia characterized by a dry, breathy hoarseness, high pitch, and intermittent pitch and phonation breaks. The patient was visibly pushing to produce voice in conversation, and was using a forced back-focus and often spoke on residual air as a result. This subjective judgement of voice quality was confirmed by objective measures including the following:

1. High fundamental frequency (142 Hz).
2. Limited frequency range (115 to 380 Hz).
3. High jitter measure-connected speech (26 Hz, PM Pitch Analyzer; normal jitter for sustained vowels).
4. High airflow rates (comfort, 205 mL H_2O; high pitch, 216 mL H_2O; low pitch, 320 mL H_2O).
5. Low phonation times at all voice conditions.

Patient M was evaluated in the late afternoon of a typical workday, when he was very symptomatic. Because he had never experienced vocal difficulties prior to suffering bronchitis, it was speculated that the persistent harsh coughing had strained the laryngeal musculature. Presence of the anterior glottal gap, the unusually high pitch, and the inability to produce a more normal lower pitch range suggested the possibility of weakness of the bilateral thyroarytenoid muscles. Indeed, patient M's attempts to sustain lower tones during the stroboscopic examination yielded a larger anterior glottal gap. The presence of this gap during low-pitch production was confirmed by the unusually high airflow rate of 320 mL H_2O/sec. Continued efforts to produce voice by forcing the weakened laryngeal system was causing the symptoms not only to persist, but to worsen.

The management approach developed for patient M included the following facilitating techniques:

1. Education.
2. Relaxation of laryngeal area musculature during phonation.
3. Direct training in respiratory support and frontal focus.
4. Vocal function exercises.
5. Evaluation-modification of telephone voice.
6. Elimination of throat clearing.
7. Hydration program.

Education

The video recording of the stroboscopic examination was used to demonstrate the relationship between the glottal gap, high airflow rate, and increased effort to produce voice. Patient M was made to understand that even with the increased effort, the voice remained weak and breathy; therefore, the effort was useless and indeed harmful to the laryngeal mechanism. The patient's understanding of why his voice was failing was a key to his becoming a willing participant in the therapeutic process. The patient had seen two laryngologists who had reported that his vocal folds were normal. He was frustrated because he knew he had a problem, but no one could "find" it. The relationship between his symptoms and his physiology "made sense," and he was ready to proceed to eliminate the bothersome problem.

Relaxation

As patient M's voice began to fatigue, his response was to tense his neck and shoulders in an effort to help force a more normal sounding voice. This effort, of course, had the opposite effect causing more laryngeal tension and fatigue. The education process was a major step in modifying this tensing behavior. The patient, however, needed a cue for when he was too tense. Once cued, he needed a simple technique for reducing unwanted tension.

The cue established for the patient was to set the alarm on his watch to sound every hour. When the alarm sounded, his task was to physically relax his neck and shoulders by rolling his head and by stretching his arms back and forth, up and down. This task took less than 1 minute, but was quite effective for this patient in reducing physical tension.

The patient had found that neck and shoulder tensing often occurred while he sat over his CRT, even when he was not talking. He noticed that, on occasion, he would not speak for 2 to 3 hours while working at the computer. Then, when he did speak, his voice was weak. The relaxation exercise was helpful in eliminating this problem.

Respiratory Support and Frontal Focus

Because of the increased airflow necessary to drive the weakened vocal folds, patient M often felt breathless while talking. One reason for this breathless feeling was his inability to complete a phrase on a normal expiration without pushing and using residual air. The use of residual air added to laryngeal tensing, which contributed to a backward tone focus. Symptomatic therapy was therefore utilized to modify these behaviors.

To develop more appropriate breathing and focus, the therapist introduced exercises utilizing phrases graduated by length. Beginning with two-word phrases such as

oh no   my no
oh my   no way
oh me

the patient was instructed to "sing" each phrase on a comfortable tone and to exaggerate a nasal focus. He was to over exaggerate both the articulation and resonation, all the while breathing between each phrase. When the appropriate tone focus and breathing pattern were demonstrated consistently, he was asked to modify the singing from one note to an overinflected "chant." The task was to maintain focus and breath support.

From the overinflected, forward-focused chant, the patient was asked to "speak" the phrase. The phrases were then gradually expanded in length to a maximum of eight to nine syllables. Negative practice, utilizing residual air and tight back focus, was used to confirm the patient's understanding and control of these concepts.

Vocal Function Exercises

Concurrent with the other therapeutic tasks, patient M was instructed in Vocal Function Exercises (VFE) (see Chapter 1). In my clinical practice, these exercises have proved extremely effective in dealing with obvious laryngeal muscle strain and weakness disorders. With an airflow volume of approximately 4,000 mL H_2O, patient M should have been able to sustain a tone for 35 to 40 seconds. His baseline VFE measures were:

Note	Seconds
E/F	22
C	15
D	16
E	24
F	26
G	30

The patient was instructed to do the VFE two times each, twice daily, in the morning and evening.

Evaluation/Modification of Telephone Voice

During the evaluation, patient M indicated that his voice fatigued more quickly when he was required to talk on the telephone at work. To determine why this occurred, a telephone scenario was utilized. The patient was instructed to call the therapist during the morning, before the onset of typical voice fatigue.

The phone call revealed that the patient artificially lowered his pitch and talked louder than normal on the telephone. Many of us have "telephone voices" that differ from our normal speaking voices. Patient M created more tension and strain, thus fatigue, by talking with his "telephone voice."

To modify this behavior, the patient was instructed to imagine that the person with whom he was talking was sitting directly in front of him. In addition he was instructed to hold the receiver to his ear only when listening and to move it 3 to 4 in. away when he was talking. By holding the receiver away from his ear, he would be monitoring his voice in the same manner as if the listener were present. His auditory feedback system would not be distorted by the receiver.

Eliminate Throat Clearing

Throat clearing became more and more evident as the patient's voice fatigued. Behavior modification and the hard swallow (described in Chapter 3) were utilized to eliminate this behavior.

Hydration Program

Patient M's liquid intake was inadequate for promotion of laryngeal lubrication. He was instructed to drink six to eight 8-oz glasses of noncaffeinated, nonalcoholic liquids per day. Water and fruit juices were the preferred liquids.

Results of Therapy

Three months of therapy were required to complete this program successfully. During this time, the combined therapy approaches were practiced, monitored, and modified as needed. Patient M first began to notice that his voice fatigue began later and later in the day. He then began to develop more of a downward range in his VFE and timbre in his speaking voice. By the middle of the month he proclaimed his voice to be normal.

Post-therapy stroboscopy demonstrated a tiny anterior glottal chink only at low pitches. All other observations were within normal limits. Perceptually, his voice quality was judged to be normal. Objective measures were as follows:

1. Fundamental frequency = 128 Hz
2. Frequency range = 98 to 560 Hz
3. Jitter measures = normal for all voice conditions
4. Air flow rates = all less than 200 mL H_2O/sec
5. Phonation times for vocal function exercises = average, 36.5 seconds.

The original complaints of voice which lacked strength and tired easily were resolved. Patient M was placed on a maintenance program of modified vocal function exercises and discharged from therapy. A 3-month recheck revealed that the patient had successfully discontinued the maintenance program and maintained normal voicing. Combining direct symptom modification with laryngeal muscle strengthening and vocal hygiene training proved successful in resolving voice fatigue.

MANAGEMENT FOR VOCAL FOLD BOWING

Another cause of vocal hypofunction is bowing of the true vocal folds. This condition occurs when the intercartilaginous portions of the vocal folds are adducted while the membranous portion fails to adduct (Aronson, 1990). This condition yields a spindle-shaped glottal gap. The degree of voice disturbance will be determined by the size of the gap.

Aronson (1990) lists five causes of bowing:

1. Atrophy of the thyroarytenoid muscle caused by denervation
2. Bilateral cricothyroid muscle weakness due to superior laryngeal nerve lesions
3. Loss of vocal fold tissue due to aging
4. Iatrogenic lesions
5. Idiopathic.

Bowing of the vocal folds is common in the elderly population. Historically, these individuals have been told that this condition is part of aging and they would "just have to live" with the voice changes. Adequate communication is of vital importance in maintaining social contacts as an individual ages. A well-preserved voice helps maintain self-respect and self-image (Greene and Mathieson, 1989).

BOWING OF THE VOCAL FOLDS

Contributed by Dawn Lowery, Ph.D.

The elderly patient presents a complicated case in which normal aging changes may be complicated by functional and/or organic problems. In the case of bowed vocal folds in the geriatric speaker, it is important to determine if the bowing is functional, acquired, developmental or a combination of the three. Functional bowing can be seen in all age groups and is generally the result of vocal misuse. This type is highly responsive to voice therapy. Second, acquired bowing of the vocal folds is noted in cases where paralysis of the recurrent or superior laryngeal nerves results in muscle atrophy of the affected vocal fold muscle. Atrophied muscle does not generally respond to voice therapy alone because of the underlying neurologic impairment, although vocal retraining in combination with various surgical procedures can improve voice quality. Finally, developmental bowing is noted in the aging larynx when neurologic degeneration results in the progressive atrophy of the vocalis muscle. The difference between acquired and developmental bowing is the rate at which the muscles degenerate, with the muscle in the former case usually deteriorating at a faster rate.

The geriatric speaker presents with an interesting case of an individual who can experience vocal fold bowing from more than one cause. Although physiologic bowing resulting in muscle atrophy is not reversed with voice therapy, functional bowing in the younger client can be reversed, and in the case of the elderly speaker, can be improved. The following case study examines the problem of vocal fold bowing in an elderly client.

Dawn Lowery, Ph.D., presents a case study demonstrating functional therapy approaches for bowing vocal folds.

CASE STUDY: PATIENT N

Patient N, a 74-year-old retired nurse, was referred by an otolaryngologist with complaints of vocal fatigue, laryngitis "not related to an upper respiratory infection," and "airiness." The otolaryngologist had diagnosed bowed vocal folds but could not find any underlying physiologic cause for the problem. According to the patient, voice symptoms had progressively increased over several years and were always worse after prolonged use of her voice or later in the day. The patient was very active and participated in exercise three times weekly, volunteered twice weekly at the hospital, and routinely participated in numerous social events. Her medical history included osteoarthritis, borderline osteoporosis, and pernicious anemia. Routine medications included aspirin (40 grains daily), calcium (1,000 mg daily), and vitamin B_{12} injections (monthly). She also reported being fitted for bilateral hearing aids, which she declined to wear because she found them bothersome.

Voice Assessment

Auditory-Perceptual

Voice quality was moderately harsh and strained. A mild hyponasal resonance was also noted. Visible tension was evident in her face, jaw, and neck. Frequent throat clearing and coughing behaviors were present. Voice quality had deteriorated by the conclusion of the voice testing.

Acoustic

The speaking fundamental frequency was reduced and the phonatory range was reduced for the highest frequency (Table 4–1). In addition, the habitual sound pressure level was elevated, with a normal intensity range. Perturbation measures revealed excessive mean percent jitter and shimmer, and a reduced signal-to-noise ratio.

Aerodynamic

The intraoral air pressure and mean airflow were excessive (see Table 4–1). Assessment of air volume revealed subnormal values. In addition, the maximum phonation time was markedly reduced in duration.

TABLE 4–1.

Acoustic and Aerodynamic Measures for Patient N

Measure	Pretherapy	Following Therapy
Mean Fo, Hz	160	190
Highest Fo, Hz	370	600
Lowest Fo, Hz	120	135
Mean sound pressure level, dB	75–79	71
Mean percent jitter	.12	.06
Shimmer, %	12	4
Signal-to-noise ratio	17	25
Intraoral pressure	17.33	11.43
Mean airflow, cc/sec	739	110
Maximum phonation time, sec	12	27
Air volume, mL	800	2,050

TABLE 4–2.

Videostrobe/Laryngoscopic Measures in Patient N

Measure	Pretherapy	Following Therapy
Videostroboscopic		
Glottic/closure	Moderate-severe bowing	Midmembraneous touch closure, posterior glottal gap
Amplitude	Moderately decreased	Slightly decreased
Mucosal wave	Moderately decreased	Normal
Symmetry	Always asymetrical	Symmetrical
Periodicity	Always aperiodic	Aperiodic at low pitch
Laryngoscopic		
Ventricular fold hyperfunction	Moderately compressed	Absent
Vocal fold edema	Mild, bilaterally	Slight, bilaterally
Laryngeal mucous	Excessive stranding/pooling, thick viscosity	Normal viscosity

Videostroboscopic

Examination of the vocal fold vibratory pattern revealed moderate-to-severe bilateral vocal fold bowing along the membranous vocal fold during all tasks except low pitch. A moderately decreased amplitude of vibration was noted bilaterally. Mucosal wave movement was similarly decreased. Asymmetrical and aperiodic vibration were present across all tasks. These results are shown in Table 4–2.

Laryngoscopic

Other laryngeal conditions were also noted during the examination (see Table 4–2). Moderately compressed ventricular folds (ventricular hyperfunction) were observed during all phonatory tasks. Mild, bilateral vocal fold edema was evident and may be a normal variant for a woman of this age. In addition, excessive and thick mucus stranding and pooling were evident in the glottic region.

Diagnostic Therapy

Diagnostic therapy procedures were used to determine if the vocal fold bowing was modifiable. This was important in determining the prognosis of vocal recovery. The rigid endoscope attached to the stroboscopic unit and video monitor were used to assess vocal fold bowing. The client was asked to sustain /i/ at a comfortable pitch and loudness. Vocal fold bowing was again evident (see "Videostroboscopic," in the earlier section). In addition, marked ventricular fold hyperfunction was apparent. The client was then asked to produce /i/ on inhalation, producing the sound as soon as she began to inhale. Phonatory inhalation was very difficult for this patient to perform. Therefore, she was asked to sustain /i/ on exhalation and then reverse the pattern, producing /i/ on inhalation. The exhalation phase was gradually weaned out of the task and the patient developed the ability to sustain an inhalation sound for a few seconds. This phonatory inhalation task demonstrated that glottal adduction could be improved and that ventricular fold hyperfunction could be decreased.

Based on this initial voice evaluation the following recommendations were made.

Hearing

It was advised that patient N consult with an audiologist about her hearing. Audiometric testing should be completed if necessary, and the hearing aids should be evaluated in order to optimize hearing. The client was informed of the potential effects of poor hearing on voice quality.

Hydration

1. **Steaming.** Use of steam as therapy was recommended twice daily to reduce throat dryness, to decrease nasal crusting, and to thin the mucous. The patient was instructed on different ways of steaming. One method included sitting in her bathroom with the door closed, inhaling the steam from the running shower for 10 to 15 minutes. Another method included the use of a commercial facial steamer or simulating a steamer by boiling water, pouring it into a bowl, and tenting a towel over the head and the bowl, inhaling the steam for 10 minutes, twice daily. The client was cautioned about placing her face too close to the water to avoid burns.

2. **Increasing water consumption.** The purpose of this recommendation is to increase internal hydration, which can modify the viscosity of the mucous secretions and result in less throat irritation. Patient N was instructed to increase her water consumption to six to eight 8-oz glasses of water daily, pending approval from her physician. It is advised to check with the client's physician, as increasing water consumption in an older individual can be dangerous. The elderly individual has more difficulty handling excessive fluid if blood pressure is high, or if other conditions such as cardiac or kidney problems exist.

3. **Room humidification.** The use of a humidifier in the bedroom at night can provide essential room moisture, especially for a mouth breather who experiences a dry throat in the morning.

Diet

The patient was advised to reduce caffeine consumption and to substitute decaffeinated beverages. The purpose of this suggestion is to facilitate a reduction in muscle tension, as caffeine is a known stimulant. Patient N admitted to drinking the equivalent of 250 to 400 mg of caffeinated beverages daily.

Voice Therapy

Voice therapy was recommended to provide education about the laryngeal mechanism and the effects on voice production; to eliminate throat clearing and coughing behaviors; to reduce muscular tension, which was most evident in the patient's face, jaw, neck, ventricular vocal folds, and upper chest, in order to improve breath support for speech; and to improve vocal fold closure. Four of the vocal techniques used for Patient N are described in the list which follows.

1. **Respiratory training.** Although patient N was involved in three times weekly aerobic exercise, her air volume was markedly low, coupled with the upper chest breathing and jaw and neck tension. The goals of respiratory training included relaxation and subsequent reduction in visible muscle tension, and improving breath support and control for speech. Training procedures included monitoring respiratory movement by use of a mirror and the client's placement of her hands. When the appropriate respiratory pattern in this stage is established, a client can progress to phonatory tasks. Three tasks were emphasized for Patient N.

Two-stage breathing. The client was asked to place one hand on her upper chest and the other on her lower abdomen. She was asked to inhale and describe which hand (and consequently, which body part) moved first and which hand had the greatest excursion. The goal was to achieve a two-step inspiratory pattern with the lower abdomen moving outward first and most, followed by a less obvious movement of the upper chest.

Lower rib expansion. A second technique requires the client to stand, placing her hands on her lower ribs and extending her fingers toward the spine. She then inhales, keeping her shoulders low as the fingers passively spread apart due to expansion of the lower rib cage.

Breath counting. When the appropriate respiratory pattern has been established this technique can be used to improve respiratory control. The patient was asked to inhale over 5 counts and hold the inhalation for 5 counts, then exhale over 5 counts and hold the exhalation for 5 counts. The cycle is then repeated once during this session, and the patient was asked to practice two cycles of the patterns two to three times daily. When the patient could easily master the pattern at five counts, the task was increased by one count at each stage. Over the course of a few weeks a client should be able to eventually master a maximum of ten counts at each stage.

The patient was advised to practice respiratory exercises throughout the day in a variety of settings. For example, she could practice while driving her car by allowing the lap belt to provide her with kinesthetic feedback.

2. **Relaxation.** Several relaxation techniques should be introduced to a client, as he or she may find only one or two beneficial. The interested clinician should read texts describing various relaxation techniques for an understanding of how to use them in therapy. Techniques include respiratory training, visual imagery, autogenic phrases, and progressive relaxation. Respiratory training was described earlier. Visual imagery is the use of images to invoke physical and mental relaxation. Often an individual will imagine a peaceful setting such as a walk along a beach or through a meadow. This can be stimulated by listening to a prerecorded tape which thoroughly describes the relaxing scene. Autogenic phrases, which can be prerecorded, use suggestive phrases to invoke relaxation. These include such sentences as "My breathing is slow and relaxed" and "My right arm is heavy and warm." Finally, progressive relaxation is a technique that requires a client to tense, hold, and then relax an isolated body part. Often a clinician will begin with the top of the body and work down, asking the client to wrinkle the forehead and hold this posture for 5 seconds and then relax the forehead, noticing the absence of muscle tension during the relaxed state.

Each technique was thoroughly instructed to patient N during therapy and recommended for daily home practice. After 2 weeks she was asked to select the technique(s) which were most beneficial in achieving relaxation. She chose visual imagery and progressive muscle relaxation, initially using an audio tape as stimulus.

3. **Visual-Auditory Feedback Training.** Biofeedback, using the rigid endoscope and television monitor, were used as described previously in the section "Diagnostic Therapy" to reduce ventricular fold hyperfunction and increase true vocal fold approximation. Visual, auditory, and kinesthetic cues were available to patient N as she learned the task. Gradually the visual stimulus was removed as long as she was able to achieve the appropriate movement patterns.

4. **Phonatory Training.**

Sustaining vowels. The first task included sustaining isolated vowels at habitual, highest, and lowest comfortable pitch levels. The client was asked to vocalize from mid-range to highest comfortable pitch, beginning with the easier to produce vowels and progressing to more difficult vowels. The goal is to gradually change pitch at a comfortable intensity level without experiencing voice breaks. Many geriatric clients have reported that the tense vowel /i/ is easier to produce, noting that the lax vowels reveal excessive voice breaks. Mirror training was used to maintain the appropriate mouth opening during the vowel production. The tendency was to close the jaw at either end of the phonatory range. The mirror was also beneficial for minimizing visible tension in the face, jaw, neck, or shoulders.

Following ascension, the patient was asked to repeat the task, singing from mid-range to the lowest comfortable pitch level. The client was then asked to gradually extend her phonatory range while sustaining a variety of vowels.

Singing. Singing combines respiratory and phonatory exercises. Songs that the patient enjoys and are within his or her vocal range should be selected for practice. The client can begin by substituting a single vowel for the lyrics in order to assist in monitoring the respiratory and phonatory patterns. When vowels are easily mastered, the lyrics can be sung. Again, mirror practice as well as hand placement on the lower ribs or chest and abdomen can benefit this technique. The goals developed for the other techniques should be combined during singing to produce phonation that has the appropriate respiratory support, has no voice breaks, is free of visible muscle tension, and maintains the appropriate open posture of the mouth.

Summary

Patient N was enrolled in therapy twice weekly for 3 weeks and then once weekly for 5 weeks. Therapy initiated with relaxation and respiratory training, which were immediately used for practice. When these techniques were mastered in therapy, visual-auditory feedback and phonatory exercises became the focus of therapy. The patient received audiologic treatment by the second week of therapy and wore her hearing aids consistently following her appointment. She also followed the hydration procedures and felt that the twice daily steaming was the most beneficial in managing the thick mucous secretions. Patient N noted significant improvement in her voice by the end of the eighth week of therapy. A voice reevaluation was repeated at that time. The post-therapy results are presented in Tables 4–1 and 4–2. All instrumental values improved from the initial evaluation, although the mean percent jitter and intraoral pressure values were above the normal limits. Vocal quality was mildly harsh following prolonged talking but considerably improved over the initial evaluation. Patient N was satisfied with her voice and was discharged from therapy. She was contacted 3 months later by telephone and reported that she continued with the steaming and phonatory exercises and had not noticed regression in her voice.

MANAGEMENT FOR UNILATERAL VOCAL FOLD PARALYSIS

Controversy regarding the efficacy of direct voice therapy for unilateral vocal fold paralysis is present. Indeed Colton and Casper (1990) argue that the long-held belief that effort closure will strengthen the nonparalyzed fold and encourage the fold to cross the glottal midline improving closure and voice quality, may be fallacious.

Although the notion of the cross-over effect is an appealing one, we have been impressed by the lack of its occurrence in patients we have examined fiberoptically, whether or not they exhibited return of voice. (Colton and Casper, p. 265).

Others support the notion of direct therapy for vocal fold paralysis (Aronson, 1990; Boone and McFarlane, 1988; Case, 1984). My own clinical experience has demonstrated mixed results with these patients. I'm never quite sure whether improvement in voice quality can be credited to the management techniques or to natural physiological changes such as muscle fibrosis and contractures (Ballenger, 1985). It is my belief, however, that the speech pathologist may play a valuable role in helping patients deal with this disorder. This role will include aspects of education, emotional support, environmental manipulation, and direct therapy.

CASE STUDY: PATIENT O

Patient O was a 42-year-old orthodontist who was referred by the laryngologist with the diagnosis of a left unilateral vocal fold paralysis. The paralysis was idiopathic in that all appropriate diagnostic testing, including a computed tomographic scan and chest radiograph, proved negative for disease.

Patient O became symptomatic 1 month prior to the voice evaluation. At that time he was suffering with a cold and awakened one morning with aphonia. The whispering lasted for 3 days. The patient was not overly concerned, as he thought the "laryngitis" was related to the cold. He became concerned when the voice remained very weak and breathy following resolution of the cold. He therefore sought the opinion of the laryngologist, who diagnosed the left vocal fold paralysis.

It was obvious during the voice evaluation that patient O was extremely concerned and emotionally distraught as a result of the paralysis. Although his voice quality was moderately severely dysphonic, characterized by breathiness, strain, pitch, and phonation breaks, he continued to work, following a normal schedule. He reported that it was increasingly difficult for him to communicate with patients with his voice fatiguing significantly by the end of the day.

Most individuals are justifiably concerned about any medical/physical problem. Patient O's response went beyond concern and seemed to border on hysteria. It was evident that solid information regarding this disorder was missing and must be quickly offered to this patient. The patient knew his test result had shown no serious disorder, but **"something"** was causing the problem. "What's to stop my other vocal fold from going out? Then what am I supposed to do?" At that point patient O broke down emotionally. The implication, of course, was that he would lose his livelihood if he couldn't communicate.

Videolaryngoscopy, including the laryngeal stroboscope, was used to show patient O his vocal folds and to demonstrate why his voice quality was dysphonic. (Line drawings may also be used.) The left true vocal fold was paralyzed in a paramedian position, yielding an incomplete closure. The left ventricular fold was strongly compressed toward the midline. The vibratory pattern was extremely distorted, as the left fold seemed to simply flap in the airstream while the right fold could not establish a normal vibratory pattern. It was explained to patient O that many paralyses are idiopathic and spontaneously resolve within 6 to 12 months. It may be speculated that since his paralysis began during a cold that nerve damage may have been the result of viral infection or neuritis. The fact that diagnostic testing had been negative, though it didn't give him the answer he sought as to cause, was certainly better than the alternative result. The likelihood of the right vocal fold becoming paralyzed was extremely slim.

This information appeared to calm the patient somewhat. Objective measures were then completed, which yielded the following results:

1. High fundamental frequency = 160 Hz
2. Limited downward frequency range = 126 to 480 Hz
3. High jitter measures = steady state vowels at all pitch levels and connected speech
4. High air flow rates = all pitch levels + 300 mL H_2O/sec
5. Low phonation times at all pitch levels.

Once the stroboscopic examination and objective measures were completed, the interview with the patient was finally conducted. Patient O had practiced dentistry for 12 years as an orthodontist in an upscale neighborhood. He was very busy, and his practice was successful. He had developed a personal lifestyle that reflected this success.

The patient's medical history included a tonsillectomy and hernia repair as a child, with no other hospitalizations noted. The only chronic disorders reported were frequent sinusitis for which he used terfenadine (Seldane) and borderline high blood pressure, which was monitored but not medicated. Patient O stopped smoking at age 30 following 12 years of smoking one pack of cigarettes per day. His liquid intake was adequate. He reported that prior to the onset of the paralysis, he "felt great."

The social history indicated that the patient was married for 12 years and had two daughters; aged 9 and 6 years. His wife was a homemaker. His work schedule included office hours from 8 A.M. to 5 P.M. 5 days/week and every other Saturday. In addition, he lectured at the medical school for 1 hour, once a month.

Nonwork activities included an active social schedule of parties, dinners, and benefits. His wife was active in volunteer groups, and the patient was obligated to attend many of these activities. In addition, he played tennis three times per week. The patient was distressed because playing tennis made his voice weaker, and he couldn't call out game scores. Other activities involved his daughters' school and extracurricular activities.

Following the interview, patient O continued to express his concerns regarding the paralysis. He was upset with not only the prospect of a permanent paralysis but also having to wait 12 months for alternative surgical treatments, as explained by the laryngologist. The basic rationale for a trial direct voice therapy program was explained. The concept of effort closure was described, and the following therapy plan was devised:

1. **Goal 1.** Patient O was taught to produce each vowel utilizing a glottal attack. He was instructed to (1) breathe in, (2) posture the vowel while building air pressure, and (3) release the vowel, as follows:

a	eat	ooze
e	it	oats
i	ate	ought
o	etch	out
oo	at	up

Each vowel and vowel/consonant was produced twice each, three times per day, using the glottal attack.

2. **Goal 2.** Same as week 1, with the addition of stretching the vowel sound for 2 seconds.

3. **Goal 3.** Same as week 2, with the addition of pushing the palms of the hands together to add an isometric push and to increase effort closure.

4. **Week 4.** Monitor results of therapy with stroboscopic observation and objective measures.

In addition to direct therapy, patient O was to build at least three vocal rest periods into his daily work activities, use amplification for an upcoming lecture, and ask his competitor to call out tennis scores.

Only minor improvement was noted during the first 3 weeks of direct therapy. The glottal attack/pushing exercises were simply seen as a possible way of increasing right vocal fold adductory strength. The patient was not taught to produce conversational voice in this manner. During conversational voice, the patient was demonstrating far too great laryngeal area, neck, and shoulder tension as a compensatory behavior. Not only was the resultant voice quality weak and breathy, but also strained in its production.

It was also evident that the patient continued to be deeply depressed by his vocal condition. This emotional conflict contributed to musculoskeletal tension and thus to vocal strain. The need for professional counseling was discussed, and the patient agreed to a psychological referral. He was eventually hospitalized for 2 weeks and placed on an antidepressant medication. The patient stabilized emotionally and was able to return to voice therapy with a clearer perspective and realistic expectation. Strengthening exercises continued for 3 more weeks in combination with relaxation exercises utilized to eliminate unnecessary tension. Progressive phrase production was practiced to identify the appropriate pitch and loudness level that would maximize voice quality, given the limitations imposed by the paralysis.

Patient O's voice quality did indeed improve perceptually to a mild dysphonia characterized by breathiness and occasional pitch breaks. Objective measures improved somewhat but remained abnormal. For example:

1. Fundamental frequency dropped 160 to 148 Hz, still abnormally high.
2. Jitter measures improved for comfort level and high pitches, but remained high for low pitch and connected speech.
3. Airflow rates dropped below 300 mL H_2O/sec, remaining well above 200 mL H_2O/sec, but so did patient O's effort to produce voice.
4. Phonation times remained low for all pitch levels.

Stroboscopic observation of the vocal folds demonstrated a greater compression of both ventricular folds, but the approximation of the true vocal folds did not appear to be improved. The vibratory pattern of both true folds was improved, again, as a result of a more relaxed effort and steady airflow used to produce the voice.

Did patient O improve in overall voice quality because of the effort closure exercises? The objective measures demonstrate improvement, but it is unclear whether these exercises had a positive impact. My clinical sense was that decreasing tension and finding and stabilizing the "best" voice were the keys to voice improvement in this patient.

The combination of direct voice therapy and psychological support were keys to this patient's recovery. Spontaneous recovery was not to be patient O's good fortune. One year following the onset of his paralysis he underwent Teflon injection. We did not have the opportunity to follow his progress through this procedure, but understand that he continues to practice quite successfully as a busy orthodontist.

GLOTTAL GAP REDUCTION

Contributed by Jack Gluckman, M.D.

In the following case study, Jack Gluckman, M.D., describes the most common surgical procedure for reducing the glottal gap: injection of Teflon suspension.

CASE STUDY: PATIENT P

Patient P, a 55-year-old woman, underwent surgical excision of a paraganglioma arising from the left vagus nerve (glomus vagale tumor), which necessitated resection of a portion of the main trunk of the nerve. Her immediate postoperative course was uneventful other than obvious breathy dysphonia and mild to moderate dysphagia, particularly for liquids, characterized by aspiration and coughing. These symptoms improved over the ensuing months, but continued to represent a social embarrassment to the patient. At 6 months following the surgery, laryngeal examination revealed minimal pooling of secretions in the piriform sinus on the left and an ipsilateral vocal cord paralysis with the cord lying in the cadaveric position. A contrast esophageal study revealed mild esophageal dysmotility and mild aspiration which could easily be cleared by coughing. Radiography of the chest failed to reveal any permanent changes from the aspiration.

Because of the dysphonia and aspiration, it was elected to perform injection of Teflon into the paralyzed vocal cord. This was performed using the endoscopic technique under local anesthesia in the operating room, with dramatic improvement in voice and elimination of the aspiration.

Discussion

Vocal cord palsy results from vagal nerve damage, with the position of the cord being dependent on the site of involvement. In a recurrent laryngeal nerve palsy, the cord usually assumes in the paramedian position, resulting in a weak and breathy voice with poor projection because of the air leak. Aspiration is rarely a problem. The severity of the dysphonia depends on the ability of the contralateral vocal cord to compensate and the degree of atrophy of the vocalis muscle that results from the paralysis. In vagal trunk injury, both the recurrent laryngeal nerve and superior laryngeal nerve are affected, and the cord lies in a more adducted position (the cadaveric position). These patients have a significantly breathy and weak voice, with aspiration being a major problem because the contralateral cord is really unable to compensate adequately and the cough is weak.

Injection of the laterally positioned vocal cord in order to medialize the cord and straighten its vibrating edge is not new. Bruning (1911) first reported this technique using paraffin, but this fell into disrepute of the potential risk of developing a paraffinoma. The technique was revitalized by Arnold (1955), who with others experimented with a wide variety of substances including cartilage particles, collagen, ground-up tantalum, silicone, and bovine bone paste, before settling on Teflon paste.

Teflon is a trade name for a polymer of tetrafluoroethylene which has been shown both in animal and human experiments to be extremely well tolerated by the body. It is walled off by a foreign body reaction and within a few months is noted to persist at the injection site as a rubbery mass.

Indications

Essentially, Teflon injection should be considered only if one is certain that the nerve has no hope of spontaneous recovery, for example, in cases of a severed nerve. Even in this situation, one should, if possible, wait at least 3 months before injection, as the symptoms tend to improve significantly due to compensation by the contralateral cord or spontaneous medialization of the cord. If the cause is idiopathic or if it is possible that the vocal cord may spontaneously recover, one should wait at least 1 year from the onset of the paralysis before using this technique.

Teflon injection should, therefore, be considered if the voice is breathy and weak, or if aspiration is present. In evaluating the patient, it is not necessary to see a chink between the cords during adduction to warrant the use of this technique.

Technique

There are essentially three different techniques for Teflon injection, with each technique having advantages and disadvantages:

1. Indirect laryngoscopic technique
2. Transcutaneous technique
3. Direct laryngoscopic technique.

Indirect Laryngoscopic Technique

This is performed in an outpatient setting with the patient sitting in front of the surgeon. Usually topically applied local anesthesia will suffice, but occasionally the anxious patient may require a mild sedative to augment this. With the patient retracting the tongue, the larynx is visualized by a laryngeal mirror held in the oropharynx, and the Teflon-loaded Bruning's syringe with a specially fitted 19-gauge laryngeal needle is used to inject the vocal cord transorally. The correct amount of Teflon to be injected is assisted by asking the patient to phonate after each injection; the amounts are increased until a satisfactory voice is obtained. This technique does require considerable expertise and is not as popular as the direct laryngoscopic technique.

Transcutaneous Technique

This technique consists of injection of Teflon into the vocal cord by way of the cricothyroid membrane. It is particularly useful in patients where the other techniques are not feasible because of trismus, neck rigidity, or other anatomic reasons. The patient is treated in the sitting position, and a topical local anesthesia is applied to the mucosa of the larynx by means of a spray. The skin over the cricothyroid membrane through which the injection will be performed is infiltrated with local anesthesia. A number 18 spinal needle attached to the Bruning's syringe is used to inject the vocal cord. The injection is then monitored by the placement of a fiberoptic laryngoscope attached to a video monitor. The correct amount to be injected is assessed by the voice obtained as the patient phonates during the procedure.

Direct Laryngoscopic Technique

This is the preferred technique of the author. It is performed in the operating room. The larynx, pharynx, and oral cavity are anesthetized using topical local anesthetic and sufficient intravenous neurolept anesthesia to permit suspension microlaryngoscopy, but at the same time, allowing the patient to cooperate by phonating on demand. Once suitable anesthesia has been obtained, the laryngoscope is suspended, the endolarynx is visualized under the microscope, and the paralyzed cord is injected using the Bruning's syringe. The patient is asked to phonate, allowing one to determine the optimum amount of Teflon to be injected.

While this remains the most popular technique for Teflon injection, it is thought by some to be inferior to the other techniques in that the larynx is distorted by the suspended endoscope and it is more difficult for the patient to phonate properly during the procedure.

Results

Irrespective of the technique used, the key to obtaining a good result is the positioning of the Teflon within the vocal cord. There are multiple approaches, with each surgeon having his or her own preferred technique. In general, one should inject in the paraglottic space as opposed to the free edge of the cord, as the latter method will result in lumps of Teflon on the free vibratory surface of the cord, giving an unsatisfactory result. In addition, care should be exercised not to inject too much Teflon into the anterior half of the cord, as this will prevent adequate glottic closure posteriorly. Finally, it is almost impossible to close the posterior glottic chink satisfactorily, and one should accept this in performing this procedure and not over inject in this area with the potential for airway obstruction.

While one attempts to gauge the optimal result intraoperatively as the patient is phonating, there is always some edema after the procedure, and the maximum effect can only be gauged at 5 days. While much debate exists as to whether Teflon injection results in as good a voice as the more contemporary thyroplasty, in the end, if the patient is able to obtain a clearer, stronger voice with limitation of aspiration, this should be regarded as a success; using these criteria, the success rate approaches 90%. That one is not able to replicate the preinjury voice should not be regarded as a sign of failure.

Complications

Without doubt, the most common feared complication with Teflon injection is overinjection, with airway compromise. This should be avoided at all costs, even to the point of planning repeated procedures with small incremental injections until the desired effect is obtained. If airway compromise does occur, the patient should be observed overnight and placed on steroids and, if absolutely necessary, a tracheostomy performed. Occasionally, too much Teflon may be injected anteriorly, resulting in a worse voice. In this situation, the Teflon may need to be extracted under microlaryngoscopy, but this can be technically very difficult to achieve. Teflon granuloma and Teflon inadvertently placed in the subglottis are occasionally described complications.

In conclusion, Teflon injection for unilateral vocal cord paralysis is a simple, tried, and tested method for medialization of the vocal cord. It is easy to learn and, in experienced hands, the results are extremely successful.

UNILATERAL VOCAL CORD PARALYSIS

The management of unilateral vocal cord paralysis has evolved over the past 5 to 10 years from injection therapy for both acute and chronic vocal cord rehabilitation with absorbable gelatin foam (Gelfoam) and Teflon, to vocal cord medialization as introduced by Ishiki et al. (1975). Medialization by injection improves glottic closure for cough and prevention of aspiration. Injection also may improve voice quality by decreasing air escape through

the glottis, but has limitations in the degree of vocal improvement. The amorphous injected substance provides bulk and mass, which basically renders a medialized cord with abnormal and poor vibratory characteristics compared with the normal vocal folds. Medialization by laryngoplasty, however, provides improved glottic closure for laryngeal protective function and allows excellent and near-normal vibratory quality of the medialized cord when viewed with stroboscopy. Limitations still exist related to intensity of speech or resistance to forceful air flow through the glottis. When the site of nerve damage is superior to the superior laryngeal nerve, limitation of vocal range may exist because of the inability to alter length, tension, and mass of the medialized cord.

Acute rehabilitation of a paralyzed vocal cord is strongly dependent on the underlying cause of the paralysis and expected time course of recovery, if anticipated. Patient factors, particularly the loss of laryngeal protective functions of cough, and of closure to prevent aspiration, weigh heavily in the decision-making during the acute phase. Generally, if vocal quality is the only acute problem, then vocal therapy should be instituted to strengthen the mobile cord while the patient is observed. Frequently, spontaneous medialization will allow return of good vocal quality without surgical intervention.

Teflon injection is considered useful for short-term permanent rehabilitation in debilitated terminal cancer patients who are aspirating and in whom a general anesthesia or even heavy sedation for a neck procedure may place the patient at high risk. The airway is maintained during suspension laryngoscopy, and allows for a safe approach and Teflon injection in these unfortunate patients.

Vocal cord medialization laryngoplasty also allows for acute rehabilitation of the glottic closure. Laryngoplasty has the advantage over Gelfoam injection of lasting for a prolonged period of time for temporary rehabilitation, and when left intact, provides a permanent rehabilitation. It also retains a reversible quality needed for potential recoverable lesions.

LARYNGOPLASTY FOR VOCAL CORD MEDIALIZATION

Contributed by Thomas J. Kereiakes, M.D.

In the following case study, Thomas J. Kereiakes, M.D., discusses the technique and use of external laryngoplasty for vocal cord medialization. The case presentation is followed by the author's comments regarding the usefulness of this form of rehabilitation for unilateral vocal cord paralysis.

CASE STUDY: PATIENT Q

Patient Q, a 39-year-old phlebotomist, underwent total thyroidectomy with partial left neck dissection at age 19 years for thyroid carcinoma. This resulted in a left true vocal cord paralysis. Voice quality was high-pitched and breathy, generated by overclosure compensation of the supraglottic larynx. Her voice was frequently mistaken for that of a young child, with a limited vocal range, level of intensity, and limited breath support that allowed only four- to five-word sentences (see Table 4–3). There was no aspiration with swallowing, and her cough mechanism was adequate for clearing her tracheobronchial tree. In this situation, treatment for vocal quality was the primary emphasis of rehabilitation.

External laryngoplasty with vocal coard medialization was recommended for her rehabilitation. The technique outlined by Koufman (1986) was utilized. Modifications were made in the technique to allow intraoperative monitoring of vocal cord position through fiberoptic examination and subjective vocal quality assessment. In addition, the mechanism of laryngeal measurements was adapted by this author to allow for accurate stent creation to maintain the medialization.

Procedure

Under intravenous sedation, the neck was injected along the anterior sternocleidomastoid muscle border for regional anesthesia by use of an anterior cervical nerve block. The patient was then injected locally in the midneck overlying the larynx. Through a horizontal midline neck incision placed over the thyroid cartilage, the strap muscles were elevated and retracted from the left lateral thyroid lamina. Prior thyroid surgery created adhesions of these muscles to the cartilage, requiring sharp dissection to expose the thyroid lamina. Measurements of height and width of the lateral lamina were used to calculate the window size (Fig 4–1). The window was incised in the cartilage just below the midline, with the posterior edge tilted slightly superiorly to match the natural "incline" of the vocal fold.

At this point in the procedure, a fiberoptic endoscope was passed through the patient's nose, which allowed observation of the vocal cord position. While the cartilage window was depressed inward with a small, right-angle hemostat, a measurement was taken to determine the stent size. Measurements were taken at the posterior and anterior edges of the window during the medialization to determine the stent thickness. Both posterior and anterior measures were required because the degree of medialization of the anterior and posterior

TABLE 4–3.

Preoperative Acoustic and Aerodynamic Measures

Preoperative frequency range (cycles/sec)	Jitter	Frequency (cycles/sec)	Flow Rate (mL/sec)	Maximum Phonation Times (sec)
		223.7*	315	7.9
162.7–514.1	2.08	316.7†	422	5.8
		200.5‡	350	6.4

*Comfort.
†High.
‡Low.

portion of the window may be different. In addition, vocal quality was tested while the patient counted and the window was gradually depressed. While the patient counted, a small ruler was used to measure the amount of window displacement. Visual observation and auditory perceptual judgments were used to determine final measurements.

The distance from the outer table of the window to the inner table of the thyroid lamina determined the thickness of the "T," or inner flange of the prosthesis which fits inside the larynx. This thickness determines the amount of medial displacement of the cartilage window when the stent is in position. The vocal quality is subjectively monitored and is heard to pass from a breathy quality, to normal-sounding quality, to a compressed or forced-sounding speech. By repeating this maneuver several times, it can subjectively be determined what degree of medialization is· needed for good vocal cord closure for voice. This is usually less than the measurement taken when the vocal cord is placed in the midline. To ensure both good airway and good voice, the stent is designed to medialize the cord between these two measurements by averaging the degree of

medial displacement obtained by the two techniques.

The stent is further designed to fill the entire window with a "T" flange position under each of the long sides of the opening. Its thickness varies based on differences in the anterior and posterior measurements taken (Fig 4–2). The prosthesis was inserted for patient Q and held securely by the flanges, requiring no suturing. The strap muscles were reapproximated in the midline over a suction drain. Antibiotics and intravenous steroids were utilized. The suction drain was removed from this patient on the subsequent hospital day when she was discharged. Recovery was eventful only on the 2nd postoperative day when the patient felt some limitation of her airway as the steroids wore off. Examination demonstrated the vocal cord to be in the midline; however, she complained of restriction and the sensation of shortness of breath and suffocation. This resolved with steroids. The final vocal cord position was just lateral to the midline, and the patient had no airway complaints.

Postoperative aerodynamics and vocal studies are indicated on Table 4–4. In summary,

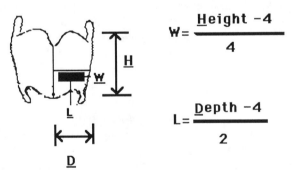

$$W = \frac{Height - 4}{4}$$

$$L = \frac{Depth - 4}{2}$$

FIG 4–1.
Measurements of the height and width of the lateral thyroid lamina, used to calculate the location and size of the prosthesis window.

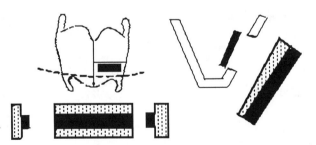

FIG 4–2.
Prosthetic stent demonstrating the "T" flange for securing the prosthesis without suturing.

TABLE 4–4.

Postoperative Acoustic and Aerodynamic Measures

Postoperative Frequency Range (cycles/sec)	Jitter	Frequency (cycles/sec)	Flow Rate (mL/sec)	Maximum Phonation Times (sec)
		226.9*	193	14.2
141.9–619.2	0.61	370.0†	174	15.7
		196.1‡	100	29.8

*Comfort.
†High.
‡Low.

patient Q returned to a normal vocal quality with normal airflow and a normal vocal range.

Discussion

This case highlights several points which influenced the author to modify previous techniques. The use of both visual and subjective functional measurements allows for a prediction of vocal cord placement and leaves a maximal airway as well. This technique of measurement and vocal cord placement was adapted by the author following experiences with several women patients with unilateral vocal cord paralysis. These women experienced airway limitation when their paralyzed cords spontaneously medialized to the midline. Because of the smaller size of the female larynx it is felt that the residual airway was sensed by the patient to be inadequate. This is similar to the finding in children with a unilateral vocal cord paralysis, and was evidenced in this patient when edema placed her cord in the midline. This measurement technique was also found to be useful in a medialization performed on an 18-year-old man who played full-court basketball. He was medialized to what amounts to paramedian position, allowing for both a good vocal improvement and a high flow rate through the glottis for exercise.

In addition to vocal quality improvement, videostroboscopy has demonstrated an increased resistance to lateral movement in the medialized fold, allowing for improved forcible closure by the contralateral cord. This increased resistance keeps the paralyzed vocal cord from being pushed by the mobile cord, thus preventing the vocal cord from blowing out of the airway when subglottic pressures are increased. The last two points would seem to

be as important as the degree of medialization.

In summary, the advantages of medialization laryngoplasty are the excellent vocal quality, predictable results, and the technical ease of performing the procedure. It is felt that the surgical techniques for the procedure are within the realm of the general otolaryngologist and do not require specialty tools or training. Other advantages of the procedure are its reversibility if vocal function returns, or if contralateral paralysis should develop. In addition, no special equipment is necessary other than the fiberoptic endoscope which is, in a modern otolaryngology practice, a common in-the-office instrument. The only difficulty encountered in doing this technique was in a densely calcified larynx in an elderly man. This larynx required both oscillating and reciprocating saws to cut the window, which was found to be cumbersome under a local anesthesia with sedation. As compared to the irreversibility of Teflon injection, and the poor predictability and occasional need for reinjection secondary to redistribution of the Teflon, it was found that this technique was extremely effective for unilateral vocal fold paralysis, with a prolonged successful result.

The technique of vocal cord medialization has therefore become the first-line therapy for vocal cord paralysis rehabilitation for both the occasional case of acute rehabilitation, as well as for chronic and long-term unilateral vocal cord paralysis rehabilitation.

RESONATION DISORDERS

A wide variation of acceptable voice resonation patterns exist, with acceptability often determined by geographic location (Stemple, 1984). Resonation disorders may be classified as either functional or organic. Shanks (1983) believes that functional voice/speech therapy for resonation disorders may be helpful in cases of hearing loss, regional twangs, assimilative nasality, nasal snort, and nasality where mild physical inadequacy of the palate/pharynx is compensable. Functional nasality problems may be the result of habit and imitation. They might result from anatomic changes from adenoidectomies or may result from extreme emotional reactions, as in psychological conversion behaviors.

Organic causes of resonation disorders may include cleft palate, submucous cleft palate, and velopharyngeal insufficiency caused by neurologic disorders and diseases affecting the peripheral cranial nerves (V, IX, X, XI). Medical/surgical intervention and speech therapy are the treatments of choice for organic causes of resonation problems.

Resonation disorders may include hypernasality, which occurs when vowels and voiced consonants receive excessive nasal resonance due to failure of the velopharyngeal sphincter to adequately close. Hypernasality may be accompanied by excessive nasal air flow during the production of pressure consonants. This excessive emission may also be called a nasal snort. Hypernasality may also be accompanied by facial grimaces as the patient attempts to compensate for lack of closure. Assimilative nasality occurs when the phonemes adjacent to /m/, /n/, and /y/ are nasalized along with these sounds.

Hyponasality or denasality is the absence of normal resonation on /m/, /n/, and /y/ caused by overclosure of the velopharyngeal sphincter or blockage of the anterior nasal cavity. Cul-de-sac or dead-end nasality describes a type of hyponasality in which all the vowels and nasals are produced with excessive nasal resonance because of anterior obstruction.

When considering functional therapy for resonance disorders it is important for the voice pathologist to be certain that the disorder is, in fact, functional and does not have an organic basis. Organic causation may be determined through medical examination, cinefluoroscopy, and manometric measures. The major characteristic of functional resonance

disorders is the lack of consistency and stimulability of the nasal quality.

The following suggestions from Stemple (1984) are made for dealing with functional resonance disorders.

Hypernasality

As usual, the first step in the modification of any vocal component is to identify the problem and to describe it in detail to the patient. Illustrations demonstrating the relationships between the resonance cavities are helpful. Tape-recorded samples of the patient's voice compared with the voice of the voice pathologist are helpful for ear training. Other suggested modification approaches include the following six methods.

1. **Articulation therapy.** Often, maximizing the precision of articulatory movements and decreasing any articulation errors will increase the intelligibility of the speech and decrease the perception of hypernasality. This will involve activating all the articulators in a somewhat exaggerated manner, with special emphasis placed on a wider mouth opening.

2. **Pitch and loudness modification.** Boone and McFarland (1988) discussed a positive decrease in the amount of nasal resonance in some patients who were taught to speak with an increased intensity at a lower pitch level.

3. **Non-speech phonation.** The patient plays with the voice, making various non-speech vocal sounds, such as animal and engine noises. If any of the non-speech sounds demonstrates reduced nasality, then work from this sound by comparing it to hypernasal sounds, training with similar sounds, and expanding into speech sounds.

4. **Utilize articulation deep test.** A deep test of articulation is used to determine if any sounds in any phonetic contexts are made with normal or near-normal amounts of nasal resonance. If so, these productions are expanded into similar sound clusters, first, then into words, phrases, and conversational speech.

5. **Do the obvious.** The patient's ability to produce a voice ". . . like you have a cold" is explored. Some patients with functional hypernasality can easily produce a hyponasal voice when speaking in this manner. They simply

were not aware that a slight modification of the "cold" voice would yield the normal nasal quality. It pays to explore this ability early in the therapy program.

6. **Negative practice.** Negative practice may also be an effective therapy tool used with resonance disorders. When the new normal resonance is first being produced, purposeful productions of the same sounds utilizing the "old" hypernasal voice may reinforce and strengthen the use of normal resonance. The patient's ability to use **both** voices upon dismissal from therapy shows a true mastery of the therapeutic goals.

Hyponasality

Functional hyponasality may occasionally occur, especially following the removal of nasal obstructions. In this case the patient's auditory feedback system does not quickly adjust. It continues to attempt to maintain the status quo even though the nasal cavity is no longer obstructed. Once the disorder has been identified and described in detail, approaches used to modify the behavior include:

1. **Utilizing the normal nasal sounds.** In this approach the speech pathologist should determine the patient's ability to produce /m/, /n/, and /y/ with normal resonance. If this is possible, /m/ and /n/ may be combined with vowel sounds and expanded through words, phrases, and the like.

If the nasal sounds are also produced with a hyponasal quality, attempts may be made to train the nasalization of /m/ using the singing voice. Humming, with the lips closed in the /m/ position, forces the production of normal nasal resonance. These productions may be slowly modified by opening the mouth while humming and saying /ma/, expanding to other vowel sounds, eliminating the hum, and then expanding into other sounds, words, phrases, and the like.

2. **Utilizing hypernasal resonance.** Some patients who demonstrate a functional hyponasal voice are readily able to produce an exaggerated hypernasal voice quality. If this is so, then different gradients of velar closure may be demonstrated and stabilized, leading to normal velopharyngeal functioning.

3. **Nonspeech phonation.** (Explained under Hypernasality.) This approach may also be an effective means of initiating normal voice resonance.

4. **Negative practice.** (Explained under Hypernasality.)

Because of the effect of resonation disorders on phoneme distortions, it is debatable whether resonation disturbances are problems of voice or articulation.

TEAM APPROACH TO REPAIR AND THERAPY OF CLEFT LIP AND PALATE

Contributed by Ann Kummer, Ph.D.

Organic causes of nasal disorders often require both medical/surgical, orthodontic, prosthodontic, and speech pathology services. In the following case study, Ann Kummer, Ph.D., describes this team approach in a child with cleft lip and palate.

CASE STUDY: PATIENT R

Patient R was born with a bilateral complete cleft lip and wide complete cleft palate. The premaxilla and prolabium were also markedly protuberant. A cleft lip repair was done at the age of 2 months. Following this initial surgery, patient R and her family were referred to the regional craniofacial anomaly team for consultation and follow-up.

Patient R was seen at the infant/toddler meeting of the craniofacial anomaly team at the age of 7 months. At the meeting, the speech pathologist gave a lecture to all the parents regarding the cause of defective communication skills in children with a history of cleft lip/palate. Methods of speech and language stimulation were discussed and demonstrated, and a written home program was given to the parents. It was explained to the parents that prior to palate closure, language stimulation should be the primary focus of intervention. Once, the palate is repaired, attention can be given to speech and resonance.

Although cleft palate is usually repaired around the age of 12 months, patient R's surgeon was reluctant to close the palate at that time because of its width and severity. Instead, he referred her back to the craniofacial anomaly team for further consultation.

Patient R was seen by the team for the second time at the age of 22 months. The cleft palate was still unrepaired. Upon informal evaluation, language skills were judged to be age-appropriate. Speech was severely defective, however, and consisted of a predominate use of glottal stops as a substitution for all pressure-sensitive phonemes. Resonance was characterized by severe hypernasality and consistent nasal emission due to the lack of a velopharyngeal valve. The team members were in agreement that immediate palate repair was indicated, and one of the team's plastic surgeons assumed management of patient R's case at the request of the previous surgeon. The palate was finally repaired when the patient was 2 years, 3 months, of age.

A complete speech, language, and voice evaluation was done at the age of 2 years, 8 months. The results of that evaluation revealed language skills to be well within normal limits. Although the mother reported some improvement in speech following the palate repair, the speech was still severely defective. Articulation was characterized by the use of glottal stops, nasal phonemes, and some glides as a substitution for all oral phonemes. Poor stimulability was still noted for the production of pressure-sensitive sounds.

Resonance at the time of that evaluation was characterized by a moderate to severe degree of hypernasality and consistent nasal emission. Nasometric testing was attempted, but cooperation was not sufficient to obtain valid results. An intraoral inspection revealed evidence of the cleft palate repair. Velar mobility was judged to be poor during phonation, and the velum also appeared short relative to the posterior pharyngeal wall.

The results of this evaluation suggested significant velopharyngeal insufficiency, making patient R a probable candidate for a pharyngeal flap. However, further evaluation of velopharyngeal function through videofluoroscopy was recommended prior to surgical intervention. This study is important so that the pharyngeal flap can be designed to fit the gap and make the best use of lateral pharyngeal wall movement. Unfortunately, the speech study is difficult to obtain in young children. Considering this patient's age, it was decided to delay the videofluoroscopic speech study. Regardless, it was felt that the surgery should be deferred in view of the fact that the palate repair was done and had been done recently. Speech therapy was felt to be indicated at some point, but considering her age, the evidence of velopharyngeal insufficiency, and the fact that language skills were normal, this recommendation was also deferred for the time. It was decided to have the parents continue working on language stimulation at home and have the patient return in 5 to 6 months for the videofluoroscopic speech study.

The videofluoroscopic speech study was done when patient R was 3 years, 6 months, of age. Her cooperation was excellent, and a very good study was obtained as a result. Following completion of the study, it was reviewed and interpreted by the speech pathologist and radiologist.

The videofluoroscopic speech study consisted of a lateral view, a frontal view, and a base view. For each view, patient R was asked to repeat standard sentences containing pressure-sensitive phonemes. On the lateral view, the velum and posterior pharyngeal wall were visualized during rest and during speech. In patient R's case, the velum was noted to be short, and it moved only slightly. It remained well below the level of the hard palate during maximum movement, resulting in a wide opening. There was no evidence of either a Passavant's ridge or an adenoid pad to assist with closure. For the other two views, barium was injected in the pharynx so that the lateral pharyngeal walls could be visualized. On the frontal view, both lateral walls were seen as if looking through the nose. Although symmetrical movement of the lateral walls was noted during speech, overall movement was very poor, causing a wide gap in the midline. The base view is a way to look up through the port and see the sphincteric action of all the structures. This view confirmed a large midline gap. Because lateral pharyngeal wall movement was symmetrical but very poor, a wide midline pharyngeal flap was suggested. The flap was done when the patient was 3 years, 10 months, of age.

Two months following placement of the flap, patient R was enrolled in speech therapy. At the initial visit, speech was still characterized by the use of primarily glottal stops for oral phonemes. A moderate degree of hypernasality was noted in connected speech.

An assessment of nasalance was done using the Nasometer (Kay Elemetrics). The nasalance score is a ratio of nasal acoustic energy to total acoustic energy (nasal plus oral) during speech. Using the zoo passage, the patient's nasalance score group was 45.17. (The mean of the normative group is 15.53, with a standard deviation of 4.86.) This confirmed a moderate degree of nasalance.

Given these observations, the goals of therapy were established as follows:

1. Produce plosive phonemes (p, b, t, d, k, g) with good oral pressure in isolation and in single words.
2. Produce fricatives (f, s, sh) with good oral pressure in isolation.
3. Decrease the hypernasal tone indirectly by developing the use of glottal stops, which results in a pharyngeal or hypernasal resonance.

To accomplish these goals, the following procedures were implemented.

1. In working on the correct production of plosives, articulatory placement was first established. For the bilabial phonemes (p, b), this was an easy task because these sounds are easily visualized. For lingual-alveolar sounds (t, d), placement was established by associating the nasal /n/ with these sounds. The velar sounds (k, g) were the most difficult for patient R, but placement was established by associating these sounds with the /ng/. In order to increase pressure, an "air paddle" made out of a thin piece of paper was placed in front of the girl's mouth during the production of the phonemes. The patient was asked to use enough force so that the paddle would move with each sound. She also placed her hand in front of her mouth and the clinician's mouth for

the tactile feedback that it could provide. Once placement and pressure were obtained for these sounds, a transfer to syllables and words was attempted.

2. For fricative phonemes, correct articulatory placement was established first. In order to encourage adequate intraoral pressure, patient R was asked to take a deep breath, then sigh. This was done with dental closure for /s/ and /sh/, and labiodental closure for /f/.

Although patient R's cooperation in therapy was excellent, her progress was very slow. She was able to achieve correct articulatory placement, and she showed improved ability to build up intraoral breath pressure. However, there was nasal emission and an inconsistent nasal rustle with the production of plosives and fricatives. It was decided to send her back to the craniofacial anomaly team for assessment of the flap.

Patient R returned to the craniofacial anomaly team 4 months following placement of the flap. The flap appeared to be intact, but there was still evidence of velopharyngeal insufficiency. It was decided to continue speech therapy for another 6 months considering the late palate repair and the fact that some patients are slow in adapting to the change in structure with a flap.

The patient was seen 6 months later and found to have improved articulation, but persistent hypernasality and nasal emission. It was decided to evaluate the pharyngeal flap by observing its function directly through nasopharyngoscopy.

The nasopharyngoscopy procedure involves using a 3-mm endoscope that is passed to the pharynx by way of the nose. Through the scope, the nasal surface of the velum can be observed as it relates to the lateral and posterior pharyngeal walls. This procedure is particularly useful for evaluating the effectiveness of a pharyngeal flap, since the scope can be passed down to directly observe each lateral port. In patient R's case, the left port closed completely during speech. The right port remained partially open, however. Bubbling of saliva was noted due to the escape of air through the port. A pharyngeal flap revision was done soon after this discovery, when the patient was 4 years, 10 months, of age.

When the patient returned for therapy following the flap revision, significant improvement in speech was noted. Resonance was judged to be normal, and the nasal emission had been essentially eliminated. The only concern at that point, aside from the remaining articulation errors, was an inconsistent nasal rustle. The nasalance score on the zoo passage was 31.07, reflecting the nasal rustle.

A nasal rustle, often called nasal turbulence, is a very audible form of nasal emission. It is usually the result of the friction that occurs when air is forced through a small velopharyngeal opening. Although the nasal rustle is very loud and distracting, it usually indicates a very small, inconsistent gap and is therefore amenable to therapy. For patient R, the following procedures were used to eliminate the nasal rustle:

1. The patient was made aware of the nasal rustle through auditory, visual, and tactile feedback. To develop her auditory awareness, the clinician imitated a nasal rustle so that the patient would recognize it. Her speech was then tape-recorded, and the nasal rustle was pointed out to her. She was soon able to identify these occurrences on her own.

Visual feedback was given through the use of an air paddle. By placing the paddle under the patient's nostrils during speech sound production, she was able to see evidence of the nasal emission through the movement of the paddle. The nasal emission was also visualized through the use of a See Scape (C.C. Publications). The nasal olive was placed in a nostril during phoneme and word production. Movement of the foam rubber stopper in the tube indicated the occurrence of nasal emission. Finally, the bar graph of the Nasometer was used to provide visual feedback.

Tactile feedback was given by having the patient touch the sides of her nose very lightly with her index fingers. The vibration from the nasal emission, especially when in the form of a nasal rustle, can usually be felt somewhere near the juncture of the nasal cartilage and the bone of the nose.

2. Once the patient was able to identify the nasal rustle and was aware of its occurrence in her own speech, she was asked to produce individual sounds, then words, and later sentences without allowing the nasal rustle to occur. That instruction alone is usually sufficient to elicit improvement from the child. She was given help in monitoring this through the use of the visual feed back modes.

3. The patient was taught to use light, quick, articulatory contacts for consonants, as she had been in the habit of using extra force for pressure sounds. This extra force, in combination with a slight delay in the release, caused a back-up of the air into the nasopharynx and contributed to the nasal rustle.

With the use of these techniques, patient R was able to eliminate the nasal rustle, even in connected speech. At the age of 5 years, 2 months, less than 4 months following the pharyngeal flap revision, her nasalance score on the zoo passage was 18.11, which is well within normal limits. She was discharged from speech therapy with age-appropriate articulation skills and normal resonance. There was no evidence of the previous problem with velopharyngeal insufficiency at the time of discharge.

REFERENCES

Arnold GE: Vocal rehabilitation of paralytic dysphonia, *Arch Otolaryngol* 62:1, 1955.

Aronson AE: *Clinical voice disorders*, ed 3, New York, 1990, Theime.

Ballenger J: *Diseases of the nose, throat, ear, head, and neck*, ed 3, Philadelphia, 1985, Lea & Febiger.

Boone D, McFarlane S: *The voice and voice therapy*, Englewood Cliffs, N.J., 1988, Prentice-Hall.

Bruning W: Uber eine neue behandlungsmethode der rekurrenslahmung, *Verh Dtsch Laryngol* 18:93–151, 1911.

Case J: *Clinical management of voice disorders*, Rockville, Md, 1984, Aspen.

Colton R, Casper J: *Understanding voice problems*, Baltimore, 1990, Williams & Wilkins.

Greene MCL, Mathiseson L: *The voice and its disorders*, ed 5, London, 1989, Whurr.

Ishiki N, Okamura H, Ishikawa T: Thyroplasty type 1 (lateral compression) for dysphonia due to vocal cord paralysis or atrophy, *Arch Otolaryngol* 80:465–473, 1975.

Koufman JA: Laryngoplasty for vocal cord medialization: an alternative to teflon, *Laryngoscope* 96:726–731, 1986.

Shanks JC: Treatment of resonance disorders. In Perkins WH, editor: *Current therapy of communication disorders: voice disorders,* New York, 1983, Thieme.

Stemple JC: *Clinical voice pathology,* Columbus, Ohio, 1984, Merrill.

Willatt D, Stell P: Vocal cord paralysis. In Paparella M et al., editors: *Otolaryngology,* ed 3, Philadelphia, 1991, WB Saunders.

CHAPTER 5

Management of Functional Voice Disorders

MANAGEMENT APPROACHES FOR

- Emotional dysphonia
- Conversion aphonia
- Conversion dysphonia
- Functional falsetto — male (hearing impaired)
- Functional falsetto — female
- Functional upper airway obstruction
- Pseudo-asthma.

MANAGEMENT STRATEGIES, INCLUDING

- Emotional counseling
- Patient education
- Progressive relaxation
- Electromyographic biofeedback
- Thermal biofeedback
- Laryngeal massage
- Non-speech phonation as facilitators of voice: cough, throat clear, glottal attack, grunting, um-hum
- Use of "falsetto" voice for remediating conversion voice disorders
- Speaking situations hierarchy
- "Gargle" as a facilitator of voice
- Laryngeal hydration
- Elimination of throat clearing.

When viewed from a strict physiologic point of view, hyperfunction and hypofunction of the laryngeal mechanism are not difficult to understand. The management approaches outlined all seek an equilibrium of the respiratory, laryngeal, and resonatory systems. However, when personality, emotions, psycho-social behaviors, and relationships are thrown into the mix, these factors tend to complicate the therapeutic process. It is well known that a person's physical condition and emotional status may be directly reflected in the quality of voice. With this in mind, presentation of the following group of disorders focuses on management techniques for functional voice problems.

The term "functional" has been chosen to describe a group of voice disorders that present with perceptual voice changes, often in the presence of normal-appearing vocal folds. Various texts have classified these disorders as psycho-social, psychogenic, conversion, personality-related, psycho-sexual, and so on. Because of disagreement concerning the causes of these disorders, the term functional is used here. Agreement does exist however, for the premise that the person cannot be separated from the voice disorder. Case studies with this premise in mind, focusing on voice change and personal awareness are presented for disorders of

- Environmental stress
- Conversion dysphonia/aphonia
- Functional falsetto
- Functional upper airway obstruction
- Pseudo-asthma.

ENVIRONMENTAL STRESS

Many occurrences in human life can lead to emotional and physical stresses that may provoke vocal disorders in some individuals. Unknown by the individual, these stresses often lead to extreme musculoskeletal tension. Laryngeal area tension, whether caused by hyperfunctional behaviors as previously described (see Chapter 4), or emotional stress, is a primary cause of vocal disturbances. The following case study describes the management approach utilized for a patient who suddenly found herself in the middle of an unpleasant life occurrence.

CASE STUDY: PATIENT S

Patient S was a 45-year-old nurse, wife, and mother of two sons, ages 16 and 20 years. She was referred from the laryngologist with a moderate to severe dysphonia characterized by a strained, raspy phonation. Videolaryngoscopy yielded grossly normal appearing vocal folds bilaterally. Stroboscopic examination of the vocal folds demonstrated a significantly decreased amplitude of vibration and a strongly dominant closed phase of the vibratory cycle.

Visually, patient S presented a very well-groomed, pleasant appearance. Her smile, however, was rather fixed and forced. It was one of those smiles where the mouth went up at the corners, but the eyes were hollow. Her breathing was shallow, with occasional deep sighs. Her neck and shoulders appeared very stiff, with the larynx being elevated and the tongue retracted.

The patient became symptomatic with hoarseness approximately 3 months prior to the examination. She reported that she thought she must have had a cold when the symptoms first started, but she wasn't quite sure. Over the past 3 months, the voice quality had worsened. Not only was she hoarse, but she also had the laryngeal sensations of extreme dryness, a "lump-in-the-throat" feeling, and actual aching that occasionally ran from her larynx, up to her neck, and to her ears. When the pain was greatest, the patient experienced what she described as "blocked hearing."

Patient S's medical history involved a complete hysterectomy at age 40, frequent D & C's prior to the hysterectomy, and a tonsillectomy as a child. Chronic disorders included frequent headaches (daily), sinusitis, and stomach pain. In addition, she had begun to experience a "shortness of breath" when speaking. Medications included estrogen (Premarin) for hormonal balance, acetaminophen (Tylenol) for headaches, terfenadine (Seldane) for sinusitis, and antacid preparation (Mylanta) for stomach pain.

Patient S had recently begun smoking again after not smoking for 5 years. Her liquid intake was adequate. She reported that on a day-to-day basis she felt only "fair" because she was "always tired."

Obviously this patient was demonstrating many signs of emotional tension and stress. During the interview section of the voice evaluation our patients are always asked, "On a day to day basis, how do you **feel**?" Medical history may tell physical condition, but this question explores the patient's emotional condition. When patient S answered "fair," this was the therapist's opportunity to explore the emotional side of the problem.

Patient S was asked, "Why only fair?" Her response was that she was so busy that she was always tired. She couldn't seem to get enough sleep. This issue was then explored while probing the patient's social history.

The patient had been married for 21 years. Her husband was a manufacturer's representative and was on the road 50% of the time in covering a multistate territory. Her 20-year-old son was an honor student attending an out-of-state university. The 16-year-old son attended a local high school. Patient S was a licensed practical nurse who worked part-time at a nursing home.

When speaking of her 20-year-old son, the patient's entire demeanor changed. Her voice quality improved somewhat, and her tension visibly diminished. However, the opposite response was noted when questions focused on her younger son. Noting this response, the patient was probed to talk about his schooling and his outside activities such as sports, clubs, and so on. The patient became visibly agitated and finally, in tears, told of the problems this son was having.

Three months before the examination, not coincidentally at the same time as the onset of her voice problems, patient S's son had been arrested at the high school with two other boys for selling and using various drugs. He was presently in a residential rehabilitation program as required by the juvenile court. The stress of this problem had caused marital problems which had "always been there" to surface. Instead of being able to rally support for their son and each other, the patient and her husband were discussing divorce. The husband was now constantly working, and the patient felt alone in her efforts to deal with these problems.

After releasing this extreme tension by verbalizing the problem and crying, the patient's voice quality was actually very much improved. This fact was pointed out to the patient. The relationship of stress and tension to voice strain was described and discussed in detail. Understanding the problem was the first step in remediating the symptoms.

Though patient S now understood why she was hoarse, she could not automatically decrease the musculoskeletal tension in the manner that her catharsis had permitted. Subsequent therapy sessions introduced a means of decreasing tension known as digital massage (Aronson, 1990).

Several methods of laryngeal tension reduction have been suggested. Some of these may include progressive relaxation (Jacobsen, 1938), chewing exercises (Froeschels, 1952), electromyographic and thermal biofeedback (Stemple, Weiler, Whitehead and Komray, 1980), and direct digital massage. Aronson (1990) suggested the latter method as a means of decreasing laryngeal musculoskeletal tension. The steps include:

1. "Encircle the hyoid bone with the thumb and middle finger, working them posteriorly until the tips of the major horns are felt.

2. Exert light pressure with the fingers in a circular motion over the tips of the hyoid bone and ask if the patient feels pain, not just pressure. It is important to watch facial expression for signs of discomfort or pain.

3. Repeat this procedure with the fingers in the thyrohyoid space, beginning from the thyroid notch and working posteriorly.

4. Find the posterior borders of the thyroid cartilage just medial to the sternocleidomastoid muscles and repeat the procedure.

5. With the fingers over the superior borders of the thyroid, begin to work the larynx gently downward, also moving it laterally at times. One should check for a lower laryngeal position by estimating the increased size of the thyrohyoid space.

6. Ask the patient to prolong vowels during these procedures, noting changes in quality or pitch. Clearer voice quality and lower pitch indicate relief of tension. Because these procedures are fatiguing, rest periods should be provided.

7. Once a voice change has taken place, the patient should be allowed to experiment with the voice, repeating vowels, words, and sentences." (Aronson, pp 314–315.)

The patient is then taught to do his or her own massage. Patient S was quite successful in decreasing laryngeal tension with this technique. Eventually, all she had to do was touch her neck with her fingers to trigger relaxation. It should be noted, however, that not all patients respond well to being touched. The therapist must explain the technique and then ask permission to proceed.

Patient S's voice quality improved to normal within 3 weeks of the evaluation. Recommendations were made for family counseling, which were automatically begun as part of her son's rehabilitation program.

Environmental stress led to extreme tension in the patient's laryngeal area, causing functional voice strain. A management program involving education, tension reduction, and counseling was successful in remediating the voice component of this stress-related disorder.

CONVERSION APHONIA/DYSPHONIA

At times, environmental tension and stress may become so severe that in the attempt to draw attention away from the real problem, people may develop various avoidance behaviors. These behaviors may be psychological conversion reactions that permit individuals to deny awareness of the stress or emotional conflict. The behaviors are unconscious methods of avoiding strong interpersonal conflicts that cause stress, depression, or anxiety. Two such behaviors are functional whispering and functional dysphonia, again in the presence of normal vocal folds.

Often, by the time patients seek help from the laryngologist and/or speech pathologist, the need for the conversion reaction has passed, and they are ready to have the voice problem resolved. The event that precipitated the need for the conversion reaction has passed. It must be stressed, however, that these patients are not malingering. They do not know that they have the capability of producing normal voice. Some patients may continue to receive secondary gains from the disorder and resist all therapy modifications, but the majority will respond quickly to direct voice therapy.

The vast majority of patients who whisper indeed present with conversion aphonia. Even the most dysphonic individual usually attempts to produce whatever voice is possible. Conversion dysphonias, on the other hand, may be more difficult to diagnose. The voice pathologist will recognize unusual vocal presentations as being conversion dysphonias when the medical examination yields normal vocal folds, when the history of the problem yields no strong evidence for the occurrence of a hyperfunctional voice disorder, when the voice quality produced is not typical of "normal" dysphonia, and when the patient demonstrates the ability to produce normal phonation during non-speech voicing behaviors such as coughing, throat clearing, or laughing.

The majority of conversion voice disorders occur in women (Herrington-Hall et al., 1988). However, we have treated men, women, and children with this diagnosis. The following case study will present some general principles of therapy used with both conversion aphonias or dysphonias.

CASE STUDY: PATIENT T

Patient T, a 13-year-old eighth-grade student, was referred with a 4-week history of "voice-loss." The patient and her mother were interviewed together, and then the interview was continued when the mother was asked to leave the examination room. As is the case with many functional voice problems, the onset of whispering was associated with a cold. The patient's mother reported that her daughter had developed "laryngitis" 4 weeks prior to this examination and then "lost her voice totally" 2 days later. The cold quickly resolved, but the patient's voice had not yet returned.

The patient was reported to be a rather shy child who succeeded reasonably well in her academic activities. Socially, she had two "best" friends and participated in the school choir, library club, and 4-H activities. Her medical history was unremarkable as related to this problem. Though she had never experienced vocal difficulties before, her mother reported that the girl had experienced a "chronic cough" 1 year earlier for which no diagnosis could be found. Following several weeks of excessive coughing, the behavior suddenly stopped. The child's mother was hoping the voice would come back in the same manner.

Laryngeal videostroboscopy was performed at this point of the evaluation as a means of educating the patient about the anatomy and physiology of the vocal folds. Patient T presented with very normal-appearing vocal folds. The whisper, of course, did not permit slow-motion observation of fold vibration, but the folds were shown to adduct toward the midline, only to stop in an incomplete closure. The lack of approximation of the folds was pointed out to the patient with an explanation similar to the following:

"Your vocal folds look very good and healthy. For some reason, the muscles that pull them together are simply not pulling the way that they should. Therefore, the vocal folds are not closing all the way; and when they do not close all the way, they do not vibrate and we hear whispered speech. Our goal in therapy, therefore, is to do whatever is necessary to force those muscles to pull hard enough to make the vocal folds come together."

With this approach, the voice pathologist has given the patient a nonthreatening explanation as to why phonation is not occurring. No comment is yet made regarding the patient's inherent ability to phonate. In fact, the "blame" for lack of phonation has been removed from the patient and placed squarely on the faulty mechanism.

Traditional management approaches then examine the patient's ability to phonate during non-speech phonatory behaviors such as coughing, throat clearing, laughing, crying, or sighing. When clear phonation is identified on one of these behaviors, it is then shaped into vowel sounds, nonsense syllables, words, and short phrases. The voice pathologist must demonstrate much patience at this time. Most patients have not phonated for several weeks. The possibility of proceeding too quickly and frightening the patient away from phonation is present. Once good, consistent phonation is established under practice conditions, the voice pathologist begins to insist gently that it be used during the therapy conversations. When voice is regained in this manner, it is seldom lost again, and patients do not substitute other conversion symptoms (Stemple, 1984).

Another management strategy was used with patient T: that is, the use of falsetto voice as a facilitator of normal voicing. It was explained to the patient that we were going to manipulate her vocal folds in a manner that would force her muscles to pull the folds together. The therapist then produced a high-pitched falsetto tone on the vowel /ai/. The patient was told, in a matter-of-fact manner, that by stretching the vocal folds for this high pitch, the folds are more closely approximated. Everyone, even those with vocal problems, can produce this tone. The falsetto was again demonstrated, and the patient was told to produce the same sound.

Following several unsuccessful attempts, the patient produced a high-pitched squeak. This was promptly reinforced with praise and repeated several times. As the falsetto voice strengthened and the sound became clearer, other vowel sounds were introduced and stabilized at this pitch level.

It was explained to patient T that we were going to use the muscle tension created by producing the falsetto tone to force the vocal folds to pull together normally. The patient was given a list of 150 two-syllable phrases and asked to read them in the falsetto voice. During this exercise she was constantly encouraged to

read swiftly and loudly. After the voice stabilized in a relatively strong falsetto, the patient was halted and asked to match the clinician when singing down the scale about three to four notes from the original falsetto tone. The patient was then asked to continue reading the phrase at this new pitch level. The same procedure was repeated two to three more times until the child's pitch closely approximated a normal pitch level. She was continually encouraged to produce these phrases louder and faster until eventually her voice "broke" into normal phonation.

Occasionally the patient will approximate normal phonation but then hesitate as if somewhat reluctant to produce normal voice. When this occurs, the patient is asked to "drop way down" and produce a guttural voice quality while reading the phrases. This will "produce more tension." After a few minutes, the patient is taken back to the falsetto voice with the break into normal phonation usually occurring soon after.

It is extremely important that the voice pathologist be patient when utilizing this technique. The normal time frame from aphonia to normal voice is approximately 30 to 45 minutes. The voice pathologist must not only be patient but also must present a very matter-of-fact, confident manner. Voice pathologists are not cheerleaders. They are simply presenting a technique that they **know** will work.

Why do these techniques work?

1. The patient is ready for change.
2. The voice pathologist has given a reasonable explanation for what the vocal folds are doing.
3. The voice pathologist has demonstrated confidence in the therapeutic techniques.

Following return of voice, it is necessary to explore the actual cause for the conversion. It is desirable to do this in a direct manner. For example the voice pathologist could say:

"I'm very pleased that the muscles are all functioning well now and that your voice has returned to normal. It sounds really good. The thing that still puzzles me somewhat is why the muscles stopped closing the folds in the first place. I can tell you quite frankly that with a lot of other patients we have seen with the same problem, the cause has been something that has happened that has been very upsetting or emotionally draining. Can you think of anything that has been going on lately that has been quite upsetting to you?"

By this time the patient has developed strong confidence in the voice pathologist and quite often opens up a floodgate of information about deaths, family problems, work problems, and the like. In discussing these problems, the voice pathologist attempts to accomplish two major objectives: (1) give the patient total and final control over the laryngeal mechanism; and (2) determine the patient's general emotional state to decide the need for further professional counseling. Up to this point the speech pathologist has been manipulating the voice. The patient now must understand that despite the ultimate cause of the aphonia, he or she is in total control of the voice and does not need to permit the problem to recur. If it does, the patient knows how to regain control of the voice.

Finally, just because the need for the conversion reaction may no longer be present, this does not mean that formal family, psychiatric, or psychological counseling would not be helpful. If the voice pathologist feels the problem is not resolved and further counseling is in order, the suggestion should be discussed with the patient and appropriate referrals should be made (Stemple, 1984).

In discussing the problem with the patient's mother, it became evident that patient T had experienced other episodes of possible conversion behaviors, most notably several long-term coughing spells. Patient T was shy. She lacked confidence. Physically she was overweight and had, in the past year, become very sensitive about her appearance. Her mother reported that around the onset of this voice problem, her daughter had come home from school very upset about being teased by some classmates about her weight. Like many children in this age group, she was very sensitive to comments by her peers and was struggling to find her own identity. Suggestions were made for further counseling.

In a follow-up voice therapy session, patient T had maintained normal voicing. As a matter of fact, she was looking forward to singing with her school choir in a concert that week. Her ability to control her voice production was reinforced. She was told that if she felt the whisper returning all she needed to do was to produce the falsetto tone and most likely her voice would return to normal. That was our last contact with this patient.

FUNCTIONAL DYSPHONIA

Contributed by R. E. Stone, Jr., Ph.D.

In the next case study, R. E. Stone, Jr., Ph.D., demonstrates the advantages of imagination and experience in developing and implementing a "speaking situations hierarchy" for functional dysphonia.

CASE STUDY: PATIENT U

Patient U was only 10 years old but represented one of the greatest intervention challenges I have encountered in nearly 30 years of clinical practice. At the mother's telephone contact for an appointment I learned that patient U came home from school one day with extreme dysphonia after attending a soccer game. She thought that he had developed laryngitis. When supper was over he produced no voice and indicated that he couldn't talk. Professional help from various disciplines over a 7-week period was unproductive in restoring normal voice and communication.

When we met, patient U's only vocalizations were utterances of vocal fry but with no accompanying lip, jaw, or tongue movements needed for word formation. These movements were not elicited even when the boy was asked to whisper. If it weren't for the vocal fry productions he might have been thought to show elective mutism. One got the impression that his talking was reduced to a series of vocal-fry grunts that may have showed syllabification, thought pauses, and interphrase silences. Additionally, the pitch and loudness of the grunts varied within restricted limits but seemed to suggest his attempts at prosody.

Patient U was adopted during infancy into a home of two older female siblings. The family life seemed healthy. The parents were well educated, and the father was a vice-president of a large company in a large metropolitan midwestern city. Both parents were energetic and had outgoing personalities that would incline them to head a successful Amway distributorship (which later they did). They did not give the impression of being overbearing or unreasonably demanding of their children.

A history provided to the clinician (C) by the mother (M) follows:

C: "Tell us a little bit about when patient U started talking this way
with a real tight voice?"

M: "O.K. He came home from school
hoarse; they had a soccer game; he
had some voice, but it sounded
like he had been screaming a lot.
Within maybe 2 hours the voice
was completely gone."

C: "All he could do then was produce
this vocal-fry–like sound?"

M: "He did not even do that; there
was just nothing."

C: "Did he mouth his words then or
did he stop talking altogether?"

M: "He stopped talking, and when I
would ask him to try he would just
make indications that there was
nothing there."

C: "How long after that before he
started pushing air through the
larynx but just a little bit" (strained
sounding voice-making that vocal-
fry kind of voice)?

M: "I would say it was like a week.
He went to a pediatrician the following day and he thought it was
laryngitis, so he told him not to try
to talk. So he made no attempt of
any kind to talk for a week until he
went to a throat specialist who
then got him to make that vocal-fry
noise. That was when he started
with . . . ."

C: So he kind of learned to produce
the sound then, huh?"

M: "Yes, I think so, yes."

C: "What other things has he done in
trying to get voice back again. You

have been to the pediatrician and
to an ear, nose, and throat specialist."

M: "And he was hospitalized for a
week and was treated then by a
psychologist, a throat specialist,
and a physical therapist. All who
were trying to make him relax
enough to be able to make his vocal cords work. They said they
were too tight."

C: "What kinds of things did they do
for relaxation?"

M: "They did hypnotic suggestion,
they put him in whirlpool baths,
they played games with him, they
just talked to him about other
things, anything that was unrelated
to his being unable to talk."

C: "You spent a deal of money pursuing this then haven't you?"

M: "Yes, about $7,000."

During the intake interview with patient U's parents a colleague met with the patient in another room. They unproductively probed the child's potential for voice production using a variety of facilitative techniques (Boone and McFarlane, 1988) including inspiratory voice, yawn, sigh, humming, throat clearing, cough- ing, and chewing.

My involvement with patient U was gov- erned by a model I have called **erg.** In physics, an erg is a unit for measuring work. It involves moving a mass through a certain distance in a given unit of time. Applied to the therapeutic setting, one might consider taking a client (mass) from one point of behavior to another (distance) within an individual therapy session (or segment of it) divided into three parts:

1. **Evaluation** of behavior or skill that is needed or (needs to be abandoned) to bring the person closer to normal.
2. **Recommendation** of desirable behavior through verbal instruction and mod- eling.
3. **Getting** on with developing the use of the desired skill (or absence of the un- desired behavior) in a hierarchy of speaking situations.

After the client achieves success criterion at one level of the hierarchy the erg is repeated at another level. Each recycling would involve a new bit of behavior. The bits are designed to shape the individual's eventual performance into the use of normal physiology for phonation, finally in normal proposition communication.

Evaluating patient U initially, I first sought to recognize those behaviors he brought to the task of communication that obviated normal voice production. Hollien (1982) has reviewed the characteristics of vocal fry (pulse register) productions, suggesting there is increased glottal resistance and decreased air flow. Patient U, consequently, needed to reduce muscle effort and increase air flow to the task of voice production. Teaching muscular relaxation (Jacobson, 1970) of the interarytenoid, lateral cricoarytenoid, and thyroarytenoid muscles to a 10-year-old child within 1 or 2 days (before he and his parents returned home several hundreds of miles away) seemed an unrealistic clinical undertaking.

Recommendation, therefore, deemphasized formal relaxation training and focused on increasing airflow. Quickly I learned that asking patient U to change behavior during speechlike activities led to failure. When a client fails at a task that I recommend, I am obligated to assume the responsibility for the error in asking something that is too difficult or in not adequately communicating what I want of the person. Because failure tends to foster undesirable thoughts in a client and unproductive consequences of my guidance, I must present requests that are understandable and accomplishable. What task could I expect patient U to succeed in to help teach increased air flow? Finally, I merely asked him to blow against his upheld index finger as if blowing out a match. This was nonpropositional use of air flow and was a request of a behavior with which he had previous experience. It was behavior that easily could be molded by later instruction, and was a task with a simplicity that anyone with normal anatomy could do. The component or partial behaviors to which patient U's attention was drawn through verbal instruction included unimpeded inspiration, no holding of the breath between inspiration

and expiration, and lack of work (muscular action) in the neck area (and consequently in the larynx) on exhalation. These partial behaviors were adopted, then, as the recommended behaviors to be employed repetitively (that is, practiced, which constitutes "getting on with the behavior") in a variety of tasks one might consider as constituting a speaking situations hierarchy.

Lowest on the hierarchical ladder was purposeful flow of air through the untensed speech mechanism. Next patient U practiced flow of air while his mouth and lips were placed in various static positions. This was done by requesting that he produce a relaxed flow of air with his mouth open, then somewhat closed with the corners of the lips pulled back, then with lips rounded, and so forth. (These positions resulted in the production of different whispered vowels; however, this fact was not pointed out to patient U because of the need to avoid the chance of failure that might have accompanied a request to "whisper /i/, whisper /a/", for example.) After the boy successfully produced multiple events, meeting at least 80% success in the desired partial behaviors while instruction (discriminative stimulus) and positive feedback were withheld, it was pointed out that he indeed produced many tokens of various vowels. He then was asked to practice production of airflow (no voice) on vowels that he read from flash cards. (This represented another level of the hierarchy: purposeful vowel production with flow of air through an untensed mechanism).

The use of unvoiced flow of air through a relatively relaxed speech mechanism was eventually shaped through carefully graded increments of a speaking hierarch into employment for propositional speech. At this point, after approximately 1 hour of intervention, patient U was whispering normally. Mouth, lip, and tongue movements had become reestablished communication behaviors along with unimpeded flow of air. Not only had an erg been accomplished, but the idea of elective mutism as a diagnostic label no longer was an appropriate consideration.

The second session began with an evaluation of what behavior was needed to bring patient U a step closer to normal communication. Even the uninitiated clinician would recognize the patient's need for vocal fold activity superimposed on the flow of air through a relatively relaxed speech mechanism. But how could vocal fold activity be recommended without a statement such as, "O.K., now produce the airflow like you did last hour, but this time with voice?" The reader may ask, also, "What's wrong with asking for voice?" Maybe nothing would be wrong. But, I submit that it risks his adopting behaviors similar to those he demonstated when he first entered therapy (which was vocal fry). Guarding against this possibility, I was compelled not to refer to "voicing." Also, I did not want to ask the patient to do any of the activities my colleague requested earlier, because he failed at them. What could I do that might rely on referents that the child knew, that were not requests "to produce voice" (because he "knew" he couldn't produce voice) and that would assure success?

I decided to approach voice production by recommending gargling. Unvoiced gargling really wasn't much different from the activity patient U had engaged in during the previous hour. The recommendation proceeded as follows, where C is the clinician and P is the patient.

> **C:** "I know you can let air flow out of your mouth. This time I'd like you to do so while gargling a small mouthful of water." (Clinician models, tilting the head backward and gargling with voice.) "Now you do it."
>
> **P:** The patient tried. He produced the bubbling sound, but no voice.
>
> **C:** "Okay, you kept the air flowing out all the time. That's a good thing, too! If you hadn't, you'd have done a lot of choking. Keeping the air going is pretty important. Now, this time let's have you gargle like your Dad might do—with a lot of sound." (Clinician models vocalized gargling.) "Now, you do it."
>
> **P:** The patient tried. He produced the bubbling sound louder than before, but still no voice. But after he swallowed the mouthful of water,

he gave a little laugh with one short period in which the voice was produced in a high-pitched squeaklike sound.

> **C:** Immediately the clinician remarked, "Hey, did you notice that part of your laugh had some voice to it? Here, gargle another sip of water and make that little squeak sound as you gargle."
>
> **P:** Patient U succeeded.
>
> **C:** "Do that again, but this time make the sound longer."
>
> **P:** Again, patient U succeeded.
>
> **C:** "This time, make your gargle sound bigger, like your Dad might sound."
>
> **P:** Again, patient U succeeded.
>
> **C:** "Okay, this time make that sound, but without using a sip of water."
>
> **P:** Again, the patient succeeded. Voice was produced, and the gurgling sound probably resulted from interruption of the voice airstream by repetitive action of the uvula against and away from the base of the tongue.

Practice followed until the client and the clinician both felt assured that this behavior could be repeated any time the client wished.

The next evaluation established the need to alter the boy's head position to an upright posture. Accomplishing this was done in three trials in which gradual increments of head position change minimized the potential for failure that might have accompanied moving the head in a single trial to a position more suitable for communication.

Next, the evaluation established the need to alter the gurgling of sound to a continuous voice production by eliminating the tongue-uvula vibration. The recommendation to the patient was a simple instruction to open the mouth widely (separating the tongue from the uvula) accompanied by providing a mode of sustained /a/. Five trials were done before the patient indicated that he felt able to consistently do this whenever he wanted.

The next intervention step needed to establish patient U's ability to maintain continuous voice while moving parts of the speech mechanism without triggering his dysphonic behaviors conditioned to the act of speaking. The recommendations involved leading the boy, by modeling, through a sequence of behaviors starting with opening and closing the mouth (vowel productions) with continuous voice. Next, vowel-like utterances were made individually rather than the continuous vowel series. Following this, individual vowel productions each were terminated with an articulatory valving; then, vowels were initiated and terminated with consonants. Even though patient U was producing nonsense and finally meaningful syllables at this time, the fact that he merely was copying the model set by the clinician seemed to keep him from recognizing that he was using voice in speechlike units. Finally, after the boy had produced several CVC units that would have resulted in meaningful words if they had been uttered in reverse, it was pointed out that the patient had been saying words backward. For example, /tub/ said backward would be "boot." "Since you have been speaking backwards, let's now say some words forward," was the recommendation used to elicit meaningful words.

Use of words to form phrases and sentences was based on increasing the length of utterance, word for word, and then finally uttering the entire unit. For example:

> **C:** "Say 'I'."
> **P:** "I."
> **C:** "Say, 'I want'."
> **P:** "I want."
> **C:** "Say, 'I want some'."
> **P:** "I want some."
> [etc., etc.]
> **P:** "I want some eggs for breakfast."

By the end of this session (2 hours) patient U was able to engage in dialogue, maintaining voice that was different from what initially he presented with and was closer to normal. The voice still had a falsetto-like quality and was produced with guarded participation. I decided to accompany patient U and his parents to lunch and observe the degree to which the boy maintained his present skill outside the clinical setting. He did admirably. Not once did he lapse into vocal fry, and during lunch he even seemed to modify voice production to be more normal. After lunch, intervention resumed and constituted a review of the processes the boy had used in reacquiring use of voice. With a trend during lunch for him to improve voice toward normal, formal activities focusing on voice normalization were deferred until the next day.

Patient U returned the next day, and his parents vouched for the accuracy of his contention that he had maintained use of the improved vocal function established during the previous afternoon and evening. Although he presented this morning with normal voice, I was uncertain of his awareness of the clinical processes and goals. To test this, I asked the boy to demonstrate the way he talked before we started intervention. He did. Then, he successfully switched at will between normal voice and that which he used previously.

One last evaluation seemed necessary. Because patient U lived nearly 300 miles away and he could not conveniently return to the clinic, I needed satisfaction that he knew what to do to reestablish normal voice if he ever began speaking with his preintervention behaviors. Notice the absence of the term "remission." Within a behavioral model of intervention the use of medical terms such as "remission", "exacerbation," and "cure" tend to be used in ways that do not foster a client's development of the awareness that the behavior brought to the task of speaking is the responsibility of the client. I was seeking indication that this client had become his own clinician, and that he had an appropriate plan of approach to solving future problems of voice of a similar nature should he exhibit them. Patient U reiterated and successfully demonstrated the intervention steps he used to reestablish normal voice.

Because his parents participated in the therapy sessions it seemed important to sample the parent's understanding of how their son implemented a change to normal and the implications of this change. This was assessed on the second morning through interview at the end of the patient's hour-long session.

> **C:** "What thoughts went through your mind as you and the family were experiencing this?"

M: "Well we were told that our son's problem was purely psychological, that until he could learn to cope with a lot of the fears and things that were going on inside of him he would not be able to produce a voice, that his subconscious would not allow him to speak. So we went through a whole lot of guilt and embarrassment. I think that each one of us wondered . . . were we the ones who caused that kind of trauma and what have we done when we thought that we had a typical normal family. You know there was a lot of self-doubt and wondering if he would ever get over this."

C: "Pretty spooky!"

M: "Yes, it was very scary, yup."

C: "Do you have any concerns or questions now that you know he is producing voice again?"

M: "No, I don't think so; I guess I would be, if he comes down with laryngitis I will be very nervous. I think I am real satisfied with the psychological end of it and . . . ."

C: "Explain what you mean."

M: "Well, I guess I worried about a lot of deep-seated problems and, you know, I don't think I am worried about that anymore. In the beginning I would have said if he had gotten his voice back maybe there would be another time when if a traumatic experience occurred, he would lose it again. I see it now more as a physical thing that he can deal with and we can help him if he, you know, if it would come to a point where there was a problem with voice, I think we would know how to handle it."

FUNCTIONAL FALSETTO

Contributed by Robert Peppard, Ph.D.

Another functional voice disorder most often associated with postpubescent males is functional falsetto. In the next case, Robert Peppard, Ph.D., presents principles of a management approach involving a hearing-impaired young man with functional falsetto.

The Problem

The use of inappropriately high-pitched voice beyond puberty by boys has often been described in the literature on voice disorders (Wilson, 1979, Aronson, 1980, Stemple, 1984). This relatively rare problem has been variously termed mutational falsetto, persistent falsetto, or puberphonia. Though sometimes reported in adult men, puberphonia is most often seen immediately following puberty when the male vocal mechanism has undergone dramatic changes in size and function caused by hormonal changes.

The vocal mechanism used in puberphonia differs from that used to produce higher pitch levels of the modal register. Young men with puberphonia actually produce a different vocal register in which the suprahyoid muscles elevate the larynx, accompanied by excessive contraction of the cricothyroid muscle. To maintain this register, respiration is usually shallow, with minimal subglottal air pressure (Aronson, 1980).

Several simple diagnostic tests can help determine if puberphonia is present. These include throat clearing, coughing, and hard glottal attack, which should all result in a dramatic downward pitch descent into the modal register. Digital manipulation of the thyroid cartilage, moving the entire larynx downward, can also be used to test for the presence of puberphonia.

Clinical experience demonstrates that in most cases this problem is readily treated by short-term voice therapy.

Causation

The current author's clinical experience differs from those who suggest that puberphonia is the result of such psychogenic factors as failure of an adolescent male to accept an adult male role, overidentification with the mother, or social immaturity (Aronson, 1980). While some psychogenic factors may play a role in this disorder, a more likely explanation is that it results from attempts to stabilize unstable pitch and quality characteristics present in the male pubescent voice (Colton and Casper, 1990).

High Risk in the Hearing Impaired

Clinical experience further suggests that hearing impairment may be a risk factor which makes persistent high-pitched voice use more likely. It has been reported (Boone, 1966, Zaliouk, 1960) that deaf children, who lack normal auditory feedback mechanisms, may not develop the lower-pitched voice of normal postadolescents. Thus the incidence of puberphonia, fairly rare in hearing males, may be more prevalent in the hearing impaired. Hearing-impaired children, having only tactile and kinesthetic feedback to direct them, may attempt to stabilize the variable function of the mutating larynx by consistently using the falsetto mode. While such use is less efficient than a lower-pitched register, it may at least provide some measure of vocal stability. Further, the focus of speech treatment for the hearing impaired is often perfecting articulation to assure intelligible speech, and the speech clinician may not feel comfortable in addressing the voice needs of these children.

CASE STUDY: PATIENT V

At the time of the evaluation patient V was a 15-year-old hearing-impaired boy. His height was 68 in., and his weight was 135 lb. He had a bilateral, symmetrical, moderate-profound sensorineural hearing loss (pure tone average, 95 db HL) which was acquired postlingually following meningitis at age 3 years. He wore binaural, ear-level aids at volume levels of 2 for both ears. He had an aided speech reception threshold of 42 dB (Audiogram, Fig 5–1). Patient V was mainstreamed and doing well in a ninth-grade public school classroom. His expressive and receptive language skills were excellent, and he communicated primarily through good oral speech, aided hearing, and lip reading. He also used American Sign Language with his nonspeaking deaf peers.

With the exception of a few phonetic distortions, his speech was quite intelligible and he had not been enrolled in speech therapy since fourth grade. During a recent hearing reevaluation, his audiologist noted that patient V's voice was quite high pitched and had a strained quality. She recommended that he be seen for a voice evaluation.

Voice Evaluation

Patient V was seen in a university hospital voice clinic by a laryngologist and a speech-language pathologist specializing in voice disorders. A complete medical evaluation, including otolaryngological examination and voice evaluation, was performed. He was accompanied to the evaluation by his mother, who reported that she was pleased with her son's academic and communication abilities. The family was aware of their son's high-pitched voice, but assumed that it was a consequence of the hearing loss and they had come to accept this pitch level as normal for their son.

Vocal Symptoms

Patient V's only voice complaints were occasional voice fatigue and periodic voice breaks. He reported that classmates sometimes teased him about his high-pitched voice. He was aware that his voice varied from his peers, but did not believe anything could be done about it. He was unaware of being capable of producing any other voice.

Medical/Laryngeal Examinations

Medical examination revealed a normal, healthy, postpubescent male with no hormonal abnormalities. Indirect laryngeal examination was normal, with the larynx appearing normal in size for a boy of his age, with no abnormalities in structure or function. Larynx height was noted as elevated, with a good deal of tension in the neck muscles.

Videostroboscopic Examination

Patient V's vocal folds were difficult to visualize as a result of tension and high laryngeal position. A topical anesthetic was used to reduce the gag reflex, which then permitted the following observations.

Glottic closure pattern was incomplete. The vocal folds appeared stretched and tense, with

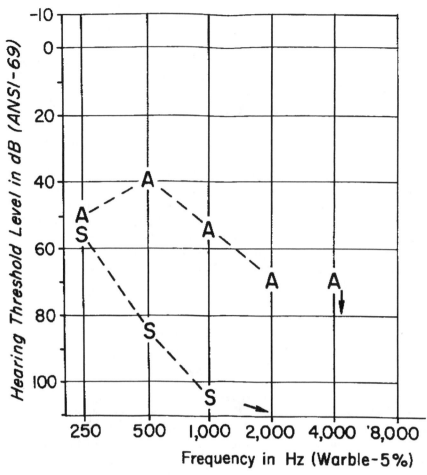

Sound Field   S---S Unaided Thresholds
              A---A Aided Thresholds

FIG 5–1.
Audiogram of aided and unaided hearing thresholds.

reduced mucosal wave. The vocal folds exhibited light contact, with thin edges. Vibration was characterized by long open phases and very short closed phases. Reduced amplitude of vibration was also noted.

Auditory Perceptual Signs

Patient V's voice was high pitched with occasional downward pitch breaks. He sounded strained, breathy, weak, and low in intensity, with little range in either intensity or pitch.

Acoustic Signs

The patient's fundamental frequency averaged 260 Hz in both sustained vowels and contextual production. His frequency range was restricted to less than one octave.

Intensity was reduced, averaging 60 dB sound pressure level (SPL) in both sustained and contextual situations. SPL range was also limited, with maximum voluntary production being 75 dB SPL.

Diagnostic Therapy

Some young men with puberphonia are aware of their ability to produce another voice. With assurances that this second lower-pitched voice is desirable, they are able to quickly shift to the new voice in all situations. Because patient V reported no knowledge of a second voice, several non-speech vocalizations were used to test for the presence of puberphonia. These included coughing, throat clearing, and hard glottal attack.

These vocalizations all demonstrated the dramatic downward shift of pitch characteristic of puberphonia. Similar descents in pitch were obtained with shouted productions, because falsetto cannot be sustained at maximum volume levels. When questioned, the patient reported that he could feel differences in his habitual mode of voice and these new lower-pitched productions, though he felt the lowered productions were not appropriate.

Somewhat reluctantly, the patient agreed to begin an intensive schedule of voice therapy to determine if the lower-pitched voice was more efficient. His reluctance was due in part to concerns that therapy would interfere with his other school and social activities and in part to his doubt that the new lowered voice was appropriate.

Therapy

In some cases of puberphonia, the more appropriate pitch levels discovered during diagnostic activities can be quickly carried over into conversational speech, and a permanent change in pitch level may be possible after one session.

Since hearing impairment limits the person's ability to monitor the changed pitch level, a longer period of therapy is usually required in which nonauditory methods such as visual feedback are used to achieve consistent use of the new voice. To account for these additional needs, multiple therapy sessions were scheduled for patient V to establish use of the new, lower-pitched voice.

Caution: If too little time is alotted for each session or if the sessions are far apart, the client may revert to the habitual falsetto pattern, which, while less efficient than the mutational voice, may especially for the hearing impaired, be more comfortable because of its familiarity.

Goals for treatment included (1) teaching patient V the method of producing the lower-pitched voice, including the ability to move voluntarily between modal and falsetto registers; (2) consistent use of a more optimal vocal

register in all speaking situations, and (3) acceptance of the new voice mode as appropriate.

Session I

The initial therapy session was scheduled for a 3-hour block with two rest breaks, 2 days after the initial diagnostic visit. It was during this session that the clinician began the process of persuading the patient that a mode of vibration that felt quite different from his habitual mode was actually optimal.

The first goal of this session was for patient V to consistently use the lower-pitched voice in sustained vowels, in reading of single words and short phrases, and in spontaneous speech consisting of short replies to simple questions. These limited contexts gave the patient many opportunities to practice the new voice register. Occasionally he would revert to his habitual pitch level, especially in spontaneous utterances. At those times the clinician would signal the patient to produce the utterance again, using a lower pitch. If the higher voice persisted, the patient was asked to initiate voice with hard glottal attack or louder volume, which almost always resulted in an appropriate downward pitch shift.

A PM Pitch Trainer, which displayed real-time measures of pitch levels on a monitor, was occasionally used as visual feedback to show the patient his ability to achieve target pitch levels. While such feedback was seldom needed for patient V, this visual feedback may be a highly desirable method for other hearing-impaired persons with falsetto.

During this first session the patient occasionally exhibited some behavioral problems. At times he would refuse to try a task, he avoided looking at the clinician, and he would say, "What's the point?" Such resistance to change should be expected even by clients with no psychogenic component, since — especially for the hearing-impaired person — the new register may feel very uncomfortable.

An analogy proved useful in helping the patient accept the discomfort he was experiencing in shifting to his new voice. It was suggested that shifting to his new voice was "like learning to use a stick shift on a car after having driven an automatic transmission." He was told that "with the new voice system you will occasionally 'stall out.' However, with practice you'll soon learn to use your new voice system and that as with a stick shift, your new voice will be a very efficient method of voice production, requiring less effort and vocal fatigue than your old voice."

Toward the end of the first session, the patient used negative practice in which he voluntarily shifted between the optimal and falsetto registers. This shift demonstrated the control which he had over the two voices and prepared him for any involuntary upward shifts he might have outside the therapy room.

By the end of the first session, the patient was successfully producing a more optimal pitch level, averaging 140 Hz at the 90% level. He had also begun self-monitoring and correcting inappropriate pitch productions without clinician prompting.

In planning for the next session, patient V chose his mother and younger brother as two people with whom he would begin using the new voice during the next therapy session, which was scheduled for a 2-hour block on the following day.

Session 2

The goal of this session was to stabilize and expand the number of situations in which the new voice was used. At the beginning of the session patient V was consistently using the lower-pitched register with the clinician. The new voice was also noted to be louder than the pretreatment voice. Some slight dysphonia and glottal fry quality were noted in the lower-pitched voice, as was some slight decrease in patient V's overall speech intelligibility, due to an increase in phonetic errors.

Such decreases in intelligibility have been noted in other hearing-impaired young men who dramatically lower their pitch. This articulatory change may be related to posterior tongue position which often accompanies the lowering of the larynx necessary for production of the modal register. Additional speech therapy may be needed to decrease these errors and increase intelligibility.

Patient V selected from a number of practice options for carry-over of the new voice. He used the new voice in telephone calls to other university departments and an airline. Very important was use of the new register outside the therapy room in a conversation with the clinic receptionist and while ordering lunch in the hospital cafeteria. The clinician provided positive feedback at patient V's consistent success in using the new voice in these situations.

At no time did the patient revert to the pretreatment voice, and after completing these assignments, he reported that, while he was still self-conscious about using the new voice, he was feeling increasingly comfortable with the new register.

The patient's mother and brother then joined the session for a short conversation about family vacation plans, in which patient V consistently used the new register. Finally, the patient agreed to utilize the new voice as much as possible outside the therapy room until the next therapy session.

It should be noted that following this session, patient V's mother reported some unease with her son's new voice quality. She said that her son's lower-pitched voice sounded unfamiliar and asked was it really appropriate for his age. She accepted assurances that indeed this was an appropriate mode for her son.

The next session was scheduled 2 days later, to give patient V time to practice the new voice.

Session 3

The goal of the third session was to evaluate the progress patient V had made in the consistent use of his new voice. The patient was much more relaxed at the start of this session that at any previous meeting. His pitch had descended even further and averaged 130 Hz. His voice was less dysphonic and displayed little glottal fry quality.

The patient reported that he was using the new mode in all situations and that only twice had he reverted to the high-pitched voice, both times when he had become excited while playing tennis. He had immediately known that the pitch was too high and quickly shifted to the optimal level. He further reported that he was becoming much more comfortable with the new voice and that friends and family seldom commented about the pitch change as he had feared they might.

The patient tried some additional negative practice and laughed when he found it difficult to shift back into the higher register. With some effort, he succeeded in doing so and reported that the higher voice now was more uncomfortable to produce than his new voice. The patient agreed with the clinician that the new pitch level was appropriate. He further agreed that additional speech therapy to improve his intelligibility would be desirable.

Therapy was terminated with an agreement that the patient would continue to use his new voice in all situations and that he would be contacted for follow-up evaluation in 3 months.

Follow-up

A phone contact was made with patient V's mother 3 months following termination of voice therapy. She reported that her son had continued to use the lowered pitch voice in all situations. He had also been seen by the public school speech pathologist, who helped him reduce phonetic errors, and it was reported that the patient's intelligibility was again at the excellent pre–voice change levels.

Conclusions

It has been suggested that puberphonia may have a higher incidence in the hearing-impaired population because of their altered feedback mechanism. It is strongly recommended that adolescent male speakers with hearing impairment be carefully monitored and screened for the presence of this voice disorder by communications disorders specialists. As the preceding case study demonstrates, with some additional time and some variation in treatment and the use of feedback, puberphonia in the hearing impaired is a highly treatable voice disorder. Successful treatment results in a more efficient voice, which also more closely compares with the speech of hearing peers. Research is currently under way to determine the incidence of this and other voice problems among the hearing-impaired population.

FUNCTIONAL FALSETTO IN THE ADULT WOMAN

CASE STUDY: PATIENT W

As previously mentioned, functional falsetto is most often associated with the postpubescent male. The author, however, has treated several adult women with this disorder. In the most recent case, patient W was a 52-year-old third-grade teacher who was referred by a friend with the complaint of having a "weak voice." The weakness was something that she had noticed all her life, but she never thought that it could be modified.

Stroboscopic examination of her vocal folds revealed normal appearing folds which approximated in a near-parallel relationship. Glottic closure was complete, but the amplitude of vibration was severely decreased. The open phase of the vibratory cycle was dominant; however, the symmetry of vibrations was regular.

Perceptually, patient W's voice quality was mildly dysphonic, characterized by a high-pitched, weak phonation. Objectively, she presented with a fundamental frequency of 220 Hz. Her pitch range was 205 to 860 Hz. Most interesting was the fact that she could not shout without overdriving the vocal folds into a high-pitched explosion of sound. Even with young men, one diagnostic sign of this disorder is the inability to shout. The positioning of the vocal folds for falsetto will not permit an appropriate buildup of subglottic air pressure to support a shouting behavior. The tenseness of the folds will not permit the greater amplitude of vibration required for the louder phonation.

How does one tell a 52-year-old woman who has always used this voice that it is not her real voice? First, you explore her knowledge of other voices. Patient W was asked if she could produce voice in any other manner. Her only response was a puzzling look that, without words, questioned the sanity of the therapist.

The next attempt to describe the problem was the intellectual approach. Through the use of the stroboscopic videotape and line diagrams, functional falsetto was explained in some detail to the patient. Patient W showed an intellectual understanding of the disorder, but was still somewhat skeptical of the diagnosis as related to her weak voice.

The clincher turned out to be the direct approach. Patient W was instructed in how to produce a hard glottal attack on the vowel /ae/. Her first attempt resulted in the deepest, loudest tone that she had ever heard emanate from her mouth. The sound also shocked and puzzled her. The therapist, looking smug, explained, "That was normal vibration of the vocal folds."

Once the shock diminished, patient W was most interested in pursuing this form of voice production. Because of the deep sound, she was not yet interested in permitting anyone else — office staff, family or friends — to hear her speak in this manner. Indeed, desensitization is an important step in dealing with functional falsetto. This patient had a lifetime of using her "old" voice. Her auditory feedback system kept repeating, "That's not me, that's not me." Systematic practice from words, through phrases, paragraph readings, and directed conversations were necessary to stabilize the "new" voice. Tape recordings were liberally used to demonstrate the normalcy of the "new" voice.

Once stabilized in therapy, patient W had to begin using the new voice with others. She started with a most sympathetic ear, my secretary, who had learned long ago when to positively reinforce. We then developed a hierarchy of situations to be tackled with the new voice, including:

- Ordering food at a drive-through restaurant
- Ordering food in a restaurant
- Calling for information about a store product
- Talking directly to her daughter
- Talking to her husband
- Talking to her class (who she was sure would laugh and giggle).

At the following session, which was 2 weeks later due to a well-deserved vacation for the doctor, patient W returned to report on her progress. Her new voice was very stable and demonstrated remarkably improved inflection and flexibility. Now it was my turn to be puzzled. Patient W reported that the day after our last session she developed a bad cold. In the past, she reported becoming aphonic during the initial stages of a cold and indeed, using her falsetto voice, she lost her voice.

"So, I decided, what have I got to lose? I tried to talk the new way and my voice came out fine. So, I've been using it everywhere ever since. I just tell people my cold changed my voice."

So much for brilliant hierarchys and desensitization plans. Final stroboscopic observation yielded a normal amplitude of vibration and phase closure. The patient's fundamental frequency stabilized at 196 Hz. Her pitch range expanded to 159 to 880 Hz. Most important, her voice was strong, easily produced, and heard.

FUNCTIONAL UPPER AIRWAY OBSTRUCTION

Contributed by James Case, Ph.D.

The laryngeal structures may also be affected by functional disorders of the respiratory system. James Case, Ph.D., presents an interesting study of functional upper airway obstruction. In this study, Dr. Case describes this unusual condition and the management approach utilized to resolve this disorder.

The medical literature is replete with case studies and group data regarding patients with acute and chronic organically based upper airway obstruction. The causal factors are numerous, and include obstruction from asthma, trauma, tumor, laryngeal paralysis, and following Teflon injection for treatment of laryngeal paralysis (Vincken et al., 1984; Chaten et al., 1991; Solomons and Livesay, 1990). Many of these cases of upper airway obstruction have compromised the airway sufficiently to require tracheostomy (Newlands and McKerrow, 1987).

Less commonly reported and understood is the phenomenon of **functional upper airway obstruction,** which often involves a significant laryngeal component. Many of these functional cases have also resulted in tracheostomy because no treatment was successful in eliminating the respiratory difficulty (Kellman and Leopold, 1982; Skinner and Bradley, 1989).

Christopher et al. (1983) reported on five patients who presented with functional disorders of the vocal folds that mimicked attacks of bronchial asthma. Laryngoscopy on these five patients confirmed that wheezing was the result of adduction of the true and false vocal cords throughout the respiratory cycle. This report followed the initial report by Rogers and Stell (1978), who described two similar cases. The first such case was of a 30-year-old woman with hoarseness, noisy breathing, and tightness in the throat. The second case was a 19-year-old nursing student with a 1-week history of cough, noisy breathing, and inspiratory stridor without hoarseness. The stridor was described as due to paradoxical vocal fold movement, which was functional. These vocal and upper airway functional obstructions were identified in the medical literature as a unique syndrome by Appelblatt and Baker (1981).

VOICE THERAPY FOR HOARSENESS AND STRIDOR

Several authors have commented that the laryngeal component of hoarseness and stridor can be helped by voice therapy. No documentation is present in the literature on specific techniques that might be helpful to such cases of functional upper airway obstruction to eliminate or reduce the vocal and laryngeal symptoms. The following case study outlines specific details of voice therapy management in a case of functional upper airway obstruction.

CASE STUDY: PATIENT X

Patient X, a 33-year-old woman, was seen January 3, 1991, at the Arizona State University Speech and Hearing Clinic for an evaluation of her voice and respiratory functions in speech. She was referred from the Mayo Clinic Scottsdale by her otolaryngologist, who described her condition as "functional upper airway obstruction." All vocal structures were within normal limits.

Patient X reported that shortly before Labor Day, 1990, she was admitted to the emergency room of her local hospital in Michigan because of respiratory difficulty. She was wheezing and experiencing some laryngeal stridor. Her voice was "raspy and harsh." According to the patient, the attending physician could see no obvious obstruction with endoscopic inspection. She was given oxygen support. She was later seen by a pulmonologist who did "deep bronchoscopy into the lower bronchial tree." She stated that "he could see no obvious obstruction until he began to withdraw the scope, at which time he saw a tracheal and laryngeal spasm."

In the next few days, several medications were provided in an attempt to eliminate the symptoms of wheezing, stridor, and hoarseness, including bronchodilators (Alupent and Ventolin), without improvement. Her physician did not offer any reasons for her difficulty but thought it might be related to nasal drainage, viral irritation, noxious gas inhalation, or allergic reaction. Patient X reported that "eventually it dissipated and went away."

In the 2nd week of December, 1990, patient X was driving behind a car with significant exhaust fumes, which triggered another spasm. She was again admitted to the emergency room and no cause was found for her symptoms, which were the same as the previous episode, nor was anything successful in treatment. These symptoms persisted and she was told to seek help at the Mayo Clinic. Because she had family in Arizona, she made an appointment to be seen by the pulmonary and otolaryngology departments at the Mayo Clinic in Scottsdale, who referred her to me. They were unable to find any organic reason for her symptoms and diagnosed "functional upper airway obstruction."

Patient X indicated that stress did not appear to be related to her symptoms. She had recently been married and went through the stressful stages of wedding planning without triggering any difficulty. She was also a student in respiratory therapy and often was involved in emergency treatments under stress and performed well without difficulty.

Presenting Symptoms and Treatment Processes

Patient X manifested a significant dysphonia. Her quiet breathing was labored and wheezy. When she was breathing quietly, no laryngeal stridor on inhalation was noted, but after talking for a few sentences, she would apparently get behind on her breathing and manifested some stridor. Figure 5–2 shows a broadband sonograph (Kay Elemetrics Digital 5500 Sonograph) of inhalatory stridor which occurred shortly after prolonging an /a/ sound. During the entire case history and early therapy moments, each breathing cycle manifested significant wheezing.

The patient's voice parameters would be described perceptually as significantly rough and breathy. Diplophonia was also inconsistently manifested. On a scale of perceptual severity, I would rate her dysphonia as a 6 on a 1 to 7 scale in which 7 is most severe. Figure 5–3 is a broadband sonograph of an /a/ prolongation, acoustic waveform, and power spectrum. The sonogram shows aperiodic glottal pulses, indistinct formants, and excessive noise in the upper frequencies. The waveform display manifests this aperiodicity clearly on this steady-state vowel.

Because of the roughness of patient X's voice, no attempt was made to elicit a habitual speaking pitch. I felt strongly that the vocal symptoms could be eliminated rather quickly and therefore spent most of this evaluation time in therapy to change her voice. Other than the baseline sonographic records, case history information, and video baseline and therapy recording, little standard documentation was obtained.

Twice during the case history, I noticed that the patient cleared her throat with a near-normal voice. She was not aware of the difference between her speaking dysphonia and the clear voice I heard as she cleared her throat. It was this throat-clearing voice that encouraged me to begin therapy to eliminate the symptoms rather than do an extensive voice evaluation with all its documentation. Also, I knew she was from out of town and I would not have long to make a difference.

Therapy

The next few minutes were spent in attempting to elicit normal voicing. Because she was overvalving during phonation, a hyperfunctional form of phonation, I approached normal voicing by having her produce a very

light and effortless grunt. After several attempts to obtain clear voicing with this light-grunt technique, without success, I asked her to clear her throat gently. After a few unsuccessful efforts, a very clear voice devoid of her dysphonic symptoms was heard. When she was asked to repeat the sound, inconsistent results were obtained. Some of her sounds were clear, others were dysphonic but not to the baseline degree. All the time I was working with these voice efforts, patient X continued her wheezing.

I felt her laryngeal structures and noticed considerable neck tension during quiet breathing and voicing efforts. The patient also stated that her neck was sore and hurt when I put any pressure on it. I explained that the soreness was likely from all the extra musculoskeletal tension involved in breathing and voice. I continued to ask her to produce the voice heard when she gently cleared her throat.

As these clear instances of voice occurred, I became increasingly concerned about the continued wheezing. I decided that this must be addressed soon in order to establish laryngeal relaxation during both biological functions of breathing as well as voice.

The next 15 minutes of therapy involved attention to her wheezing and breathing. The following language was used in therapy to achieve laryngeal relaxation for the elimination of her wheezing. It was a technique of body relaxation using the monologue as follows:

"I want to work on body relaxation. I want to teach you to control the tension in your body, particularly in your chest and neck area. While sitting as you are, I want you to close your eyes so you can concentrate on my suggestions. You will not fall asleep, but closing your eyes will help you to relax and focus.

"First, focus on the muscles around your eyes and in the area of your forehead. Completely relax those muscles. By concentrating on the muscles around your eyes entirely, you can better relax them. Make them completely limp and relaxed. No tension whatsoever. Now focus on the top (crown) of your head. Pretend you have a little point on the top of your head. Focus on it. Now sweep your mind from that point down over your head, over your forehead, over the back of your scalp. Completely relax the muscles of your head. Now sweep your mind over your face into your neck area. Move your head around very gently and then relax the muscles

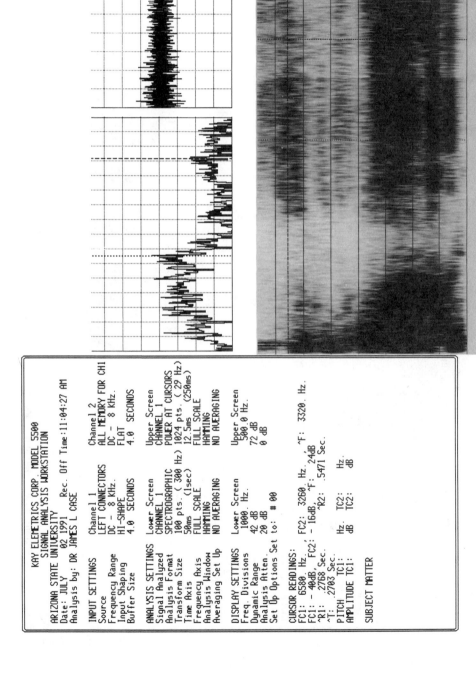

FIG 5–2.
Broad-band sonogram of inhalatory stridor.

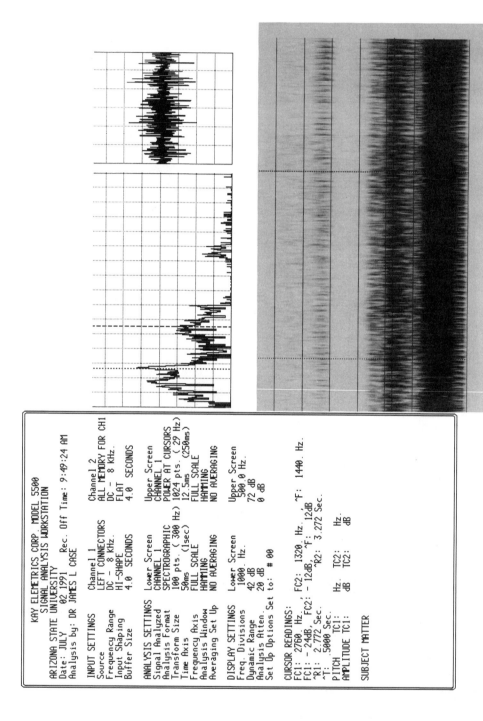

FIG 5–3.
Broad-band sonogram of /a/ prolongation, acoustic waveform, and power spectrum.

of your neck. Keep your head in an upright position, but otherwise completely relax your neck muscles. As you do this, let your breathing be deep and easy. Completely relaxed. Every part of your body must be completely relaxed."

As I continued this relaxation step of therapy, I noticed that the patient's breathing became quieter. After approximately 15 minutes of relaxation direction, her breathing was devoid of wheezing. I then asked her to open her eyes and just listen to me talk. I went on to explain that she was completely relaxed in the neck area and was not wheezing. She nodded that she noticed that. She then whispered lightly and said, "The soreness is gone."

I then asked her to maintain that feeling of relaxation, without wheezing, as she once again worked on producing effortless voice. She was able to do that well. Clear and consistent instances of voice were produced as she spoke the phrase, "uh hum."

After a few minutes of simple phrases, such as "uh hum," "one, two, three," and "I'm fine," were produced with consistent and clear phonation, I moved to more elaborate sentences and phrases, simple language such as counting from one to 20, naming the days of the week and months of the year, while constantly reminding her that her wheezing was absent and her voice was clear. I also constantly reminded her to remain relaxed and to keep the feeling of "effortless" voice production. I kept saying encouraging phrases, such as:

"Notice when you are producing voice this way, you can hardly feel anything happen in your neck and larynx effort . . . it is effortless. Your breathing is calm. Good voice production is not a vigorous process . . . it is an easy process. Don't overwork your speech structures. They are working fine with hardly any effort."

The patient had now been speaking and breathing normally for about 15 minutes. Next I wanted her to see that she could challenge her laryngeal system and still keep it working well. I said to her, "I want you to notice that you can take a quick inhalation and the system will work very well. You will not wheeze. Do it." She then took several quick inhalations without wheezing. I reinforced her action with verbal approval (I doubt that she really needed it, but old habits die hard). Then I wanted her

to realize that her new vocal control was not a delicate process, that she could yell, cough, clear her throat, speak softly, and speak loudly. The final important test came when I asked her to try to speak with the voice she had used for the past few months. She made a rough and approximate attempt to do it, but it was not the same. I felt that was fine that she could not duplicate her old voice. If she had been able to do it well, I would have told her that now she was completely in control of her voice, when it was good or bad, and should she feel that same constriction come on her again, which I did not expect to happen, she would know how to get out of it.

The next few minutes were spent in conversation centered on what had happened to her, why it was so easy to fix, and what the future meant. I also wanted others in her life to hear her voice so she would not feel any pressure returning to her family members in Arizona and Michigan. I had her make some telephone calls to those people as well as to her otolaryngologist. She then left and returned to Michigan. A follow-up telephone call revealed that her voice and breathing were stable. She was given an open-door policy to call or return anytime she had any questions or difficulty.

Figure 5–4 shows a broadband sonogram of patient X prolonging an /a/ sound after therapy voice. Her glottal pulses were normal, her formants were clear, the power spectrum is normal, and the acoustic waveform shows regular and periodic pulses. This is the objective documentation of what is clearly a successful therapy session lasting approximately 1.5 hours from the beginning of her evaluation to the successful resolution of her dysphonia stemming from functional upper airway obstruction. The entire session was videotaped except the short time I was working on relaxation, during which time I turned the camera off. I felt she might be more relaxed since her eyes were closed the entire time and she could not monitor what was being recorded.

Functional upper airway obstruction is a vocal and respiratory disorder that the speech-language pathologist must recognize. It would be easy to confuse with the more common disorders of organically based upper respiratory obstruction. When recognized and man-

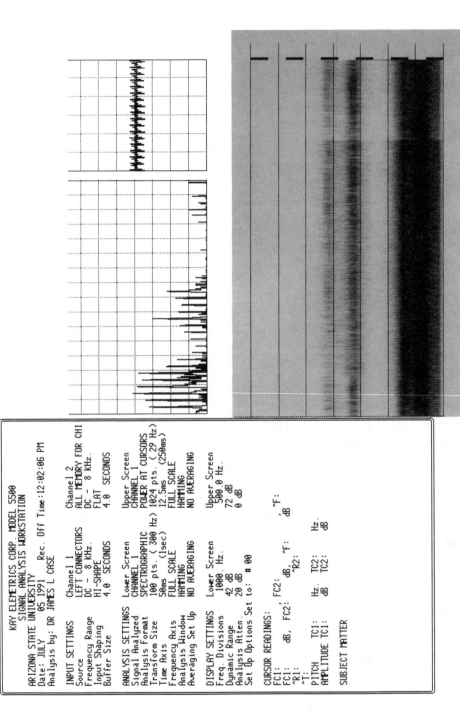

FIG 5-4.
Broad-band sonogram of /a/, posttherapy.

aged well, a relatively quick and easy resolution of this disorder can occur.

PSEUDO-ASTHMA

CASE STUDY: PATIENT Y

The final case study describes treatment of a patient with what was diagnosed as pseudo-asthma. Patient Y, a 48-year-old woman, was known personally to the author for 20 years. During this time she had exhibited significant allergic symptoms to airborne allergies, exhibiting watery eyes, nasal congestion, a dry hacking cough, and occasional wheezing, which had been diagnosed as asthma. The symptoms had become so common that they were mostly ignored by her friends in social situations.

I was therefore surprised to receive a referral for a laryngeal stroboscopic examination for patient Y from a well-known pulmonary specialist at a leading university medical school. Apparently in the past 6 months, her symptoms had worsened. She was experiencing shortness of breath, and the frequency of wheezing had significantly increased. She was using two different inhalers, antihistamines, antibiotics, and a nasal spray. She had recently coughed so violently that she lost consciousness. She therefore sought the opinion of the pulmonologist.

Results of very thorough pulmonary testing indicated a normal pulmonary system. Patient Y did not have an asthmatic condition. The wheezing was laryngeal. It was speculated that the patient's medications were drying the mucous membrane of the vocal folds and respiratory system, causing her to cough. The edema and dryness caused wheezing which further stimulated the cough reflex. Patient Y was caught in a vicious cycle.

Stroboscopic examination revealed significant tissue change of the vocal folds, with moderate edema and erythema noted. A sticky, stranding mucus was noted in copious amounts.

The pulmonary specialist suggested that, except for an antihistamine (Seldane), patient Y should discontinue the use of all other medications. In addition, she was placed on an oral hydration program to promote mucous membrane hydration, a behavior modification program for elimination of coughing and throat clearing (see Chapter 3) and vocal function exercises for improving the strength, balance, and flexibility of the laryngeal musculature (see Chapter 1).

Within 4 weeks, patient Y's coughing, throat clearing, and wheezing had been eliminated. Her vocal fold edema and erythema were significantly improved. It was very difficult for her to believe that after all the years of suffering with significant respiratory problems, most of the symptoms were functional and self-induced. The symptoms were actually exacerbated by the drying effects of the various medications, and by a continuation of the symptoms themselves.

In our clinic, we are often asked to evaluate the voices and vocal folds of individuals with chronic coughing, throat clearing, or both. When all medical testing proves negative, then functional therapy is often the treatment method of choice. When this is the case, the therapist must encourage the patient to "buy the program." Often, these patients, for years, have been convinced that they suffer from a medical problem. The therapist must gently introduce the **possibility** of a functional cause. Most patients in this circumstance are ready to try anything to gain relief from the symptoms. Functional therapy often works well and quickly as a means of offering this relief.

REFERENCES

Appleblatt NH, Baker SR: Functional upper airway obstruction: a new syndrome, *Arch Otolaryngol* 107:305–306, 1981.

Aronson AE: *Clinical voice disorders, an interdisciplinary approach*, New York, 1990, Thieme.

Aronson AE: *Clinical voice disorders, an interdisciplinary approach*, New York, 1980, Brian C. Decker.

Boone D, McFarlane S: *The voice and voice therapy*, Englewood Cliffs, N.J., 1988, Prentice-Hall, pp 122–184.

Boone D: Modification of the voices of deaf children, *Volta Rev* 68:686–694, 1966.

Chaten FC et al: Stridor: intracranial pathology causing postextubation vocal cord paralysis, *Pediatrics* 87:39–43, 1991.

Christopher KL et al: Vocal cord dysfunction presenting as asthma, *N Engl J Med* 308:1566–1570, 1983.

Colton R, Casper J: *Understanding voice problems: a physiological perspective for diagnosis and treatment,* Baltimore, 1990, Williams & Wilkins.

Froeschels E: Chewing method as therapy, *Arch Otolaryngol* 56:427–434, 1952.

Herrington-Hall BL et al: Description of laryngeal pathologies by age, sex and occupation in a treatment-seeking sample, *J Speech Hear Disord* 53:57–64, 1988.

Hollien H: On vocal registers, *J Phonetics* 2:25–43, 1982.

Jacobson E: *Modern treatment of tense patients,* Springfield, Ill, 1970, CC Thomas, pp 379–412.

Jacobson E: *Progressive relaxation,* ed 2, Chicago, 1938, University of Chicago Press.

Kellman RM, Leopold DA: Paradoxical vocal cord motion: an important cause of stridor, *Laryngoscope* 92:59–60, 1982.

Newlands WJ, McKerrow WS: Pediatric tracheostomy: fifty-seven operations on fifty-three children, *J Laryngol Otol* 101:929–935, 1987.

Rogers JH, Stell PM: Paradoxical movements of the vocal cords as a cause of stridor, *J Laryngol Otol* 92:157–158, 1978.

Skinner DW, Bradley PJ: Psychogenic stridor, *J Laryngol Otol* 103:383–385, 1989.

Solomons NB, Livesey JR: Acute upper airway obstruction following Teflon injections of a vocal cord: the value of nebulized adrenaline and a helium/oxygen mixture in its management, *J Laryngol Otol* 104:654–655, 1990.

Stemple JC: Clinical voice pathology, Columbus, Ohio, 1984, Merrill.

Stemple JC et al: Electromyographic biofeedback training with patients exhibiting a hyperfunctional voice disorder. *Laryngoscope* 90:471–475, 1980.

Vincken WG et al: Involvement of upper-airway muscles in extrapyramidal disorders, *N Engl J Med* 311:438–442, 1984.

Wilson DK: *Voice problem of children,* Baltimore, 1979, Williams & Wilkins.

Zaliouk A: Falsetto voice in deaf children, *Curr Probl Phoniatr Logop* 1:217–226, 1960.

CHAPTER 6

Management of Spasmodic Dysphonia

MANAGEMENT APPROACHES FOR

- Adductor spasmodic dysphonia
- Abductor spasmodic dysphonia.

MANAGEMENT STRATEGIES, INCLUDING

- Patient education
- Psychological support
- Tension reduction
- Pitch modification
- Loudness modification
- Inhalation phonation
- Recurrent laryngeal nerve resection
- Botulinum toxin injection
- Regulation of airflow
- Regulation of subglottic pressure.
- Unified Spasmodic Dysphonia Rating Scale (USDRS)

Imagine developing a condition so insidious that it causes loss of self-respect and confidence; a disorder so negative as to cause depression, reclusiveness, and thoughts of suicide; a condition that can ruin careers, marriages, and friendships. This disorder is spasmodic dysphonia.

Spasmodic or spastic dysphonia is a term that describes a family of strained, strangled voices. Perceptually, the voice symptoms are classified in two primary groups: adductor and abductor spasmodic dysphonia. Adductor spasmodic dysphonia, which appears to be the most

common, is characterized by strained, strangled phonation with occasional intermittent stoppages of voice. The severity may range from very mild intermittent symptoms to a very severe, persistent struggle to produce phonation. The abductor type is characterized by abductor vocal fold spasms causing sudden, intermittent explosions or escapes of air. Abductor spasms appear to occur most frequently on voiceless consonants.

Though the incidence of this disorder is thought to be relatively low, the extreme negative effects it tends to have on many individuals suffering with the disorder highlight the importance of appropriate professional care. Most researchers agree that the onset of spasmodic dysphonia is usually middle age and that the condition seems to occur equally in men and women (Aronson et al., 1968; Brodnitz, 1976). My own experience has been with patients with onset as young as 15 years. Some patients experience a rapid onset of symptoms, whereas others experience a gradual onset over many years.

The cause of spasmodic dysphonia has been debated for many years. Early descriptions linked the disorder to psychoneurosis (Aronson, 1990). Indeed, Aronson (1990) believes that one type of strained, strangled voice has a psychological cause and can be treated as a conversion aphonia or a disorder of musculoskeletal tension. An argument could be made that classifying these disorders as spasmodic dysphonia may not be appropriate. Others have advocated a neurologic origin (Aronson et al., 1968; Aminoff et al.; 1978; Blitzer et al., 1985). Blitzer et al. (1986) offered strong evidence that spasmodic dysphonia should be considered a focal dystonia specific to the larynx and similar to other dystonias such as blepharospasm and torticollis. Whether neurologically or psychologically based, the onset of spasmodic dysphonia is often associated with emotional stress and/or tension.

As the debate regarding etiology continues and theories are proved and disproved, patients continue to arrive in our practices seeking information and treatment. There appears to be fair agreement that, except for those patients Aronson (1990) classifies as spastic dysphonia of conversion reaction or spastic dysphonia or musculoskeletal tension reaction, symptom relief as a result of voice therapy or psychiatric treatment has been minimal at best. [One exception to this statement has been the anecdotal claims of Cooper (1990), which have not been independently verified.]

Until recently, most patients treated in our clinic have had the disorder for many years prior to actual diagnosis. They have sought treatments from many laryngologists, speech pathologists, psychologists, and psychiatrists. They have been prescribed various drugs and have gone through relaxation therapy, biofeedback, hypnosis, and acupuncture. One patient even sought the services of a faith healer. All patients were consistent in their frustrations over the lack of relief.

With the development of new methods of symptom relief and the subsequent professional reports and lay publicity, the diagnosis of spasmodic dysphonia appears to be occurring more rapidly. Until 1976, however, most patients with spasmodic dysphonia remained untreated, that is until Herbert Dedo (1976) suggested a fairly radical treatment for symptom relief. This treatment was to create a unilateral vocal fold paralysis. Dedo and Izdebski (1983b) reported that creation of the unilateral paralysis proved successful in relieving the adductor spasmodic dysphonia symptoms 4 years postoperatively in 90% of 306 patients. Dedo and Shipp (1980) reported that spasmodic dysphonia returned in 10% to 15% of their patients within 1 month to 2 years following recurrent laryngeal nerve (RLN)

resection. Aronson and DeSanto (1983) followed 38 patients and reported that 64% had worse voice quality after 3 years postoperatively.

As you can see, RLN resection as a procedure to relieve symptoms of adductor spasmodic dysphonia has stirred controversy. However the positive effect of the procedure for many individuals, especially when supported with voice therapy, cannot be denied.

A more recent medical treatment also involves creating a paretic or weakened vocal fold condition. This is accomplished by injecting botulinum-A toxin (Botox) into the thyroarytenoid muscle (for adductor spasmodic dysphonia) and the posterior cricoarytenoid muscle (for abductor), creating a temporary paresis of the muscles (Blitzer et al., 1988). The weakened muscles do not permit the spasms to occur, and thus the vocal symptoms are relieved.

FUNCTIONAL VOICE THERAPY FOR SPASMODIC DYSPHONIA

Some patients certainly do benefit from a direct symptom modification approach of voice therapy. Indeed, as a result of the physical struggle inherent in attempting to push the voice through the spasmodic occurrences, many patients develop secondary behaviors which make the voice quality worse than the baseline spasmodic condition. For example, patients develop extreme neck, shoulder, and thoracic tension; lowered pitch-to glottal fry phonation; monotonous phonatory patterns.

This first case study involves an individual who developed these secondary behaviors. The study describes functional voice therapy that subsequently improved the symptoms significantly, albeit without eliminating the spasms.

CASE STUDY: PATIENT Z

Patient Z, a 57-year-old high-school English and drama teacher, was referred to the Voice Center by the speech pathologist serving her school. Her history was typical of many individuals referred in the early 1980s. Though she had been symptomatic for 3 years, and had consulted three laryngologists and one speech pathologist, the diagnosis of spasmodic dysphonia had never been made or explained to her.

Patient Z had never married, and was extremely independent and outgoing. She had taught for 34 years, and stated that she "lived to teach." By the time of the initial evaluation she was extremely upset, confused, and full of self-doubt. She had independently sought the counsel of a psychologist who, unfortunately, was not familiar with spasmodic dysphonia and who supported the notion that the problem was "all in my head." In school she had developed lesson plans and techniques for which she could minimize her own speaking. She suffered with these teaching modifications; previously, she had been honored as an outstanding educator, and she was convinced that she had become less than effective in the classroom.

Away from school, this normally outgoing individual had withdrawn and for at least 18 months had lived a reclusive existence. She refused to see friends and totally avoided the telephone. Several weeks into our treatment she admitted to having had thoughts of suicide. The two things most dear to her, teaching and friendship, had been taken from her as a result of her voice disorder.

The role of the voice pathologist during the initial session was that of evaluator, to confirm the presence of spasmodic dysphonia; educator, to teach the patient what was known of the disorder; and treatment planner. Patient Z presented with adductor spasmodic dysphonia of moderate severity. Phonation was characterized by intermittent glottal stops and glottal fry phonation as well as a flat, monotonous inflection pattern. It was extremely evident from her physical appearance of neck and shoulder tension and facial expression that she was very tense, nervous, upset, and depressed.

The voice problem began 3 years prior to the examination, in the fall. It manifested as hoarseness which persisted following an upper respiratory infection. Much probing regarding other possible psycho-social issues yielded nothing related to the onset. When the hoarseness persisted for several weeks she sought the opinion of an otolaryngologist who prescribed antibiotics three times over a 4-month period

of time. As the symptoms worsened, hesitations began "shutting off" her voice, requiring her to force to speak. She reported that teaching was actually causing her to be physically fatigued because of the effort to speak. She was exhausted at the end of a school day. Some days her abdominal muscles would become sore from straining to produce voice. During the 2 subsequent years she sought the opinion of two more physicians, one of whom prescribed more medication, with the other recommending psychological counseling. A speech pathologist, new to patient Z's school, heard her speak and thought the patient presented with the symptoms of spasmodic dysphonia. She then suggested that the patient come to our center for evaluation. Desperate for help, she complied.

It was determined through examining voice quality characteristics, abilities, and inabilities, that she indeed had adductor spasmodic dysphonia. She demonstrated normal phonation when humming, singing, or when speaking in lilting accents. She loved to read aloud from the writings of the American dramatist Tennessee Williams because the higher-pitched rhythm of the U.S. southern dialect reduced her effort to talk and improved the voice quality. She could laugh normally and felt that her voice was "near-normal" when she talked to her cat. The patient also thought that her voice quality was improved following ingestion of wine. This lead her to try tranquilizers, which did not improve her voice quality.

Following identification of the problem, patient Z was given much information, as it was then understood, regarding spasmodic dysphonia. She was greatly relieved that she suffered with a "recognized" disorder and that the problem was not necessarily psychologically induced. (In retrospect, patient Z also had a very mild head tremor, which is not an unusual co-occurrence with spasmodic dysphonia.) The possibility of a nonspecific central nervous system disorder was discussed. The differences between vocal symptoms of organic tremor and spasmodic dysphonia were discussed because of the patient's observation of her likeness to a popular actor.

Treatment options were then discussed. As with many patients, patient Z was distressed to learn that treatments would produce only symptom relief and not cure the disorder. Recurrent laryngeal nerve resection (to be discussed in detail later in this chapter) was described. Functional voice therapy designed to eliminate secondary tension, inappropriate pitch, and inflection was discussed. The decision was made to try functional voice therapy.

It was interesting to note the change in patient Z's entire persona from the initial session to the second session. From a tense, depressed, and beaten individual arose an encouraged, determined, and resolute person. During the first session we identified the vocal tasks that she could perform well with fair consistency. These included:

- Humming and singing
- Speaking at a higher pitch
- Speaking with a slight Southern dialect.

It was discovered that she could speak well to her cat because she was speaking in a higher-pitched, "baby" voice.

She had developed the habit of producing voice with muscle tenseness, back-focus, and at low pitch, in an effort to overcome the intermittent spasms. Because the patient had no idea when the spasms would occur, she postured her phonatory/respiratory system in a manner that produced constant tension and pressure. The first step of therapy was to introduce relaxation techniques to demonstrate the degree of tension. Progressive relaxation as well as Electromyographic (EMG) biofeedback were successfully utilized for this purpose.

Phonatory tasks were then added to this newly relaxed state, utilizing a slightly higher pitch and phrases controlled by length. Though the spasms persisted, their frequency and severity were noted by the therapist and the patient to decrease. Phrases were lengthened, and the patient was trained to breathe more normally. A mid-tone focus permitting a slightly breathy phonation was deemed acceptable by the patient. In addition, she felt comfortable in slightly overinflecting her phonation patterns of pitch and loudness, which also seemed to decrease the severity of the spasms.

Longer phrases utilizing these techniques were then expanded into paragraph readings with and the without phrase or breath markers

and finally into practiced conversational speech. Because of patient Z's background in drama, the entire therapy program was completed within 6 weeks. The spasms, of course, persisted, but were heard only as occasional hesitations during speech production. The patient learned to permit her voice to flow through and past the hesitations without redeveloping the previous strained postures. Eliminating the secondary behaviors proved adequate for this patient. She did not then choose to pursue surgical intervention.

SYMPTOM MODIFICATION FOR ABDUCTOR SPASMODIC DYSPHONIA
Contributed by Susan Shulman, M.A.

In the following case study, Susan Shulman, M.A., suggests symptom modification for abductor spasmodic dysphonia through teaching patients to speak on inhalation.

CASE STUDY: PATIENT AA

Abductor spasmodic dysphonia, according to the professional literature, does not generally lend itself to benefit from voice therapy. However, the voice disorder can be minimized, for some patients, if the client is willing to learn the process of speaking on inhalation.

The following case study describes the voice disorder and treatment of patient AA, a 63-year-old hospital administrator in Dallas, Texas. At the onset of his voice disorder, he was in charge of the construction of a new hospital in addition to his regular responsibilities as hospital administrator. He reported numerous environmental, occupational, and personal pressures. In addition, he frequently and repeatedly gave extensive tours and lectures in a noisy shell of a building, without benefit of amplification.

The voice disorder was identified by an otolaryngologist as chronic hoarseness, beginning in 1976. The patient had a second otolaryngological examination with a diagnosis of vocal fold swelling and inflammation in October, 1977. He was placed on 2-weeks' voice rest. Afterward, he reported that the voice quality was "worse." The hoarseness persisted, and even worsened following a severe gum infection. In August 1978, patient AA was diagnosed by a neurologist as having amyotrophic lateral sclerosis (ALS). A visit to a laryngologist in California produced a diagnosis of myasthenia gravis and the recommendation of a thymectomy. In September 1978, the neurologist recommended psychiatric counseling. Subsequent psychiatric counseling did not prove beneficial in remediating the voice disorder. In May 1979, myasthenia gravis was eliminated as a diagnosis. In September 1979, patient AA was diagnosed with left ventricular heart aneurysm and a motor neuron disease involving the bulbar muscles. In March 1981, the neurologist again made the diagnosis of ALS, although he was "not sure of the nature." In 1983, the patient reported blepharospasms. A laryngological report described bowed vocal folds. He underwent a Teflon injection to the right vocal fold without improvement. In 1984, magnetic resonance imaging, revealed moderate cerebral atrophy without abnormality of the brain stem. A visit to his neurologist in 1987 resulted in a "retraction of the ALS diagnosis."

With his contacts as a hospital administrator, patient AA was always referred for "one more opinion." However, the variety of opinions and the depressing nature of some of the diagnoses made it difficult for him to be consistent in his voice therapy or even to be encouraged to feel that he could significantly improve his voice quality.

The voice therapy was sporadic, but basically concurrent with the patient's other medical treatment. Vocal rehabilitation began on Oct 12, 1977. It was November 1986 before he was able to speak fluently, utilizing the alternative communication of voicing on inhalation. Weaving a cycle of improvement, leveling off, regression, and progress into eventual success was not an easy task for the voice pathologist or the patient.

In 1977, the initial voice evaluation revealed marked hoarseness, excessive laryngeal-pharyngeal resonance with low pitch, breathiness, high expiratory effort, and poor breath support. The diagnosis was moderate dysphonia with laryngeal-pharyngeal resonance. At this time voicing was hoarse, but not aphonic. From 1977 to May of 1983, the patient experienced fluctuations in the voice from aphonia to intermittent breathy dysphonia. By 1980 the voice disorder was clearly recognized as abductor spasmodic dysphonia. Patient AA also experienced occasional periods of voicing that were "essentially clear and effortless." He was seen intermittently during this period but continued to maintain that he was going to "get his voice back," no matter how long it took! He was given medical retirement from his job as hospital administrator in 1982. Almost immediately after retirement, he opened a small shop that required constant talking to customers.

Every conceivable voice therapy technique was tried in the course of this complex case. It seemed that relaxation exercises and breathing exercises reduced the patient's overall body tension, but did not result in producing the consistency of voice that we hoped to obtain. He was able to produce more frequent voicing by guiding a voiceless whisper to a voiced sound. The vowel sounds provided excellent practice with this technique. However, the only constant was his ability to produce sound on inhalation. I had tried, without success, to convince this patient that he could talk on inhalation in the early stages of therapy. Immediately following the exercises on inhalation, he was able to produce voicing for short periods on exhalation, so he was reluctant to voice only on inhalation. Inhalation as an alternative voice technique was the only option available in May, 1983. Two months later, the patient was experiencing intermittent, but consistent, voicing on inhalation. However, it was difficult to convince him that he could speak effectively on inhalation. Sporadic therapy continued, with emphasis on inhalation and attempts at controlling exhalation. The roller-coaster effect of the therapy was its most consistent feature. He discontinued therapy until August 1985, at which time he was experiencing moderate to marked difficulty with laryngeal abductor spasms. He could voice easily on the inhale, but expiratory effort was excessive with poor results. At this time, 1985, he began using a small microphone while working in the store. He reported that the amplification resulted in less vocal strain and fatigue. He came intermittently for therapy and reported "good days and bad days."

Tongue posturing exercises were helpful as well as exercises to stimulate balanced movement of the tongue, lips, jaw, and relaxed velum. Exercises for central breath support were somewhat beneficial. By January 1986, the voice was presenting itself intermittently as he continued humming on inhale, but he was still unconvinced that he could talk on inhalation. The therapy program continued to push phonation on inhalation as the only alternative possible. He began to meet required percentages set in the therapy session for speaking on inhalation: 5% one week, 10% the next, and so forth. Health problems slowed the progress somewhat. In September 1986, patient AA was introduced to a fellow abductor spasmodic dysphonia patient who was using inhaled speech 95% to 100% of the time. This proved to be a turning point in patient AA's therapy. This meeting was inspirational and reinforced the fact that it was possible to achieve his goal. In October, he was utilizing inhaled speech approximately 30% of the time with increasing quality. Breath supprt and inability to speak more than a few words at a time presented the most difficult obstacles. By November 4, he reported feeling that he was "50% of the way" as his breath improved and the overall quality became clearer with a more natural tone. On November 18, 1986, progress notes included his statement that "I'm 90% to 100% there."

Patient AA has been seen in my office once each year since 1986. In 1989, he had cancer surgery and a heart attack. He retired from his business and consequently used his voice less. The quality became "weaker," and it was more of an effort to talk. I recommended that he increase the voice exercises and use his voice on a regular basis. In June 1990, he reported that he had to do the voice exercises consistently to get optimum voice. Also, he found that regular physical exercise contributed to improved vocal quality with less effort.

At present (June 1991), patient AA continues to have other health problems, such as back trouble, which adversely effect his voice control. However, he knows exactly which exercises to do so he can recover vocal function. He does have to do his vocal exercises on a regular basis to help him phonate as easily as possible and maintain dependable, consistent voice.

The intermittent maintenance sessions reflect overall stabilization of the voice with some spontaneous voicing on exhalation as well as inhalation, 5 years after he began speaking on inhalation.

Initially, my rationale for utilizing inhalation techniques came from working with patients with ventricular dysphonia. It seemed reasonable that similar hyperfunctional compensatory techniques would be present in patients with spasmodic dysphonia as well. False vocal fold swelling and increased muscle tension are obviously factors with spasmodic dysphonia. Therefore, voicing on inhalation should relax the laryngeal musculature while strengthening true vocal fold function at the same time. I feel that voicing on inhalation can help accomplish the following goals: enhanced relaxation of the extrinsic neck musculature, relaxed tongue posturing, reduced jaw tension, and elimination of clavicular breathing patterns, while at the same time bringing the vocal folds together easily and without spasm. Depending on the severity of the voice problems, needs, and the motivation of the client, the technique can be used either as a relaxation technique or as an alternate means of communication. There is no question that this speech varies significantly from normal voice; however, the technique does provide a voice. For some patients this is a welcome improvement. During the evaluation, a voice that is stronger or clearer on inhalation than on exhalation provides a good prognostic sign that inhalation exercises will be helpful.

Inhalation techniques are also extremely powerful for working with a variety of voice disorders, including vocal fold paralysis, postoperative aphonia, and conversion aphonia. This procedure provides almost immediate success at voicing, which is frequently a strong motivator.

The procedures that I followed for working with the inhalation techniques for patient AA are the same procedures I utilize with any patient I feel may benefit from this technique. It is important to provide a thorough explanation about voicing on inhalation. Provide pictures of the vocal folds (video tapes if possible), explaining the length of the vocal folds, the action of the vocal fold muscles, and a brief explanation of the false vocal folds.

Show the patient how a full, silent inhalation lowers the larynx, which helps to speak without strain. Introduce the patient to the concept that the inspiratory muscles contract throughout inspiration and should activate the first part of the expiratory phase.

Demonstrate "donkey breathing." It may feel or sound silly, but it works to relax the tension in the vocal fold muscles. Be sure that the inhalation is supported abdominally and not with a shallow clavicular breath. If the patient complains about dryness or fatigue, the breath is too shallow. Try to explain the feeling of openness in the back of the throat as you produce the sound.

As your patient produces E on inhale (singly then repetitively), listen for a high-pitch, somewhat nasal sound that is produced with an open throat. Repeat, repeat, repeat! Next, say E on inhale followed by numbers all produced on inhalation. Once your patient has achieved this step (it could vary from one to two sessions or more) progress to attempting to match the sound on exhalation without strain. The ability to produce effortless sound on exhalation is the key to the next stage of therapy.

This point in therapy usually determines whether your patient needs to continue relaxation and speaking on inhalation only, or whether inhalation will be primarily used as a relaxation technique for speaking on exhalation with reduced strain. For most patients, it is a relaxation technique.

If the patient continues speaking on inhalation only, you simply have him or her practice phonating for longer periods on an "in" breath. Gradually, and with great perseverance, patients can speak longer phrases on inhalation. Breath support will not flow, nor will the patient's voice sound like "I used to sound"; but the patient will be able to speak. Utilize graphs and charts to monitor progress and to increase the percentage of time spent speaking on inhalation. In combination with other procedures, charting of behaviors can be a very effective therapy tool.

Voicing on inhalation is a powerful therapy technique for selected cases. The complexity of the specific case presented was offset by the determination of the patient. The array of physicians involved and the variety of diagnoses had a significant effect on the commitment of the patient to voice therapy. Imagine yourself diagnosed by one physician as having myasthenia gravis, with recommended surgery; another doctor says you're crazy; then a third says you have ALS. Then you begin to understand how difficult it was for patient AA to believe that his breathing could help him recover his voice. His achievement is truly remarkable and was characterized by progress, setbacks, progress, regression, and finally stabilization of progress to satisfactory voicing. Voicing on inhalation as an alternate means of communication was a viable option for this patient, and he has benefitted significantly from being receptive to exercising that option.

SURGICAL/MEDICAL TREATMENT FOR SPASMODIC DYSPHONIA

Contributed by Krzysztof Izdebski, Ph.D.

An individual highly involved in the original and continuing research related to recurrent laryngeal nerve section as a treatment for spasmodic dysphonia is Krzysztof Izdebski, Ph.D. Dr. Izdebski presents a detailed description of the current surgical/medical/voice therapy treatments utilized for adductor spasmodic dysphonia. These treatments include nerve section and injection of botulinum toxin. Dr. Izdebski is firm in his belief of the importance of preoperative and postoperative voice therapy with the surgically/medically treated patients. Indeed, voice therapy may be the primary determining factor for the success or failure of these treatments.

Background

Voice therapy for adductor spasmodic dysphonia (ADD/SD) is outlined and discussed here with respect to two patient populations. The first group comprises individuals who elected unilateral recurrent laryngeal nerve (RLN) resection as a form of primary treatment (Dedo, 1976; Dedo and Shipp, 1980). The second group, comprises patients who underwent intramuscular injection of botulinum-A toxin (Botox) (Blitzer et al., 1986; Ludlow et al., 1988). The surgical approach is intended to cause complete and permanent unilateral true vocal fold (TVF) paralysis, while the pharmacologic approach (Botox) causes temporary paralysis/paresis of selected intrinsic laryngeal muscle(s). Both treatment techniques are nonetheless symptomatic, leaving the basic disorder intact. Both techniques result in disruption of laryngeal sensory motor flow, reduction of vocal fold adductory collision force and glottic contact area, as well as in alterations in ways subglottic air pressures (Ps) are generated (Izdebski, 1991). These components are thought to be essential in generation of the primary symptom of ADD/SD, the so-called strained-strangled or overpressured voice (Izdebski and Dedo, 1981; Izdebski, 1984). Therefore, initiating voice therapy in surgically or pharmacologically treated ADD/SD patients necessitates a thorough understanding of treatment techniques and their immediate and long-term consequences on laryngeal anatomy and phonatory physiology. This knowledge is of utmost importance not only to the understanding of the mechanisms responsible for symptom relief, but also with regard to post-treatment voice therapy planning, maintenance of asymptomatic phonation and in explaining or treating symptom recurrence (Izdebski, 1991; Aronson and DeSanto, 1983)

Recurrent Laryngeal Nerve Resection

Recurrent laryngeal nerve resection is performed on an inpatient basis with the patient being admitted to the hospital the day before surgery. Surgery is carried out under general anesthesia. The patient is intubated with an endotracheal tube, the neck is sterilized and draped, and a horizontal incision of approximately 40 mm is created (usually within the natural crease or fold of the neck), approximately 20 mm below the inferior margin of the cricoid cartilage or just above the manubrial notch. After carrying the resection to the left side of the trachea, and inferiorly to the thyroid gland, US retractors are used to move the gland laterally. Careful tissue dissection toward the anterior surface of the esophagus then continues, to locate the main trunk of the RLN, which is usually found 10 to 20 mm lateral to the tracheoesophageal groove. At times, it may be necessary to dissect the thyroid isthmus and to

trace the RLN toward the cricothyroid joint. Strap muscles are not sacrificed.

Following RLN identification, the nerve is stimulated with minimal electrical current, and the movement of the ipsilateral TVF is observed by direct laryngoscopy. Next, a 20- to 30-mm segment of the RLN is resectioned and removed, and a silk ligature is tied around its lower stump in an attempt to prevent regrowth. The operated site is then closed with plastic surgery techniques (using both subcutaneous and subcuticular sutures), and a small drain may be left in place. After the patient is extubated, awakened, and taken to the recovery room, the result of surgery on voice quality (relief from overpressure) can be heard immediately. Ordinarily, the patient is discharged from the hospital on the 1st or 2nd day after surgery, undergoes routine postoperative check-ups for wound infections, and begins counseling and postoperative voice therapy as soon as possible. Except in rare cases the surgical procedure itself (intubation) does not cause postoperative complications that may adversely influence the postoperative voice.

Consequences of Recurrent Laryngeal Nerve Surgery

Recurrent laryngeal nerve resectioning results in unilateral TVF paralysis ipsilaterally to the resection side. The position of the paralyzed vocal fold may be variable. RLN resectioning also causes abrupt disruption of unilateral sensory-motor flow, bilateral reduction of TVF adductory and collision forces, bilateral reduction in TVF contact area, decrease of Ps and increase of air flow (Izdebski, 1991; Izdebski, 1984; Shipp et al., 1985; Shipp et al., 1988). Denervation directly affects the working of four of the five intrinsic laryngeal muscles on the operated side that are responsible for adductory/abductory movements and phonatory adjustments of the TVFs. The muscles affected are the (1) thyroarytenoid (TA, the main body of the TVF and the main phonatory tensor), (2) posterior cricoarytenoid (the main abductor of the TVF), (3) interarytenoid (the main adductory muscle responsible for posterior closure and positioning and stabilizing of the vocal folds in midline), and (4) lateral cricoarytenoid (also the adductor responsible for stabilizing and stiffening of the adducted TVF).

The cricothyroid (CT) muscle, a primary vocal pitch elevator, remains unaffected because it is innervated by the extrinsic branch of the superior laryngeal nerve. All of the intrinsic laryngeal muscles contralateral to the RLN section remain unaffected because they are innervated by the opposite RLN. The paralysis may, however, affect indirectly (on a long-term basis) the phonatory workings of the intrinsic laryngeal muscles on the opposite side. Also, all extrinsic laryngeal muscles remain unaffected bilaterally; hence, the vertical larynx positioning, which plays an important role in voice and swallowing control (Shipp and Izdebski, 1975; Logemann, 1988), remains intact. This retained ability of laryngeal movement is useful therapeutically.

Postoperative Glottic Shape, Activity, and Relation to Voice Qualities

As a consequence of RLN sectioning, one side of the glottis (usually the left) is no longer mobile. The immediate postparalytic position of the TVF can be anywhere from the midline to a widely abducted placement (lateralization away from the midline), hence influencing the degree of postoperative breathiness, aperiodicity, and diplophonia (Thumfart, 1988). The exact postresection TVF positioning cannot be predicted accurately even with a preoperative xylocaine test (temporary RLN chemical block); hence, postoperative voice quality cannot be predicted accurately (Izdebski et al., 1979; Izdebski and Dedo, 1980). Because denervated muscular tissue is subject to atrophy, fiber loss, thinning, and other factors, (such as laryngeal shape, size, gravity, age, sex, and motions of the nonparalyzed contralateral vocal fold), the ultimate long-term position of the paralyzed TVF may change significantly over time from its immediate postoperative location. This in turn will profoundly influence the resultant voice quality. The critical time frame for this process is approximately 5 to 9 months, but repositioning may occur at times as late as 18 to 24 months (Faaboreg-Andersen, 1964). Therefore, in some cases postoperative

voice therapy may be lengthy and may require up to 9 or 12 months or longer.

Because symptoms are eliminated as long as the minimal glottic gap is preserved, it is of utmost importance to aim treatment at preserving positioning of the paralyzed TVF in such a way that the ultimate long-term post-paralytic fixation of the TVF will be somewhat between almost-median and semi-paramedian position. A plus or minus 1- to 1.5-mm glottic gap is thought to be ideal because it produces good phonatory voice with minimal breathiness or other symptoms. Therefore, voice therapy must be organized in such a fashion as to prevent undesirable and disadvantageous repositioning of the TVF on a long-term basis, and yet it must promote phonatory closure to achieve functional voice. Improper therapy ("pushing" voice exercises) leading to disadvantageous repositioning of the paralyzed vocal fold will have negative consequences on voice. It will result in either persistent breathiness if the paralyzed TVF remains too lateral to the midline, or worse, it will cause recurrence of spasticity if the paralyzed TVF is forced too close to the midline (Dedo and Izdebski, 1983a).

Acoustic Consequences of RLN Surgery

The immediate acoustic consequence of RLN surgery is the elimination of overpressured voice, and replacement of this voice quality with various degrees of breathy to normative voice (Izdebski, 1984). To understand fully the acoustic consequences of RLN surgery on postoperative voice quality and to design voice therapy properly, three main vocal qualities must be considered: overpressure, breathiness, and aperiodicity. Properly assessing the presence of these three voice qualities in the postoperative voice is crucial in interpreting the ongoing postoperative voice changes, as being due to (1) intrinsic elements (caused by expected changes in postoperative anatomy, such as atrophy, or vibratory asymmetry of the TVFs), (2) extrinsic factors (such as acoustic changes due to proper or improper voice therapy), (3) combined effects, and (4) compensatory approximation of the glottis. Final acoustic parameters therefore may not be reached before a 5- to 9-month postoperative interval, and need to be understood, evaluated, explained, and when needed, treated appropriately.

Overpressure

Overpressure is the main characteristic of ADD/SD (Izdebski and Dedo, 1981; Izdebski, 1984). This quality is understood as resulting from an increased vocal fold contact area, prolonged closed portion of the glottic cycle, increased collision force, decreased air flow, and elevated Ps (Izdebski, 1991; Izdebski and Dedo, 1981; Izdebski, 1984; Shipp et al., 1988). The degree of overpressure present in a voice sample reflects the severity of symptoms and is dependent on the interplay between those factors and compensatory behavior. Overpressure therefore, connotes increased (overadducted) midline contact of both TVFs and should never be present in the immediate postoperative period if the RLN was sectioned successfully.

Breathiness

Breathiness is an acoustic consequence of freely escaping air through a nonadducted and/or nonvibrating glottis (Izdebski, 1984). The magnitude of breathiness may be determined by the degree of unapproximated distance between the mobile and nonmobile TVF, Ps, and airflow (Faaboreg-Andersen, 1964; Zemlin, 1981). In addition, an unapproximated glottis contributes greatly to reduced vocal loudness and to decreased ability to vary pitch, the other major characteristics of post-RLN resection voice.

Breathiness is most prevalent in the immediate postoperative state, but when it persists on a long-term basis, breathiness must be treated accordingly. When voice therapy treatment fails to reduce excessive breathiness, augmentation of the paralyzed vocal fold by means of injection (usually with Teflon) is carried out (Dedo, 1976; Dedo and Izdebski, 1981). This, however, should not be undertaken earlier than 9 months postoperatively. In both treatment approaches, utmost care must be executed because aggressive treatment will bring back ADD/SD symptoms (Dedo and Behlau, 1991; Dedo and Izdebski, 1983a).

Postoperatively, ADD/SD patients— although technically now representing a case of TVF paralysis—must not be treated with voice therapy techniques that are used for treatment of classic idiopathic or iatrogenic TVF paralysis. It is therefore important to underscore again that the breathiness (unless excessive) should not be worked on directly at all. Mild breathiness is modifiable by working on other aspects of postoperative voice, particularly by eradicating aperiodicity and developing pitch flexibility. Also, as strange as it may sound, some degree of controlled breathiness is desirable in the postoperative voice to preserve long-term asymptomatic voice. Therefore, some patients need to be taught actually how to be "breathy," or how to preserve mild breathiness. Remember that presence of breathiness signifies, not-a-midline-positioning of the paralyzed TVF, the most crucial parameter in preventing recurrence of overpressure.

Weak Voice

Reduction of vocal loudness is a chief complaint of the patient who suffers from prolonged breathiness. Obviously, the classic therapeutic approach used to treat paralyzed TVF immediately comes to mind. The temptation to use this approach must however be tempered, because introducing classic exercises for paralyzed vocal folds to improve loudness may have deleterious effects on symptom recurrence. Classic "pushing" techniques, although effective for idiopathic or other causes of unilateral vocal fold paralysis, are counterproductive in postoperative ADD/SD, because maneuvers designed to force adduction of the TVFs will trigger the critical physiologic conditions that are primarily responsible for symptom occurrence. Pushing techniques may also promote ventricular approximation, and ventricular approximation is an undesirable consequence of voice therapy (Izdebski, 1990; Von Doersten et al., 1991). Half-swallow-"boom" technique, head rotation, or flexion are more beneficial (McFarlane and Boone, 1988), as are those techniques described elsewhere, designed specifically with regard to ADD SD (Dedo and Shipp, 1980).

Aperiodicity

Aperiodicity primarily reflects asymmetrical vibratory patterns of the vocal folds postoperatively (Shipp et al., 1985). Aperiodicity appears to be a combination of asymmetry between paralyzed and nonparalyzed vocal folds and of chaotic vibration within the paralyzed TVF itself. The last is a consequence of denervation, which allows for continuous vibration of the mucosa, however without direct ability to make proper mucosal adjustments by means of muscle contractions. Aperiodicity typically becomes more predominant during production of low and loud voice fundamental frequencies. This is because the asymmetry of the biomechanics is more pronounced here and the length-tension forces are most reduced at these voice levels. Again, as with breathiness, aperiodicity reflects idiosyncratic characteristics and will change over time.

Vibratory asymmetry may be reduced by activation of the CT muscle (elevation of vocal pitch), which helps to bring the paralyzed TVF toward the midline as it elongates, hence reducing its internal slack. This increases chances for proper aerodynamics, resulting in turn in decreases in vibratory asymmetry between the paralyzed and nonparalyzed TVFs. Therapy is considered successful only when it achieves improved vibratory symmetry. Improvement usually requires substantial increases in speaking vocal pitch (at least in the early therapy stage), with patients resenting this maneuvering on the grounds of improper, unnatural, and unaccustomed vocal levels and improper vocal image for their age and sex. They may simply "hate" the high breathy voice, and refuse to participate in acquisition of these skills. Careful maneuvering between voice therapy, psycho-acoustic discrimination, and psychotherapy is often needed. Therefore, a thorough understanding of diverse therapy principles is crucial.

Other Voice Qualities

In addition to the foregoing postoperative voice characteristics, unilateral paralysis causes other acoustic changes. These are present to lesser degrees and include diplophonia, vocal fry, pitch breaks, and tremor.

Diplophonia. — Diplophonia is closely aligned with the quality of aperiodicity. Diplophonia occurs when the vocal fold vibrates in such a manner that two or more strong voice fundamentals are observed simultaneously. This quality is rare but, when present, is more prevalent in men than in women, probably because vocal fold characteristics in men allow greater intravocal fold variability. Therapy is aimed at eliminating one of the fundamentals, preferably the lower.

Monotonous Voice. — A large percent of operated patients will also demonstrate a decreased ability to vary voice fundamental frequency in speech, rendering their output monotonous. This usually occurs in patients with minor breathiness and aperiodicity. There is no reason for such voice production postoperatively because of postoperative anatomy. This monotonous production is understood as persisting from the preoperative time, representing preoperative compensation voice. Voice therapy aimed at elimination of monotonicity is very successful, and usually requires only a couple of sessions.

Vocal Fry. — Vocal fry refers to voice quality produced in the lowest vocal register. It is difficult to specify precisely the postoperative vocal fry mechanism in these patients. This voice quality seems to be accomplished by inappropriate respiratory mechanics, in combination with postoperative anatomic changes at the glottic level. Should vocal fry be encountered, it is recommended to abandon working on the voice quality itself, and instead to promote therapy reinforcing respiratory mechanics, specifically avoiding talking on extremely low or extremely high lung volumes. Working on achieving more breathy phonatory states is also indicated.

At this time, it may be important to note that although faulty respiration itself is not considered to be a part of preoperative ADD/SD symptoms, operated patients may continue to show respiratory patterns similar to their premorbid conditions. These involve excessive breath holding, overinflation, and so on. These respiratory issues should be addressed early in therapeutic procedures. To promote successful speech production, respiratory biomechanics must be brought back to normal patterns as soon as possible.

Tremor. — True vocal tremor may accompany ADD/SD symptoms in some cases. If tremor is present preoperatively, it will persist postoperatively, but with reduced magnitude (Izdebski and Dedo, 1981; Dedo and Izdebski, 1983; Dedo and Izdebski, 1983b; Aronson and DeSanto, 1983; Izdebski, Shipp, and Dedo, 1979; Izdebski and Dedo, 1980). Exact mechanisms of vocal tremor generation is unknown, but tremor is assumed to differ significantly from that of ADD/SD voice (Aminoff et al., 1978; Ludlow et al., 1986; Izdebski and Dedo, 1979). While overpressure is phonotopically organized (Izdebski, 1991), tremor affects indiscriminately voice intensity and frequency, whisper, and all other pseudo-phonatory or vegetative tasks (Faaboreg-Andersen, 1964). Tremor may also involve periodic oscillations of the entire vocal tract, including both vocal folds, palate, supraglottic larynx, oropharynx, and tongue — affecting overall speech articulation. The respiratory system may also be involved. Therapeutic treatment of preoperative or postoperative phonatory tremor is extremely difficult, and success is at best minimal. Proper treatment utilizes simultaneous increases of muscle loads, changes in expiratory airflow, and altering body positioning. Physiologically, this is a difficult concept, which in addition is very difficult to execute by elderly patients, who unfortunately are typically affected by tremor (Findley and Koller, 1987; Weiner and Lang, 1989).

Steps in Adductor Spasmodic Dysphonia Voice Therapy

Therapy for ADD/SD begins before RLN surgery. In general, taking on treatment of these patients requires a working knowledge of at least the following therapy models: motor-learning, classical conditioning, psychotherapy, counseling, and self-assessment. In addition, a thorough knowledge of phonatory physiology and biomechanics, including respiratory physiology, knowledge of instrumentation, and biofeedback principles is required. The entire process involves numerous steps,

which are outlined later. The therapy outline, planning, need, and benefits, are highly variable from patient to patient and need to be tailored individually.

Therapy will fail with a "cookbook" approach. At times, therapy may be only short but concentrated (one to three sessions of 2 to 3 hours' length). In other cases, it may be very lengthy (weekly or biweekly sessions over a 6- to 12-month period). Additional literature reports up to 3 years active postoperative treatment in some cases to establish habitually normative voice (Iwamura, 1980). With some patients, concentrated daily treatments up to 4 hours in length are more effective than hourly sessions spread over time. Such concentrated "en bloc" therapy is also needed with some outpatients who come from a distance. Whatever the case, in the initial postoperative period, therapy must be continued by the patients themselves daily on a "home-bound basis" after leaving the office. The overall therapy plan is best when the plan is designed following completion of phonatory function studies.

Step I (Preoperative)

The first step of therapy includes preoperative involvement with the patient, including voice evaluation, counseling, and introduction to postoperative therapy principles. Preoperative voice evaluation is crucial to postoperative treatment planning. Evaluation comprises phonatory function studies including laryngovideostroboscopy, electroglotography, acoustics, and aerodynamics (Hirano, 1981; Izdebski et al., 1990). These studies should be conducted before and after chemical RLN blocking (Izdebski and Dedo, 1980), if such a testing is performed.

Counseling reflects concern that RLN surgery does not cure the disorder, and that surgery does not guarantee "normal voice"; therefore, the principles of RLN section and their consequences on phonation must be discussed in detail, as outlined earlier. Specifically, the importance of maintenance of asymptomatic voice, and postoperative recurrence of symptoms cannot be overemphasized. Postoperative therapy and long-term follow-up may also be planned at this preoperative counseling session.

Step 2 (Preoperative)

The second step of therapy involves visiting the patient in the hospital on the eve of surgery. This visit is very important from many points of view. First, it provides an opportunity to answer last-minute questions. These questions usually regard postoperative care, specifically involving anticipated difficulties with phonation, swallowing, and coughing. At this time it should be explained to the patient again that there will be a delay in coughing reflexes and possible choking may occur for a few days following surgery. Finally, it is important to stress again that postoperative voice quality may be very distorted or that the voice may be totally aphonic. The patient must be prepared one more time for the many postoperative "vocal surprises," which may include an almost normal voice.

Step 3 (Postoperative)

The third step of therapy involves visiting the patient in the recovery room, and in the hospital setting for the first 1 to 2 postoperative days prior to his/her discharge from the hospital. If postoperative choking occurs, modified dysphagia therapy for intake of liquids or a soft mechanical diet is applied. Also, interaction between the patient and family is of utmost importance at this time. The immediate postoperative period is also time for critical review of the new voice quality, and for outlining the remaining treatment plan.

Step 4 (Postoperative)

Step four involves actual (active) voice therapy, which starts as soon as possible after the patient is discharged from the hospital. Preoperatively acquired therapy skills and understanding of phonatory biomechanics by the patient becomes very helpful at this time. Repetition of the phonatory function studies is important, because these measures are fundamental to proper therapy design and planning. These measures show in detail the patient's postoperative glottic configuration and biomechanics. Anticipated duration of treatment will vary depending on the patient and his or her postoperative glottic configuration and acoustic characteristics based on this examination.

No matter the frequency or duration, treatment must be focused, accurate, and productive. The actual length of treatment will obviously depend on the immediate postoperative voice quality, postoperative architecture and mobility of the glottis, and the clinician's ability to predict the recovery pattern and understand the patient's needs overall.

General Guidelines of Voice Therapy for RLN Sections

As stated earlier, voice therapy begins as soon as possible following RLN section. On the first day after surgery, it is important to have the patient sustain a simple vowel (of the patient's own choice) at the most comfortable effort level and for the maximum phonation time. Maximum phonation time is measured against total lung volume (or constant respiratory setting) and Fo/dB targets. Maximum speaking time is also established. This refers to the number of words (voiced segments only) the patient is able to produce in one comfortable breath. Next, the patient produces a glissando, changing voice frequency from the lowest to the highest, and from the highest to the lowest using most comfortable intensity and effort levels. Vocal range and relative SPLs should be noted. Utilization of the Visi-Pitch system (Kay Elemetrics), sound pressure level (SPL) meters, electroglottograph (EGG) and/or air flow signals are very useful for these procedures. Laryngovideostroboscopy is also conducted and configuration of the glottis at various voice frequency and intensity levels are studied.

Typically, in the immediate postoperative period, almost all patients are able to produce rather symptom-free and clear high-frequency phonation, but will have difficulty descending to lower pitches. This difficulty is particularly noted through the mid-portion of the voice frequency range. Voicing may, however, return at the lowest frequencies, especially if the patient can produce the upward and downward glissando with relatively few breaks or moments of aphonia. A smooth glissando is a good indication of vocal fold contact area, and signifies a relatively narrow glottic gap.

In some cases the patient's voice may sound quite good. However, excellent voice quality now may signify vocal troubles later. When the patient produces no phonatory voice and is able to produce only very breathy or hissy phonation, it simply signifies a very wide positioning of the paralyzed vocal fold. This wide positioning should not be prognosticated as indicative of persistent breathiness over time. Laryngeal framework manipulation is useful here and usually is a good predictor of how much pitch and loudness control is missing.

As previously stated, when patients are experiencing persistent breathiness, and desperately want a loud voice, they must not be subjected to "pushing" exercises. Weak voice is worked on indirectly by either improving other voice quality characteristics or by manipulating the external environment to minimize the negative effects of the soft voice. For the latter, suggestions are often drawn from oral rehabilitation techniques. Such lists should include suggestions for the families as well. If the patient is planning to return to work as soon as possible after surgery, but continues to have a breathy voice and needs to communicate with groups, a portable amplifier should be arranged and its use strongly advocated. Unfortunately most of these units are of poor design, causing poor voice transmission and annoying feedback problems. With the help of a good electronic technician, these units can be easily modified. The best units are wireless systems used by street singers, such as Mouse, because they allow a hands-free operation, good sound, and portability. These are however expensive.

It is of primary importance to establish a new pitch level for the patient as soon as possible. Normally, this would be established on the first day after surgery but because of a bizarre combination of voices which may occur, and poor patient control over phonation, they are only encouraged to search for the most comfortable voice level on the first day. It is also important to push their voices upward so that they have a lot of space to fall down. Again, this fits the postoperative patterns because the lower frequencies of the voice may be lost postoperatively at this stage, and forcing or fighting the voice needs to be eliminated as much as possible.

Working on higher voice frequency also equalizes the nuisance of aperiodicity perceived as "squeakiness" by patients. There are two factors to this phenomenon: (1) "squeaki-

ness" often reflects uncontrollability of the glottic adjustments; and (2) it reflects the fact that voice is produced with relative ease and that it is a totally different voice from the one established by many years of fighting overpressure. Hence, working on elevated pitches will improve periodic vibration of vocal folds bilaterally and will decrease "squeakiness." It may be recalled that after surgery the patient has four out of five muscles paralyzed on one side. Adjustments of the folds can be produced by the nonparalyzed vocal fold on the opposite side by bilaterally working the cricothyroid muscles, by the strap muscles, and by vertical larynx positioning. Again, vocal fold adjustment lends itself well to utilization of higher voice fundamental frequencies rather than the low fundamental frequencies. Vertical larynx positioning can be of help by utilizing contraction of the nonaffected extrinsic laryngeal muscles that are responsible for laryngeal descent and laryngeal elevation.

To reduce aperiodicity of vocal fold vibration, it is mandatory that Ps be regulated. It is beneficial at this stage to use as low as possible Ps because higher Ps would necessitate overadduction of the glottis. Also, lower Ps necessitates less and easier vocal adjustments and regulations for a more periodic vibration. Therefore, immediate postoperative voice therapy is aimed at (1) producing as good as possible a high-frequency voice, (2) gradually lowering the frequency, (3) observing the levels at which aperiodicity or breathiness become most prominent, and (4) then pitching the voice upward again. You will find that when the patient decreases Ps and utilizes cricothyroid and extrinsic laryngeal muscles, he or she will be successful at producing an easy phonation, bringing pitch down just above the disturbing aperiodic level.

At this initial stage, sustained phonation is worked on extensively. Vowels, diphthongs, voiced consonant, and consonant/vowel combinations are worked later on. It is important to avoid voiceless, or voiced/voiceless pairs at the beginning of treatment. Reading material should be restricted at the very beginning to "all voiced" segments, which usually requires a clinician to prepare a large body of meaningful sentences far in advance. When these sentences are constructed in a spontaneous ad hoc manner during therapy, meaningless or nonsensical phrases are often created. This may, however, break the monotony of the therapy, making it humorous at times. Again, all sentences are produced at the highest frequency levels possible, observing that decreases in pitch do not cause increases in existing aperiodicity. Based on this therapy pattern, experience has shown for most patients that periodic phonation can be produced below the falsetto or high-frequency register rather rapidly and that this can be maintained well in the upper portion of the normative or modal registers. Through therapy, the voice quality will eventually become more periodic at the lower frequency levels. From the very beginning, patients must be trained in the ability to discriminate pitch and intensity levels. They must also learn to correlate between sound production and manner of productions (motor-learning theory). Biofeedback is of great help. This may include working on the patient's ability to monitor airflow and respiratory effort, and to visualize pitch levels.

It is also important to provide proper psychological support for these patients. For many years, they have been told different stories about the cause of their disorder and how to deal with it. Often, they have undergone unsuccessful courses of very frustrating, costly, and lengthy voice therapy or other medical and pharmacologic therapies. These "experienced" patients are specifically reluctant to undergo postoperative voice treatment, and must be counseled early on that the RLN surgical approach if not supported by postoperative voice therapy will promote failure on a long-term basis. This is evidenced by numerous reports in the literature (Dedo and Behlau, 1991; Izdebski et al., 1981; Dedo and Izdebski, 1983a; Dedo and Izdebski, 1983b; Aronson and DeSanto, 1983). These patients must understand that best long-term results are achieved with postoperative voice therapy, and that the therapy is an integral part of the surgical regimen. This understanding helps the clinician enormously in combatting the patient's reluctance to undergo therapy. It is also important to note that many of these patients may initially respond in a euphoria-like manner to their postoperative voice, regardless of the voice quality. Soon however, they may become critical of their voices, and may even find the "new voice" invasive, abusive, or unacceptable. Patients may be depressed about their inability to produce loud voice, or not being able to vary the voice at will. When this occurs, it is very helpful to play preoperative voice recordings and sequential recordings showing therapy progress. This documentation usually has enormous positive power and takes care of the anxiety and frustration of being unable to produce "normal" voice simply as a consequence of surgery. Voice recordings and phonatory function study records are also extremely crucial when recurrence of symptoms is being faced.

Typical Postoperative Voice Profiles

Specific postoperative voice therapy issues can be demonstrated with discussion of the five most typical postoperative profiles. Profile 1 illustrates patients for whom only minimal postoperative therapy is needed. Profile 2 illustrates a need for a lengthy voice therapy aimed at improvement of aperiodicity and reduction of breathiness. Profile 3 shows patients with persistent breathiness, unsuccessful voice therapy, and need of additional voice treatment after Teflon correction (underinjection). Profile 4 demonstrates patients with mild recurrence of symptoms. Profile 5 shows patients needing additional voice therapy after recurrence of overpressure and treated by staged carbon dioxide (CO_2) laser to achieve increased lateralization of the paralyzed TVF and to increase glottic gap.

Profile I

This profile represents approximately 20% of those patients whose immediate postoperative voice is almost of normative quality and loudness. My experience has demonstrated that usually this is a female patient with a rather thin neck and more or less gaunt stature. Preoperatively her voice was classified as having a mild to moderate degree of spasticity (Dedo, 1990; Izdebski and Dedo, 1990), and symptoms were usually present for no more than 3 years (Izdebski et al., 1984). The patient is usually ecstatic about her postoperative voice, the ease of its production, and reports only minor side effects which are essentially limited to "a lump in the throat" and some difficulty with swallowing liquids. The voice may be somewhat aperiodic, but there is absolutely no overpressure, hence the patient is anxious to talk on the phone, to go back to work, to interact with the family and children, and to undertake a social life as soon as possible. To protect the "new voice," patients elect to speak on a much lowered vocal pitch and in rather monotonous voice pattern. Vocal fry may be present. Initiation of sounds is abrupt and follows deep inhalation, and patterns of breath holding with many sentences produced on one breath are prevalent. The speaking rate is rapid, and maximum phonation and speaking times are extreme despite paralysis. Laryngovideostroboscopy shows bilaterally present mucosal vibratory wave, but with restricted propagation and small vertical phase. Aperiodicity is minor, glottic gap is less than 1 mm. vocal folds are under a certain degree of "tension," and the glottis is approximated posteriorly. There is no rotation of the glottis, and there is no evidence of ventricular approximation. Electroglotography shows a somewhat prolonged closed phonatory phase. The acoustic signal is essentially clean. There is no evidence of tremor. Dynamic range is narrow, but vocal loudness is elevated.

Such essentially "normative" immediate postoperative acoustic and physiologic patterns unfortunately connote concern and signify a possibility of recurrence of symptoms within 9 months or earlier. Hence, therapy is developed to introduce some degree of breathiness in these patients, to increase voice flexibility (inflection), to reduce speaking rate, and to alter respiratory patterns. Obviously, it would be ideal to preserve the immediate postoperative state of glottic physiology to continue to produce "normative" voice on a long-term basis postoperatively. Experience proves that working to maintain this "normative" voice is dangerous and, instead, exercising ability to produce controlled breathiness may be needed. This obviously introduces a high degree of disappointment in these patients and disbelief that such excellent surgical results must be thought as potentially signifying failure.

After finding proper vocal pitch and loudness range and a degree of breathiness to which the speaking voice needs to be brought,

therapy begins. Patients are shown how to decrease lung volumes for voice production and how to reduce verbal output per each breath group. Aperiodicity is usually eliminated by increasing voice fundamental frequency and decreasing SPLs. Voice flexibility is exercised by using emphatic speech patterns and rapid pitch changes. Utilization of acoustic feedback on a Visi-Pitch display is very useful for these purposes.

Because negative "vocal image" in these patients is counterproductive to the exercises designed to elevate vocal pitch toward the higher levels of the speaking voice frequency range (up to ±350 Hz for women, and up to ±150 to 200 Hz for men), ample time is spent on psycho-acoustic pitch discrimination and acceptance of this upward adjusted vocal range. Pragmatic transfer is important for building self confidence. This is done best by confronting the new vocal image and by testing the shaky confidence of the patients with telephone conversations; with conversations between the patient and office staff; and, when possible, by transferring the usage of the new voice to outside situations (such as shops). This proves to the patient that this new elevated level of voice does not arouse improper responses from strangers (which happened when overpressured voice was present).

Only then, vocal targets are placed and practiced to be retained on the long-term basis. If possible, a family member is brought into the therapy session early on and is taught how to monitor proper pitch production in day-to-day situations. Patients are encouraged to undergo this form of training in an "en bloc" therapy paradigm (2 to 3 hours per day), over a few sessions. Following the achievement of therapy goals, the patient is discharged, but is encouraged to follow-up by telephone on a weekly basis for at least 4 weeks. The patient is scheduled for a routine follow-up in the office at 1, 3, 6, 9, and 12 months. The patient is routinely referred for voice care to a voice therapist in the local area of the patient's habitat. Long-term acoustic follow-up by voice recordings is encouraged.

Profile 2

Profile 2 illustrates approximately 50% of patients, who immediately postoperatively show breathy-to-phonatory but aperiodic voice with no significant difficulty in swallowing of liquids, no lump in the throat, but poor coughing. These can be either men or women, usually between 40 and 60 plus years of age, with no specific preoperative severity profile except that they usually do not represent the severe or most severe cases (Dedo, 1990; Izdebski and Dedo, 1990). Preoperative symptom duration, onset and progression, or professional profile are insignificant correlates to postoperative voice quality (Dedo and Izdebski, 1983; Izdebski and Dedo, 1990). Postoperative phonatory function studies show bilaterally distributed mucosal vibratory wave with the paralyzed vocal fold in a slightly wider than median-to-paramedian position, but showing the ability to approximate the glottis posteriorly. Bowing may be present at rest, the glottic gap appears more prominent during upward intensity, and downward voice frequency changes. The degree of glottic gap decreases somewhat by increased frequency and increased vocal intensity; however, full contact area seen stroboscopically alongside the entire glottis is not attainable at this time. Mucosal vibratory wave is present bilaterally but is highly asymmetrical, and its propagation is wide, with wide amplitude. At times, undulating motions within one vocal fold can be observed, giving in addition a rise to diplophonic voice quality. Vocal fold impedance based on electroglotography is variable depending on voice intensity and frequency, but the closed phase is not elongated during best phonatory targets. Air consumption is extensive, allowing for only one to two short sentences or phrases (approximately seven to twelve words) to be produced per breath group. Most comfortable sustained phonation at full lung volume is usually less than 10 seconds, although maximum phonation time can be elongated somewhat by increasing voice intensity and frequency. Maximum speaking time per breath group using all voiced segments as a target usually also does not exceed 10 seconds. The voiced-voiceless pairs or randomly distributed phonemic-morphemic combinations give much shorter speaking times per breath group.

Breathing patterns are not of any consequence at this time; however, patients may have the tendency to overinflate because of phonatory air losses. Attempts to produce louder, lower voices introduce quality changes or profound aperiodicity, which is easily verified with stroboscopy or acoustic analysis. Overinflation also promotes ventricular approximation, which is understood to be a compensation mechanism for the ill-functioning glottis. This is, of course, highly undesirable. At times, patients may show reduced vocal tremor, if tremor were present preoperatively; however, vocal arrests typically present in this patient preoperatively are eliminated completely.

Like the previous group, these patients are also very pleased with the results despite the fact that their voices are not strong. They too report much easier production of connected speech and may show "normative" or improved speech timing and total elimination of vocal arrests and overpressure. When elevating pitch, their phonation typically switches into "paralytic falsetto voice," with severe aperiodicity occurring during elevated loudness levels. Others may sound funny to themselves, and some may find their postoperative voice quality offensive. Yet, paradoxically, they may be totally passive with regard to the need of improving the overall quality of their postoperative voices. Although usually pleased, some of these patients may be easily panicked by any sudden voice change (positive or negative) occurring postoperatively. Despite such an unstable vocal profile, they may be very reluctant to engage in voice therapy, partially because of earlier negative experience with lengthy and unsuccessful therapy (presurgically), or because they do not believe in this form of treatment, or because they simply doubt their own ability to make improvement. Their spouses, on the other hand, are full of encouragement and totally support the need for postoperative voice therapy; hence, they may become ideal "co-therapists," specifically with respect to monitoring improper voice production outside the medical setting. However, because they may be often elderly, spouses do not perform ideally in these roles; therefore, the therapist must not rely heavily on their support in achieving therapy goals.

To be successful with these patients, therapy must begin with perfecting the easiest vocal phonatory patterns which can be produced by them consistently postoperatively.

Usually this means focusing on respiratory tasks because these are easiest for patients to execute at this time. Elimination of aperiodicity by voice frequency maneuvering follows, with exercises to elevate pitch, and with elimination of breathiness being treated last because of difficulties in achieving productive results when working on these targets.

Because of their reluctance to engage in therapy, it is often important to construct treatment sessions in 5- to 10-minute blocks during which specific goals are targeted and exercised. Maximum single session length should not exceed 45 minutes, and even this is often too long. Again, with some patients, best results are achieved in "en bloc" settings, with a 30-minute session interrupted by a 30-minute break and repeated approximately three to four times per day. Over the following 1 to 2 weeks, therapy should be reduced to a minimum of 1 hour per day, and home assignments increased from 5 minutes per hour (four to five times per day) to 10 to 15 minutes per hour, five to eight times per day. Total length of treatment in these cases may be up to 3 months counting continued sessions on a weekly basis. Two- to 3-week reevaluations are advocated. If no satisfactory improvement is achieved at the 6-month interval, with laryngovideostroboscopy and phonatory function studies showing no reduction of glottic gap and no occurrence of ventricular fold approximation, therapy may continue for an additional 3 months. However, vocal fold physiology should be reassessed periodically during these 3 months. Should ventricular approximation be noted, therapy may be discontinued or redirected toward elimination of ventricular approximation, and Teflon underinjection may be contemplated. This should not occur, however, earlier than 9 months postoperatively.

Profile 3

This profile represents approximately 12% to 15% of patients who suffer persistent excessive breathiness despite some gains reached by lengthy therapy over a 9- to 12-month period. These individuals show no symptoms of overpressure or arrest, with occasional tremor. Their initial maximum phonation and speaking time has doubled or tripled since the beginning of therapy, but it is still extremely short (less than 10 seconds). They continue to show poor dynamic range. Loud voice production is usually of very short duration and with assistance of the ventricular folds. Ventricular phonation is also used routinely for daily communication, and their voice sound very harsh. Laryngeal videostroboscopy shows moments of approximation of the TVFs and phonatory vibratory wave bilaterally. But the glottis is predominantly open with the posterior portion showing a solid gap and the inability to approximate. Patients have difficulties in elevating voice and show a rotated or tilted arytenoid cartilage on the paralyzed side. Vertical laryngeal movement is laborious and slow. The ventricular fold may be bulging and obscuring the view of the paralyzed TVF. Air consumption and aperiodicity factors are high.

These patients are very frustrated and must undergo Teflon underinjection to correct the incompetent glottis. This must be followed by voice therapy. Teflon treatments attempt to push the paralyzed TVF towards the midline, but since this is not successful in treating a posterior glottic gap (the condition present here), voice therapy must continue. The purpose is twofold: (1) to undo the compensatory ventricular phonation, and (2) to allow achievement of the best phonatory mechanics after Teflon injection, which stiffens the vocal fold. This is a difficult process because these two components are often mutually exclusive. To reduce ventricular approximation, nonphonatory tasks are exercised. To improve phonatory motility of the injected TVF, phonatory tasks must be practiced. These include rapid pitch and intensity changes (short glissandos and crescendos) executed both in sustained and dynamic modes. Following Teflon injection, therapy must be short, precise, and nonaggressive, because the combined contributions of Teflon and therapy may result in symptom recurrence. If this happens Teflon removal is indicated, again supported by appropriate voice treatment.

Profile 4

This profile represents approximately 15% of patients whose symptoms recur within the first 9 to 12 months (described in the first example). The symptom recurrence is however less than preoperatively.

These patients usually panic at the slightest occurrence of the "vocal catch." They may now exhibit in addition to overpressure some degree of harshness, which usually connotes overcompensation by the ventricular folds. Their phonation function measures are similar to preoperative studies, but the magnitude of findings is less.

Voice therapy concentrates on "thinning out of their voices" and making them sound less loud. Unfortunately, only a few of them will succeed. Those who do owe their success to their persistence and practicing on a home-bound basis. The others will become candidates for salvage treatment, either with CO_2 laser thinning or by Botox injection (see the following section). Appropriate voice therapy must follow afterwards.

Profile 5

This profile represents approximately 5% of patients who fail postrecurrence voice therapy, and were treated with staged CO_2 laser thinning (described later). This process may stretch over 12 to 24 months or longer, with voice therapy interspersed between consecutive thinnings and aimed at restoration of "any" phonatory voice immediately after each thinning has been completed. The long-term therapy goal is to achieve as normative voice/speech as possible. Many of these patients were in the severe or extremely severe category of ADD/SD patient preoperatively and may in addition be afflicted with accompanying disorders (tremor, oromandibular dystonias, and other movement disorders). Speech therapy is therefore needed in addition to voice therapy. Post-thinning therapy requires applications of all techniques and skills needed to achieve improved glottic closure, elevated voice frequency, enlarged dynamic range, improved prosody, improved respiratory control, speech articulation, and reduced ventricular fold approximation.

Botulinum A Toxin (Botox)

In contrast to RLN section, intramuscular injection of botulinum-A toxin (Botox) is performed on an outpatient basis. It results in selective paralysis or paresis on one intrinsic laryngeal muscle, usually the thyroarytenoid (TA) muscle.

On the day of the procedure, the patient is brought to the clinical voice laboratory (surgery center, operating room, or specialty office) and is positioned in a semireclined or supine position. Injection may be carried unilaterally or bilaterally. The neck is cleaned with an alcohol pad and a small wheal is raised in the skin through the injection of local anesthetic (lidocaine) with a hypodermic needle. Following this preparation, Botox is injected intramuscularly, under EMG guidance, preferably with simultaneous voice monitoring (Ward et al., 1991). The needle used for injection is a Teflon-coated 25-gauge (1.5-inch-long) hypodermic needle with its beveled distal tip exposed to perform as a unipolar recording electrode. The patient is grounded, and a reference electrode is pasted on the patient's body in a close proximity to the recording electrode. Using a 1-mL tuberculin syringe, the desired Botox preparation (number of units) is drawn into the syringe, which is then connected to the recording needle and EMG-acoustic monitoring system. Following advancement of the needle through the skin and through the cricothyroid membrane, the needle is aimed at the target muscle (usually the TA). The typical trajectory of the needle is oblique (at a ± 30-degree angle) toward the mid-portion of the TA. Once the needle is inserted into a muscle, EMG monitoring of the generated vocal signals takes place. To assure accuracy of placement and proper muscle verification, the voice of the patient is monitored simultaneously with the EMG signal during vegetative, phonatory, and respiratory tasks. Following proper verification of electrode placement and proper targeting, Botox solution is injected into the muscle, and the needle is advanced to a different location within the same muscle. Monitoring of EMG and voice continues throughout the injection. Following completion, the needle is then left in place for a few seconds, and the muscle is activated again usually showing diminishment in its activity during execution of vocal tasks. The needle is then withdrawn fully, or if additional injection is needed on the opposite side, the needle is advanced toward the contralateral vocal fold, and the procedure is repeated. At times, it may be useful to monitor both the passage and placement of the needle within the TA muscle through the flexible fiberoptic laryngoscopy. This may however promote coughing and make injection difficult. If this is the case, the pharynx and laryngeal vestibule are anesthetized topically. Few patients may require preoperative sedation, and this can usually be accomplished with diazepam (Valium) or other sedatives. The time required for injection is extremely short (usually no more than 3 to 5 minutes); however, preparation is extensive, so that the entire procedure may take up to 1 hour.

Botox may also be injected directly (perorally or during general anesthesia) using a long, curved syringe. The vocal folds are visualized indirectly with a laryngeal mirror while the syringe is placed through the oral cavity to the larynx. No EMG voice monitoring is required. Injection is performed by a physician (ear, nose and throat specialist or a neurologist). Ideally, intraoperative monitoring should be carried out by a voice pathologist.

Intramuscular injection of Botox results in inhibition of acytecholine releases, loss of acytecholine receptors, decline of end plate potentials, and grated paralysis. Functionally, the muscle becomes denervated, it atrophies, and develops extrajunctural receptors, followed by terminal sprouting (Ward et al., 1991; Scott, 1989; Scott, 1991). In other words, for a period of time the muscle behaves like a denervated muscle (due to RLN section), but after new synaptic contacts on adjacent fibers are reconstituted, the muscle gradually reanimates (Kao et al., 1976; Simpson, 1989; Pamphlett, 1989). This is in contrast to RLN section. The initial reduction of actively firing muscle fibers results in weakening of the muscle, and hence in reduction of the feedback to the motor neuronal pools in the brain stem (basal ganglia) (Ludlow, 1990; Ludlow et al., 1988). Therefore, the intramuscular injection of Botox has similar consequences on phonation production and control as RLN section or RLN block, except that one muscle is affected selectively. In the case of the TA, this is evidenced by a decreased activation level, bowing of the injected TVF, decreased glottic

compression causing reduction of the adductory force, incomplete posterior glottic closure, reduction of Ps, and increase of airflow as long as the toxin remains active. Contrary to the consequences of RLN surgery, Botox does not affect the posterior cricoarytenoid (PCA) musculature, hence the vocal fold continues to be mobile (abductory and adductory). Unlike RLN surgery, the procedure introduces vocal fold edema, requiring the patient to observe modified voice rest for up to 3 days after injection. This delays the onset of active post-Botox voice therapy.

Botox injection also has no direct effects on the working of the intrinsic laryngeal musculature of the opposite noninjected site, nor does it have effects on the cricothyroid muscles or on the extrinsic laryngeal muscles bilaterally. Also, a glottic gap of approximately 1 to 3 mm occurs longitudinally depending on the injection effects. This gap will vary and change with time, until total recovery of the injected muscle reoccurs. This time determines the period of overpressure-free phonation. Symptoms will reoccur dependent on the time needed for the muscle to reanimate. This may be as short as a few weeks, and theoretically cannot exceed 6 months. (Scott, 1991; Jankovic and Brin, 1991). Therefore, voice therapy must relate to the state of the glottis, and postinjection voice quality.

As is the case with RLN section, voice therapy is recommended and advised for post-Botox injection. This recommendation is based on two reasons. First, because patients treated with Botox will experience a variety of unfamiliar voice qualities in degrees varied from minimal dysphonia and breathiness to severe breathiness aphonia and aperiodicity, breathiness is usually most pronounced within the first 7 days after injection and may be more severe following bilateral injections. It is not necessary, however, to spend much therapy effort on combating breathiness unless it persists over a 1-week period. Secondly, post-Botox therapy is recommended because it may prolong the asymptomatic period and ultimately reduce the frequency of injections. It is also hoped that while under injection, the patients have more chances to learn to control their glottis, and this may be beneficial on a long-term basis in combating ADD/SD.

Aperiodicity also may be more pronounced after Botox than after RLN section because the toxin introduces increased vibratory imbalance between the injected and noninjected TVFs bilaterally and causes decreased ability to adjust tension of the vocal fold mucosal covers. Differences may be even more pronounced with bilateral injections, even when equal unit dosage is given to each vocal fold.

Totality of acoustic consequences post-Botox are again directly proportional to the degree of paresis caused by the toxin, changes in glottic configuration, vibratory asymmetry, and compensatory approximation of the glottis. All of the acoustic parameters will be subject to change during active denervation and the active reinnervation period. As with RLN section, these changes need to be properly understood and evaluated in order to be explained and treated appropriately.

Principles of Voice Therapy After Botox

Principles of voice therapy after Botox injection are similar to RLN section. Some differences, however, apply. Again, it appears that best results occur in those patients who underwent intensive voice therapy before injection (albeit unsuccessfully). In general, postinjection voice therapy is acute, and aims at providing the patient with tactical guidance that can be used to improve voice quality in anticipation of symptom recurrence and during rapidly changing vocal fold biomechanics after Botox. Because the principles which maintain asymptomatic voice are explained by the SD model (that is, collision force, contact area, and Ps), production of high-frequency voice with low SPL is encouraged.

The didactic part of voice therapy is also similar to that of RLN section in that the procedure must be explained in detail, and the predicted or anticipated vocal changes outlined. Patients are warned regarding difficulties with swallowing, and usage of soft voice is encouraged. Because of edema (resulting from needle penetration and injection), modified voice rest is advocated for the duration of up to 3 days following injection.

Perhaps even more importantly than with RLN section, it must be stressed that Botox injection does not cure the disorder, nor does it guarantee a good phonatory voice. Also, the period of relatively "normal and symptom-free" voice may be very short, and full symptom recurrence may come soon and rather suddenly after the injection. Therefore, it is important to follow these patients on a weekly basis. To check their vocal status, telephone conversation will suffice, but a more elaborate evaluation requires an office visit. Patients are also instructed to keep a diary, and it is useful to provide them with a tablet on which they can score negative or positive observations regarding their voices. For sake of simplicity, the tablet may be divided into pluses and minuses ($+/-$), with the "0" line corresponding to a normal voice, "$+$" corresponding to a spastic voice, and "$-$" corresponding to a breathy voice. Patients are encouraged to mark these voice qualities accordingly over a period of time. This provides both the patient and the clinician with a summary of post-Botox vocal dynamics, and can be used effectively in planning and predicting voice treatment after subsequent injections.

Recurrence of Symptoms

Although recurrence of symptoms is not very clearly understood, the ADD/SD model (Izdebski, 1991), predicts that symptoms will recur not only after Botox (Zwirner et al., 1991), and RLN block (Izdebski and Dedo, 1980), but also after RLN section (Izdebski et al., 1981; Dedo and Izdebski, 1983a; Dedo and Izdebski, 1983b; Aronson and DeSanto, 1983), or whenever the physiologic conditions that trigger symptoms are met (Izdebski, 1991). Recurrence is not surprising because all of these treatments are symptomatic, leaving the basic disorder intact.

Clinically, recurrence happens when the paralyzed vocal fold is repositioned too close to the midline. This repositioning can be accomplished by reinnervation, overcorrection with various injectables or, may be secondary to the movement of supraglottic structures during attempts to produce loud phonation, or due to vigorous overcompensation. Similar repositioning of the TVFs applies to the patients with Botox injections. However here it is the consequence of rapidly regenerating TVF function and rapid regaining of the normative mechanics of the injected muscle.

Recurrence of Spasticity

Many techniques are used to relieve recurring spasticity. Voice therapy alone may not be efficacious, but it plays an important role in combination with surgical/pharmacologic corrective techniques. The most commonly used corrective technique is to thin the paralyzed vocal fold with a CO_2 laser beam (Dedo and Shipp, 1980; Izdebski and Dedo, 1981; Dedo and Izdebski 1983b). Through this action, a 2-mm-wide groove is created in the paralyzed vocal fold, and as it begins to heal, the scarring action pulls the edge of the TVF laterally, creating a wider glottis. The advantage of this technique is in not tampering with the integrity and elasticity of the vocal fold free vibratory margin. However, the healing process may be very lengthy, and multiple repetitions of this process may be necessary to create adequate lateralization. Voice quality during this process may be severely breathy, aperiodic, and harsh. Little can be done during this time to restore phonation to normative values, but therapy is needed and must be aimed at reducing increases in Ps, and at decreasing tension of the vocal folds so that the nonoperated and operated vocal folds can engage in phonation. Therapy also promotes recovery of mucosal membrane (cover) elasticity, and to do so, exercising low to high rapid pitch changes seems very useful. Voice treatment is not appropriate in these cases during the first 2 weeks after CO_2 laser surgery because of edema.

Other surgical techniques used to combat recurring symptoms involve resectioning of the RLN of the operated side, or by Botox injection (Ludlow et al., 1990). Reinnervation has been shown to be one possible mechanism of symptom recurrence following RLN section (Fritzell et al., 1982; Schiratzki and Fritzell, 1988), however, without restoring adductory/ abductory motion of the TVFs. If mild recurrence happens, voice therapy aimed at introducing controlled breathiness may be useful. This is, however, very difficult to achieve technically and may leave the patient with a voice that will fail in noisy situations. Remember, using voice therapy to combat recurring symptoms may be as frustrating and difficult as in a fresh case of ADD/SD.

In many instances, patients who show recurrence and are injected with Botox show improvement (Ludlow et al., 1990). These patients are treated with post-Botox voice therapy principles. They are taught how to cope with the unexpected voice changes, and how to regulate the airflow, Ps, and pitch. Therapy needs to be adjusted in synchrony with the changing functions of the glottis as Botox loses its effect.

Summary

Recurrent laryngeal nerve surgery and/or Botox approaches represent symptomatic surgical and pharmacologic treatment of ADD/SD by replacing overpressured strained/strangled voice with various degrees of breathy to normative phonation as a consequence of unilateral total or selective paralysis of the TVF. Both treatments are symptomatic, leaving the main disorder intact. Post-treatment voice therapy is therefore an integral part of the overall treatment regimen. Utmost care is executed to engage patients who are candidates for surgical or pharmacologic treatment into a systematic postoperative voice therapy program to assure maintenance of achieved results on a long-term basis.

Successful voice therapy introduces acquisition of new voicing skills and patterns that are free of overpressure and interruptions. Therapy must also eliminate the negative changes introduced by vocal fold paralysis. These new voicing patterns aim at producing phonation with elevated pitch levels, increased breathiness, and decreased loudness. In other words, therapy aims at reduction of the main components thought to be responsible for ADD/SD cluster of symptoms: TVF collision force, TVF contact area, and elevated Ps.

Therapy may be acute or lengthy but must reflect the patient's individual needs in relationship to post-treatment laryngeal physiology and resultant acoustic consequences. Therefore, for best results, therapy must be individualized, and a "cookbook" approach will fail. Treatment may be frustrating to patients and clinicians, and substantial reluctance to treatment may be expressed by patients because of a history of therapeutic failures or aversion to the newly acquired voice quality. Therefore, voice therapy must incorporate methods routed in motor-learning, counseling, self-managing, behavior modification, classic conditioning, psychotherapy, biofeedback, and auditory discrimination. Knowledge of phonatory and respiratory physiology is fundamental to proper design and execution to treatment. Clinical evaluation supported by instrumentation and phonatory function studies are of paramount benefit in designing and executing proper treatment. Therefore, voice therapy for ADD/SD is undoubtedly the most challenging task in our field.

It is important to remember that voice therapy is an integral part of ADD/SD treatment. This is crucial because, insurance companies may challenge the need of post-treatment voice therapy (specifically in view of "recently accomplished medical treatment"), and also may question the cost/benefit ratios of therapy. These grumblings must be challenged head on, on the basis of ADD/SD impact on patient's social and professional life and recurrence of symptoms in patients who were not afforded postoperative therapy. Similarly, it is hoped that post-Botox therapy will prolong asymptomatic duration of speech and will ultimately reduce the frequency of injections.

MANAGEMENT OF ABDUCTOR SPASMODIC DYSPHONIA

Contributed by Andrew Blitzer, M.D., and Celia Stewart, M.S.

While injection of the thyroarytenoid muscle has proved to be beneficial for relieving symptoms of adductor spasmodic dysphonia, like injections have not proved helpful for patients with abductor spasmodic dysphonia. Andrew Blitzer, M.D., and Celia Stewart, M.S., present a case study describing a technique for injecting the only intrinsic abductor muscle, the posterior cricoarytenoid muscle. Injection of this muscle is showing promise for eliminating the symptoms of this disorder.

CASE STUDY: PATIENT BB

Patient BB is a 40-year-old, right-handed, Irish-Presbyterian radio announcer. Twelve years prior to his examination he noticed a weakening of his voice near the end of his broadcasts. The weakening progressed, and he developed breaks in phonation, especially during broadcasts. He has also had an increased number of breaks during telephone conversations. He has learned to avoid certain words to avoid the breaks. His voice is also worse when he's fatigued or has ingested caffeine. During the examination, his laugh was normal, as was his singing, humming, and yawning. He did not have signs of dyspnea or dysphagia. Ethanol ingestion did not produce any change in the character of his symptom. He did not have any sensory tricks to make his voice better.

He had had a normal birth and normal childhood growth and development. He is otherwise healthy, and does not take any medications. He was previously told that his disorder was psychogenic and was referred to a psychiatrist. Confident that he did not have a mental disorder he never went to the psychiatrist. He had a normal MRI, ceruloplasmin level, and normal results of routine serum chemistries.

His conversational speech was characterized with moderate to severe breathy abrupt voice termination, breathy voice quality, and reduced voice loudness. The aphonic breaks in his voice reduced the smoothness and intelligibility of his speech. He frequently produced short, quick, one-word responses with normal voice quality, but the voice quality was not sustained in conversational speech. He sustained /a/ and /i/ in modal and loft register without phonation or pitch breaks. He produced a clear cough and shout. No vocal tremor was observed.

Fiberoptic laryngoscopy revealed a synchronous and untimely abduction of the true vocal folds, exposing an extremely wide glottic chink. These spasms were triggered by consonant sounds, particularly when consonants were in the initial position in words. Stroboscopy revealed a normal mucosal wave during voiced segments, with intermittent opening of the posterior glottis.

Characteristics of Abductor Spasmodic Dysphonia

Spasmodic dysphonia or laryngeal dystonia (LD) is a speech disorder characterized by breaks in speech fluency. The *abductor* type is due to intermittent abduction of the vocal folds, resulting in a reduction of loudness and aphonic whispered segments of speech. Aronson's description is "a voice in which normal or hoarse voice is suddenly interrupted by brief moments of breathy or whispered (unphonated) segments." The voice may begin to manifest nonspecific hoarseness or breathiness and over a period of days or weeks begin to show signs of intermittent breathy breaks (Aronson, 1985).

Some of the patients have a mixed abductor-adductor type, with an admixture of breathy breaks and tight, harsh sounds. Connito and Johnson (1981) proposed that both conditions exist in all the patients and the symptoms depend on whether there is more adductor or abductor activity. The disability from abductor LD may be profound. Telephone calls and stress exacerbate the disorder and make the speech pattern more unintelligible.

Evaluation of Abductor Spasmodic Dysphonia

Diagnosis and treatment of this difficult-to-diagnose voice disorder requires a team approach, including a speech-language pathologist, an otolaryngologist, and a neurologist. The four components of the evaluation are the case history, the voice and speech signs and symptoms, the evaluation and observation of the structure and function of the vocal folds, and the neurologic evaluation of the movements of the body.

Speech-Language Evaluation. — A standard evaluation of voice symptoms for spasmodic dysphonia is in the process of being validated in a combined effort between Columbia University and New York University. The evaluation is called the Unified Spasmodic Dysphonia Rating Scale (USDRS). On the USDRS, the severity of the voice symptoms is rated along several parameters, including overall severity, breathy voice quality, voice arrests, aphonia, voice tremor, and expiratory effort. We have been rating patients on a seven-point scale on which 1 = no instance; 2 = mild; 3 = mild to moderate; 4 = moderate; 5 = moderate to severe; 6 = severe; and 7 = profound. The USDRS has been used for both the initial evaluation and for measuring change following treatment. It is recommended that patients be evaluated with the USDRS and videotaped at the initial evaluation and at intervals following treatment so that adequate records can be maintained to evaluate changes over time.

Voice and speech tasks on the USDRS include reading aloud, spontaneous speech, and voice tasks that test the patient's ability to use voice at the limits of the voice and speech mechanism. The tasks are easier to perform when a patient has mild spasmodic dysphonia and more difficult when a patient has severe spasmodic dysphonia. Evaluating a patient's ability to perform the tasks and describing the

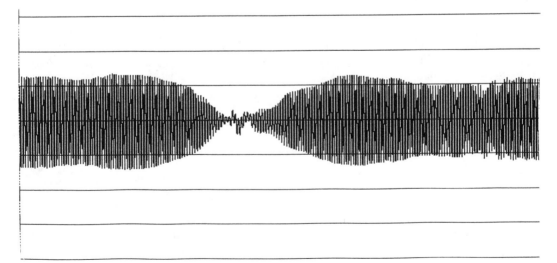

FIG 6–1.
Acoustic waveform from the DSP Sona-Graph model 5500 visually displays a breathy voice break.

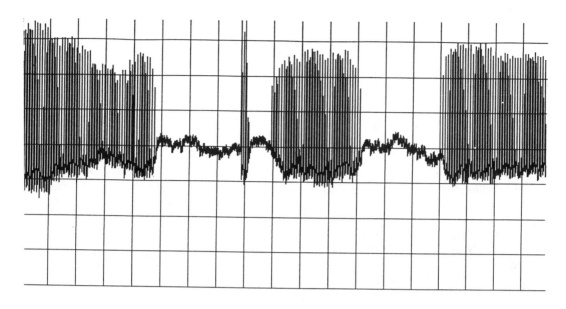

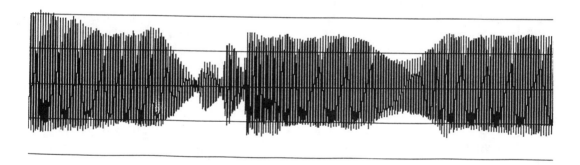

FIG 6–2.
Simultaneous recordings of /a/ as detected by electroglottography (*upper tracing*) and an air conduction microphone (*lower tracing*).

voice and speech symptoms on the tasks helps to identify the severity of the dysphonia, the effectiveness of the patient's response to therapy, and the need for further treatment.

Descriptions of voice function and changes in voice production with treatment can be further documented through acoustic evaluation. The acoustic aspects of vocal tremor and voice breaks are observed through waveform analysis and narrow-band spectral analysis (Fig 6–1). Tremor can be visualized to determine its consistency, relative frequency, and changes

with various levels of breath support. The frequency and length of voice breaks can also be visualized utilizing electroglottography (Fig 6–2).

Otolaryngologic Examination. — All patients should have a detailed history, with particular attention to other abnormal cervicocranial function. A thorough head and neck examination is performed. Fiberoptic direct laryngoscopy is performed to allow observation of the larynx while the patient speaks words and sentences, thus permitting the detection of the abductor or adductor spasms causing dysfluency. The movements can be recorded and analyzed in slow speed or stop action. This cannot be easily performed with indirect laryngoscopy, in which anterior tongue traction limits the speaking ability. Most of these patients can usually perform pure phonation of vowels without disclosing the dysphonia that produces breaks between voicing onsets and offsets (Brin et al., 1992).

Videostroboscopy is also useful in assessing dysphonia. The strobe allows analysis of the regularity and symmetry of the mucosal wave, the presence of tremor, and the degree of glottic closure. The videotaped version of this examination can be reviewed to help differentiate abductor, adductor, and the compensatory laryngeal dystonias (Hirano, 1992).

Laryngeal electromyography is performed in many patients. This allows analysis of the motor unit potentials as well as localization of active parts of the laryngeal muscles. In our initial EMG study of adductor SD patients, we found some patients with a diagnosis of spasmodic dysphonia who had other disorders including tremor, myoclonus, and pyramidal and extrapyramidal diseases (Blitzer et al., 1985).

Neurology Examination. — A complete history is mandatory for patients with dystonia. A family history of other members with dystonia, history of head trauma, perinatal or developmental abnormalities, history of another neu-

rologic disease, or exposure to drugs known to cause dystonia (e.g., phenothiazines) is imperative. Examination should find the intellectual, pyramidal, cerebellar, and sensory examinations normal. The clinical phenomenology will often be the clue to etiology. Primary dystonia is typically action-induced; symptoms are enhanced with the use of the affected body part and the region may appear normal at rest. Secondary dystonia frequently results in fixed dystonic postures. The presence of extensive dystonia limited to one side of the body suggests a secondary etiology. Dystonia may involve the muscles of the oral cavity, larynx, pharynx, tongue, and jaw. An MRI scan, SMAC, complete blood count, ceruloplasmin concentration, erythrocyte sedimentation rate, electromyogram, EEG, and antinuclear antibody assay may all be useful to rule out a metabolic or neurodegenerative disease etiology (Brin et al., 1992).

Therapy for Abductor Spasmodic Dysphonia. — Speech therapy and relaxation therapy may help to moderate the symptoms, but provide little if any long-term benefit. Pharmacotherapy provides little for the long-term relief of symptoms. Our group reported early benefit from anticholinergics in some patients (Blitzer et al., 1988), but the early success was not maintained.

Our group and others have reported impressive success in the treatment of adductor laryngeal dystonia with localized injections of botulinum toxin (Botox) into the thyroary-

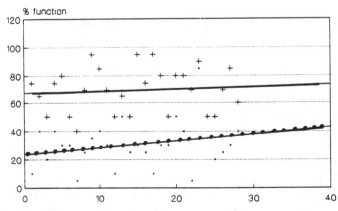

FIG 6–3.
Percentage of normal function for patients with abductor laryngeal dystonia. Series A (pretreatment) = *bulleted line*; series B (after Botox) = *solid line*.

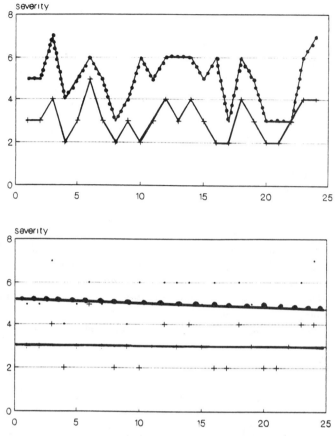

FIG 6–4.
Overall severity of abductor laryngeal dystonia plotted for each patient. *Right*, same information as in *left* grid, but presented in a linear plot to demonstrate the average improvement. Series A (pretreatment) = *bulleted line*; series B (after Botox) = *solid line*.

tenoid muscle(s) (Blitzer and Brin, 1991). In our series of more than 400 patients, voice recovery to an average of 90% of normal function was reported by patients. The injections could be given comfortably via a percutaneous route in an ambulatory setting. The side effects from such injections were minimal. The injections lasted an average of 4 months.

In abductor spasmodic dysphonia, we believed the posterior cricoarytenoid (PCA) muscle was most responsible for the breathy voice, but we were initially reluctant to treat the PCA muscle with Botox because of our concern of airway compromise. However, a severely disabled patient urged us to try treating his PCA muscle, even if it meant performing a tracheostomy.

After receiving approval from our institutional review board, one of the authors (A.B.) performed a direct laryngoscopy and an at-

tempt at injecting one PCA directly through the laryngoscope. This attempt proved difficult for the patient, had no EMG control, and did not improve voice quality. We therefore developed an EMG-guided percutaneous technique. The larynx is manually rotated, and the Teflon-coated hollow EMG recording needle is placed posterior to the thyroid lamina, through the inferior constrictor muscle, until it reaches the cricoid cartilage. This directly impales the PCA. The patient is asked to sniff, which yields maximum abduction, and the EMG signal is observed for correct needle placement. Botox is then given when the needle is in an area of brisk electrical activity.

Since this first injection 3½ years ago, we have reported 32 patients with abductor laryngeal dystonia who were treated with Botox (Blitzer et al., 1992). Initially we attempted to weaken or paralyze one PCA muscle with an injection of 3.75 units in 0.15 mL. After 1 week, a fiberoptic laryngoscopy was performed to observe the vocal cord function. In 25% of the cases, weakening or paralyzing just one PCA produced significant voice improvement. In general, such patients had less severe pretreatment symptoms. Others may need additional toxin injections. For those who still had abduction in the vocal cord, an additional 2.5 to 3.75 units were given to paralyze the PCA. If the PCA is already paralyzed and the voice is not improved, conservative serial doses of 0.675 to 2.5 units in 0.1 mL are given into the contralateral PCA. No further injections are given if there has been stridor, or the glottic chink has been significantly narrowed. If both PCAs have been treated and the voice is still breathy, despite weakening of both PCAs and narrowing of the glottic chink in those who have significant tremor, we have injected 2.5 units in 0.1 mL of Botox into the cricothyroid

muscle. The overall success rate was return to 70% of normal function in the entire treatment group (Fig 6–3).

In reviewing the graphs of data from our standardized vocal rating scale (Figs 6–4 and 6–5, Table 6–1) a clear improvement is seen in all cases in overall rating, breathy voice quality, and aphonia. When reviewing tremor, it was noted that several of the patients had a worsening of their tremor. The reason for this is that the tremor existed before, but was visual and not voiced; as phonation improved with PCA weakening the tremor became audible and the quality of speech was improved, but still disabling in some cases.

In reviewing the data, those who had a combined disorder of segmental cranial and/or axial tremor and/or respiratory involvement only had a best average improvement to 58% of normal function. Those with a tremor only had improvement to 65% of normal function.

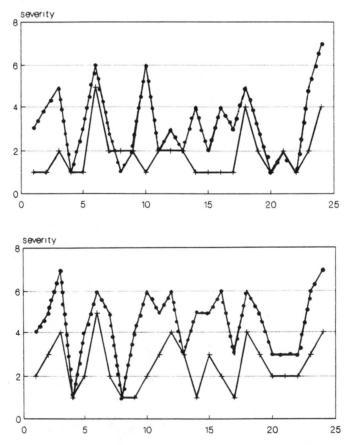

FIG 6–5.
Left, aphonia in abductor laryngeal dystonia. *Right,* breathy voice quality in laryngeal dystonia. Series A (pretreatment) = *bulleted line;* series B (after Botox) = *solid line.*

TABLE 6–1.

Abductor Laryngeal Dystonia Staging System

Stage 1	Focal disease
Stage 2	Segmental cranial or axial
Stage 3	Tremor
Stage 4	Tremor with segmental dystonia and/or respiratory dysynchrony

Many of the patients in these groups required additional treatment.

Therefore, we have devised a staging system for abductor LD patients (Table 6–1), in which stage 1 consists of those patients with focal symptoms; stage 2, those with segmental cranial or axial symptoms; stage 3, those with a tremor; and stage 4, those with a tremor with segmental axial/cranial symptoms and/or respiratory dyssynchrony. This staging system will allow better pretreatment counseling with patients. They can be prepared for the type of response expected and the possibility of other injections or procedures to achieve a functional voice. Three patients additionally have had a combination of Botox injections of the PCA and type 1 thryoplasty (see Chapter 4).

Speech therapy is helpful following injections of Botox to improve the quality and prolong the response to the toxin. Therapy should focus on decreasing expiratory drive and coordinating respiration, phonation, resonation, and articulation as described by Allen (personal communication, 1989). Improving the patient's posture and decreasing extraneous muscle activity in the head, neck, shoulders, and chest can improve control of the expiratory drive and decrease tension levels in the larynx. The patient can modify the speaking environmental noise to enhance communication.

REFERENCES

Aminoff MJ, Dedo HH, Izdebski K: Clinical aspects of spasmodic dysphonia, *J Neurol Neurosurg Psychiatry* 41:361–65, 1978.

Arnold GE, Pinto S: Ventricular dysphonia: new interpretation of an old observation, *Laryngoscope* 70:1608–1627, 19

Aronson A: Abductor spastic dysphonia. In Aronson A (ed): *Clinical voice disorders,* (ed 2.) New York, 1985, Thieme Medical Publishers, pp 187–197.

Aronson AE: *Clinical voice disorders,* ed 3, New York, 1990, Thieme.

Aronson AE et al: Spastic dysphonia, I: voice, neurologic, and psychiatric aspects, *J Speech Hear Disord* 33:203–218, 1968.

Aronson AE, DeSanto GW: Adductor spasmodic dysphonia: three years after recurrent laryngeal nerve resection *Laryngoscope* 93:1, 1983.

Blitzer A, et al: Clinical and laboratory characteristics of laryngeal dystonia: a study of 110 cases, *Laryngoscope* 98:636–640, 1988.

Blitzer A, et al: Localized injections of botulinum toxin for the treatment of focal laryngeal dystonia (spastic dysphonia), *Laryngoscope* 98:193–197, 1988.

Blitzer A, et al: Letter to the editor, *Laryngoscope* 96:1300–1301, 1986.

Blitzer A, et al: Electromyographic findings in focal laryngeal dystonia (spastic dysphonia), *Ann Otol Rhinol Laryngol* 94:591–594, 1985.

Blitzer A, Brin MF: Laryngeal dystonia: a series with botulinum toxin therapy, *Ann Otol Rhinol Laryngol* 100:85–90, 1991.

Blitzer A, et al: Abductor laryngeal dystonia: a series treated with botulinum toxin, *Laryngoscope* 102:163–167, 1992.

Brin MF, et al: Movement disorders of the larynx. In Blitzer A (eds): *Neurologic disorders of the larynx,* New York, 1992, Thieme Medical Publishers, pp 248–279.

Brodnitz F: Spastic dysphonia, *Ann Otolaryngol* 85:210–214, 1976.

Cannito MP, Johnson P: Spastic dysphonia: a continuum disorder. *J Commun Disord* 14:215–223, 1981.

Cooper M: *Winning with your voice,* Hollywood, 1990, Fell Publishers.

Dedo HH: Surgery of the larynx and trachea, Philadelphia, 1990, BC Decker, vol ii, pp 29–59.

Dedo HH: Recurrent laryngeal nerve section for spastic dysphonia, *Ann Otol Rhinol Laryngol* 85:451–459, 1976.

Dedo HH, Behlau MS: Recurrent laryngeal nerve section for spastic dysphonia: 5- to 14-year preliminary results in the first 300 patients, *Ann Otol Rhinol Laryngol* 100:274–279, 1991.

Dedo HH, Izdebski K: Problems with RLN surgery for spastic dysphonia, *Laryngoscope* 93:268–271, 1983a.

Dedo HH, Izdebski K: Intermediate results of 306 recurrent laryngeal nerve sections for spastic dysphonia, *Laryngoscope* 93:916, 1983b.

Dedo HH, Izdebski K: Surgical treatment of spastic dysphonia, *Contemp Surg* 18:75–90, 1981.

Dedo HH, Shipp T: *Spastic dysphonia: a surgical and voice therapy treatment program*, Houston, 1980, College Hill Press.

Faaboreg-Andersen K: The position of paretic vocal cords, *Acta Otolaryngol* 57:50–54, 1964.

Findley LJ, Koller WC: Essential tremor: a review, *Neurology* 37:1194–1197, 1987.

Freud E: functions and dysfunctions of ventricular folds, *J Speech Hear Disord* 27:334, 1962.

Fritzell B, et al: Experiences with recurrent laryngeal nerve section for spastic dysphonia, *Folia Phoniatr* 34:160–76, 1982.

Hirano M: *Clinical examination of voice*, New York, 1981, Springer-Verlag.

Hirano M: Stroboscopic examination of the normal larynx. In Blitzer A, et al (eds): *Neurologic disorders of the larynx*, New York, 1992, Thieme Medical Publishers, pp 135–140.

Izdebski K: Symptomatology of adductor spasmodic dysphonia: a physiologic model, Paper presented at the Voice Foundation annual meeting, Philadelphia, 1991.

Izdebski K: Acoustic and physiologic characteristics of ventricular dysphonia, Paper presented at the XIX Symposium on Care of the Professional Voice, Philadelphia, 1990.

Izdebski K: Overpressure and breathiness in spastic dysphonia: an LTAS study, *Acta Otolaryngol* 97:373–378, 1984.

Izdebski K, Dedo HH: Preoperative and postoperative voice quality in spastic dysphonia patients and clinical severity scaling: an audio tape. Supplement to Dedo HH: *Surgery of the larynx and trachea*, Philadelphia, 1990, BC Decker.

Izdebski K, Dedo HH: Spastic dysphonia. In Darby JK, editor: *Speech evaluation in medicine*, New York, 1981, Grune & Stratton, vol ii pp 105–127.

Izdebski K, Dedo HH: Selecting the side of RLN section for spastic dysphonia, *Otolaryngol Head Neck Surg* 89:423–426, 1980.

Izdebski K, Dedo HH: Characteristics of voice tremor in spastic dysphonia: a preliminary study. In Lawrence V, editor: *Transcripts of the VIII Symposium on Care of the Professional Voice* (Part III, Medical/Surgical Therapy), New York, 1979, Voice Foundation, pp 17–23, 1979.

Izdebski K, Dedo HH, Boles L: Spastic dysphonia: a patient profile of 200 cases, *Am J Otolaryngol* 5:7–14, 1984.

Izdebski K, Ross JC, Klein JC: Rigid transoral laryngovideostroboscopy (phonoscopy). *Semin Speech Hear*, 1990.

Izdebski K, Shipp T, Dedo HH: Predicting postoperative voice characteristics of spastic dysphonia patients, *Otolaryngology* 87:428–434, 1979.

Izdebski K et al: Postoperative and follow-up studies of spastic dysphonia: patients treated by recurrent laryn-

geal nerve section, *Otolaryngol Head Neck Surg* 89:96–101, 1981.

Jankovic J, Brin MF: Therapeutic uses of botulinum toxin, *N Engl J Med* 324:1186–1194, 1991.

Kao I, Drachman DB, Price DL: Botulinum toxin: mechanism of presynaptic blockade, *Science* 193:1256–1258, 1976.

Lehmann QH: Reverse phonation: a new maneuver for examining the larynx, *Radiology* 84:215–222, 1965.

Logemann J: Swallowing physiology and pathophysiology, *Otolaryngol Clin North Am* 21:613–623, 1988.

Ludlow CL: Treatment of speech and voice disorders with botulinum toxin, *JAMA* 264:2671–2675, 1990.

Ludlow CL, et al: Spasmodic dysphonia: botulinum toxin injection after recurrent nerve surgery, *Otolaryngol Head Neck Surg* 102:102–122, 1990.

Ludlow CL, et al: Effects of botulinum toxin injections on speech in adductor spasmodic dysphonia, *Neurology* 38:1220–1225, 1988.

Ludlow CL, et al: Phonatory characteristics of vocal fold tremor, *J Phonetics* 14:509–516, 1986.

McFarlane S, Boone DE: *The voice and voice therapy*, ed 4, Englewood Cliffs, N.J., 1988, Prentice-Hall.

Pamphlett R: Early terminal and nodal sprouting of motor atons after botulinum toxin, *J Neurol Sci* 92:181–192, 1989.

Schiratzki H, Fritzell B: Treatment of spasmodic dysphonia by means of resection of the recurrent laryngeal nerve, *Acta Otolaryngol* 449(suppl):115–117, 1988.

Scott AB: Mechanism of botulinum-A toxin on muscle activity, Paper presented at The IV Annual Pacific Voice Conference, San Francisco, 1991.

Scott AB: Clostridial toxins as therapeutic agents. In Lane S, editor: *Clostridial neurotoxins*, New York, 1989, Academic Press, pp 399–412.

Shipp T, et al: Subglottal air pressure spastic dysphonia speech, *Folia Phoniatr* 40:105–110, 1988.

Shipp T, et al: Intrinsic laryngeal muscle activity in a spastic dysphonia patient, *J Speech Hear Res* 50:54–59, 1985.

Shipp T, Izdebski K: Vocal frequency and vertical larynx positioning by singers and non-singers, *J Acoust Soc Am* 58:1104–1106, 1975.

Simpson LL: *Botulinum neurotoxin and tetanus toxin*, San Diego, 1989, Academic Press.

Thumfart WF: From larynx to vocal ability: new electrophysiological data, *Acta Otolaryngol* 105:425–431, 1988.

Ward R, et al: EMG electrode placement and verification for botox injection, Paper presented at The IV Annual Pacific Voice Conference, San Francisco, 1991.

Weiner WJ, Lang AE: *Movement disorders: a comprehensive survey*, Mount Kisco, New York, 1989, Fortuna.

Zemlin WR: *Speech and hearing science*, Englewood Cliffs, N.J., 1981, Prentice-Hall.

Zwirner P, et al: Acoustic changes in spasmodic dysphonia after botulinum toxin injection, *J Voice* 5:78–84, 1991.

CHAPTER 7

Management of the Professional Voice

MANAGEMENT APPROACHES FOR

- Acute upper respiratory infection
- Chronic gastroesophageal reflux laryngitis
- Improper vocal technique (singing and speaking)
- Vocal nodules
- Voice abuse
- Poor breathing techniques
- Poor posture
- Functional hypernasality.

MANAGEMENT STRATEGIES, INCLUDING

- Antibiotic therapy
- Steroid medication
- Relative voice rest
- Hydration
- Antacids
- H2 blocker
- Sleep position modifications
- Modification of eating habits
- Abdominal breathing training
- Relaxation training
- Elimination of hard glottal attacks
- Improving posture and stance
- Reduction of throat clearing
- Reduction of shouting
- Improve vocal focus
- Vocal function exercises
- Airflow biofeedback
- Vocal hygiene counseling

- Breathing training
- Linking words within phrases
- Enliven the soft palate.

The young pitcher came set, paused, kicked and released the ball. As he followed through, he felt a twinge in his pitching arm and shoulder. It was a feeling he had never felt before. It was not really pain, but a burning sensation that ran from the back of his bicep, up his arm, and through his shoulder to his neck. The pitch was low and outside, and the catcher returned the ball. The pitcher walked behind the mound, windmilled his arm in both directions, and stretched it across his body. Knowing that this was not the pitcher's normal routine, the manager became alert and stepped to the top step of the dug-out for a better look. The pitcher returned to the mound. The catcher put one finger down and tapped the inside of his left leg, signaling an inside fast-ball. The pitcher fired the ball, which sailed high over the batter's head. As he released the ball, he grabbed his arm, wincing in pain. The manager and trainer rushed to the mound. The relief pitcher was called into the game, and the starter was immediately sent to the hospital for preliminary x-rays. After the game, the manager told reporters that he didn't think the injury was serious. Nevertheless, even though the team was in a tight pennant race, he would not rush the pitcher back into a game until they were certain he was 100% sound. The pitcher was much too valuable to the team to risk further or permanent damage.

The tenor was singing in the second of three acts, in the third performance of a week-long run. The opera featured his role and the music was extremely demanding, especially for his young voice. He had felt a little under the weather that day and was physically and vocally fatigued. While singing a strenuous duet with the female lead, he reached for a climactic "A" which he reached and then suddenly released. The soprano knew something was wrong. The conductor raised his eyes to the stage. The tenor suppressed a cough caused by a severe tickle and dry feeling in his throat. He was alarmed, but knew that he must continue. Between the second and third acts, the tenor drank some warm water, which relieved the tickle. The dry feeling persisted, and his speaking voice was slightly husky. The soprano quietly asked of his condition, to which he smiled and replied that he was fine. The third act was uneventful, but the tenor's singing voice was uninspired and lacked its typical color and clarity. Though concerned, the tenor, his manager, and the conductor excused the problem as fatigue. This role was a career opportunity that the tenor did not wish to "blow." Unfortunately, his voice "blew" before the end of the week. When a medical examination was finally conducted, indirect laryngoscopy revealed a hemorrhage of the right vocal fold which likely occurred at the first sign of trouble. His continued singing had threatened permanent damage.

Khambato (1979) paralleled the experiences of professional singers and actors with those of professional athletes. Because of their physical work demands, athletes are at greater risk than the general population for developing muscular and joint injuries. Likewise, because singers and actors demand more from their voices than would the average person, they are at greater risk for developing laryngeal disorders. Despite these similarities, the mentality for seeking treatment for injuries, as shown in the foregoing examples, is often very different for the two professional populations.

The prized athlete is generally required by management to seek treatment for injury promptly so as to quickly promote healing and reduce the possibility of further or permanent damage. Singers and actors, however, often minimize the disability to avoid canceling even one engagement. Granted, the financial ramifications may be huge, but permanent injury would certainly be worse. Professional actors and singers often fear developing a reputation for unreliability and continue using the damaged voice, often risking permanent vocal disability.

Even nonperformance professional voice users, such as teachers, clergy, and lecturers, typically behave in the same manner as their more elite counterparts. In the face of vocal difficulties, teachers continue to teach, lecturers continue to lecture, and preachers continue to preach rather than risk loss of income, and damage to their reputations, or because they simply see no other alternative.

Who then are professional voice users? Professional voice users are those individuals who are directly dependent on vocal communication for their livelihood. Koufman and Isaacson (1991) suggested a "vocal usage" classification system comprised of four levels.

Level 1 is the **elite vocal performer.** Professional singers and actors for whom even slight vocal difficulty may cause serious consequences belong in this level. **Level II** is the **professional voice user,** for whom even moderate vocal difficulty would prevent adequate job performance. Clergy, public speakers, lecturers, telephone operators, airline reservationists, and so on are examples of level II.

Level III is the **nonvocal professional.** This level is comprised of doctors, lawyers, business persons, sales persons, and others who could not perform their work properly if suffering with severe dysphonia. Mild or moderate dysphonias may be inconvenient, but would not preclude adequate job performance. **Level IV** is the **nonvocal nonprofessional.** This is the factory worker, laborer, and clerk who would not be prevented from doing their work if experiencing vocal disability. The history and vocal needs of each patient will ultimately determine his or her own personal vocal level.

This chapter deals with the management of voice disorders in the elite vocal performer and the professional voice user (levels I and II). A voice disorder in this population has a dual impact. Not only does it cause the interfering vocal symptoms characteristic of the disorder, it also carries with it a high level of emotional strain and anxiety. The anxiety is caused by the disorder's potential impact on the person's reputation, ability to meet professional commitments, and ability to perform and make a living.

The multidisciplinary voice team is the recommended standard of care for all voice disorders. The team approach is even more essential for the professional voice user. Individuals who comprise the voice team must all work together to remediate all aspects of the voice disorder. These aspects include management of general health and emotional health, vocal hygiene counseling, symptom modification, and retraining of the artistic voice. Team members will include the professional voice user, the otolaryngologist, the speech pathologist, the vocal coach, and the singing coach. Occasionally the voice user's manager and producers must also be included in the rehabilitative process. Successful rehabilitation may depend on the abilities of these professionals to compromise and work together with the patient's **long-term** vocal health as the primary consideration. Ideally, the professional voice user will ultimately assume responsibility for the well-being of his or her own voice (Stemple, 1984).

It may be common to assume that because of the intimate dependency relationships that professional voice users have with their voices, that they would know how their laryngeal mechanisms work and understand general concepts of good vocal hygiene. This assumption is seldom correct. Indeed, in our practice, we find few professional voice users who have even a vague awareness of the anatomy and physiology of the vocal mechanics. Nor do they understand the consequences of poor vocal hygiene. Therefore, education becomes a very important part of any remediation program.

Many fine publications have recently detailed the evaluation and management of the professional voice user (Sataloff, 1991; Gould, 1991; Stemple, 1984; Lavorato and McFarlane, 1983). These publications cover common causes of voice disorders in this population. Causative factors include:

1. **Misuse and abuse.** Poor singing/ speaking technique, singing out of range, chronic coughing/throat clear-

ing, smoking, poor hydration, over-use of the voice.
2. **Chronic medical problems.** Esophageal reflux, allergies, sinusitis, upper respiratory infections, prescription drug use, poor diet, fatigue, illicit drug use.
3. **Environmental factors.** Performing in smoky, dry, musty environments; exhaustive schedules; dry environments such as airplanes and hotel rooms; loud back-up music; parties; poor acoustics.
4. **Emotional factors.** Stage fright, anxiety, self-confidence, depression, performance stress.

The professional voice user is also susceptible to any and all causes of voice disorders common to the general population. The case studies in this chapter examine many of these etiologic factors. The studies also illustrate the advantages of the multidisciplinary management team for the remediation of voice disorders in the professional voice user.

VOICE THERAPY COMBINED WITH VOCAL COACHING

Contributed by Robert Thayre Sataloff, M.D.

In the following case study, Robert Thayre Sataloff, M.D., combines medical treatment with voice therapy and vocal coaching to successfully remediate the threatening voice problems of a legitimate "rock star."

CASE STUDY: PATIENT CC

Patient CC, a 24-year-old rock music star was seen emergently during the second month of his first world tour promoting an album. Initially, he complained only of a sore throat and upper respiratory infection that had been present for 2 days. However, inquiry revealed several other problems that really were of greater concern to him. He reported a 3-week history of hoarseness and neck pain following singing, breathiness, decreased ability to sing softly, and diminished range (especially upper). When the symptoms first appeared, they were noticeable primarily following performances, but his voice was normal the following day. For the previous 2 weeks, his voice had remained hoarse and breathy all the time, although it became considerably worse during performances. He also had a long history of morning hoarseness, halitosis, prolonged warm-up time, and frequent throat clearing; and these symptoms seemed to have become more pronounced in the past few weeks which had also been characterized by extreme stress. He was known for clear, ballad-like high singing, and he had already had to cut some of his most famous songs from his concerts. He was performing three or four nights per week in large halls and stadiums. He had no formal training for speech or singing, although he was extremely intelligent and well educated in other disciplines. He had no other medical illnesses, used no medications or recreational drugs, and was highly motivated and cooperative.

Physical examination revealed normal ears and hearing, mild nasal congestion, moderate pharyngitis, and no neck masses. His speaking voice was hoarse and breathy. Indirect laryngoscopy showed marked erythema of the arytenoids, with no significant erythema or edema of the true vocal folds, except at the junctions of the anterior and middle thirds, where there were small nodules. Strobovideolaryngoscopy confirmed that glottic closure was impaired anterior and posterior to these soft masses. There were no hemorrhages, mucosal disruptions, or adynamic segments. Flexible fiberoptic laryngoscopy revealed supraglottic hyperfunction with decreased anterior-posterior diameter during speaking at his habitual pitch. Laryngeal architecture returned to normal with a slight voluntary increase in pitch.

Objective voice analysis revealed normal pulmonary function, with increased laryngeal mean airflow rate. Perturbation, jitter, and shimmer were mildly increased, and the harmonic-to-noise ratio and percent voiced speech were decreased. Formal evaluations by a certified speech-language pathologist and a singing voice specialist confirmed the vocal problems noted, analyzed them in greater detail, and included trial therapy that showed the patient's excellent ability to modify voice technique quickly. He had an excessive number of harsh glottal attacks. He spoke English with a British accent, although he was from a northern European country and English was not his native tongue. Examination of his singing technique revealed an unbalanced stance, with weight over his heels; ineffective abdominal support; thoracic breathing; alteration in laryngeal position with pitch changes; and excessive tension in his neck, jaw, and especially the tongue. Similar problems were present in his speaking voice, to a lesser degree. The hoarseness and breathiness were present throughout his range, but less apparent on lower notes. There was a poorly controlled break in his passagio.

Discussion

Professional singers frequently have complex, multiple medical problems (Sataloff, 1991). This patient's difficulties included (1) acute upper respiratory infection, (2) chronic gastroesophageal reflux laryngitis, (3) improper vocal technique, and (4) nodules.

The management of acute upper respiratory infection in professional singers depends on the severity of the infection, skill of the singer, importance of upcoming performances, and long-term performance schedule. In this case, pharyngeal cultures were taken, and the patient was started empirically on an antibiotic. Cultures later revealed that the antibiotic choice (ampicillin) was appropriate for his infection with *Haemophilus influenzae*. Corticosteroids have a place in the management of upper respiratory infections, but they must be used with great caution. In a technically excellent singer who has a particularly important performance followed by a period of rest, a short course of steroid medication may be extremely valuable for inflammatory or even infectious laryngitis. However, in the case presented here, signs of infection were limited to the pharynx. The arytenoid edema was caused by gastroesophageal reflux, and the nodules were caused by voice abuse. There was no significant vocal fold edema except the traumatic response around the nodules, and steroids were not used. Absolute voice rest (silence) is rarely necessary except following submucosal hemorrhage or mucosal disruption (traumatic tear), and it was not used in this case. However, relative voice rest is always helpful. The patient was counseled regarding voice conservation and hygiene, and instructed to use his voice only when he was being paid to do so. Hydration is a particularly important consideration. However, in singers with reflux, large quantities of water should not be consumed immediately prior to singing, because upright reflux during performance is common and is worsened with a stomach full of clear liquids.

Morning hoarseness, chronic sore throat, frequent throat clearing, excessive phlegm, prolonged warm-up time, a sensation of a "lump in the throat," and night coughing are common signs of gastroesophageal reflux laryngitis. Typical dyspepsia (heartburn) is usually absent. Reflux is common among singers for several reasons. First, they frequently perform on an empty stomach late at night, then eat immediately before retiring. This induces reflux by generating acid secretion and mechanically stressing the lower esophageal sphincter. Second, abdominal support necessarily includes increased intra-abdominal pressure which tends to compress the stomach, causing its contents to reflux into the esophagus and throat. Third, performing careers are stressful. Stress is commonly believed to aggravate problems associated with gastric acidity, including reflux and ulcer disease. Gastroesophageal reflux is a chronic source of vocal fold irritation that frequently underlies other vocal problems. In this case, it was treated with elevation of the head of the bed, antacids, a H2 blocker (ranitidine), and avoidance of night-time eating. The patient was willing to modify his habits so as to eat a larger breakfast and lunch, a light supper a few hours before performance, and nothing for 3 hours before going to sleep.

The small, early vocal nodules should not be diagnosed on the basis of one examination. "Physiological swellings" that resemble nodules occur in many singers, but disappear after 24 to 48 hours of voice rest. They are not believed to be significant clinically. This patient was asked to remain silent except when absolutely necessary for 24 hours and was reexamined. Slight edema around the nodules had resolved, but they were still clearly present. The proper treatment for vocal nod-

ules is voice modification, not surgery, and not silence. Because of this patient's compelling professional commitments (documented by the fact that his insurance company paid $250,000.00 for every performance canceled), only two performances were canceled for medical reasons. Emergency voice therapy and singing lessons were instituted. He received 1-hour sessions of each, once or twice daily for 1 week. Voice therapy concentrated on development of abdominal breathing and support, connection of breath support with vocal production, and relaxation of hyperfunctional muscles in the head and neck. Speaking pitch was not addressed specifically, but it increased spontaneously by approximately three semitones when the excessive tongue, jaw, and neck tension were eliminated.

Because English was not patient CC's language, he had no particular need to continue the dialect of British English (Liverpool area) he had acquired, an accent characterized by a high percentage of harsh glottal attacks. His native northern European language did not have a similar pattern, and his speech was initially much better in his mother tongue than it was in English. A limited amount of accent training ameliorated this problem. The speaking voice training was extremely helpful to him not only in daily life, but also during radio and television interviews. Traditional voice therapy was coordinated with singing voice training. This also concentrated on development of abdominal support and relaxation of head and neck muscles. He was trained rapidly to produce the sounds he needed without vocal strain, but without sounding "operatic." The voice therapy team attended his first concert in Philadelphia and subsequent concerts elsewhere over the next few weeks. He was able to incorporate the speaking and singing modifications into his performances quickly. His ability to sing his customary repertoire began returning within 2 weeks, and his nodules resolved in approximately 6 weeks.

Summary

This patient's upper respiratory infection resolved promptly, of course. He was able to complete his tour without difficulty. He has continued to use trained speaking and singing technique, and anti-reflux therapy. He has had no further voice problems.

THE DEVELOPING PERFORMER

Contributed by Barbara Jacobson, Ph.D.

In the following case study, Barbara Jacobson, Ph.D., reports the case of a young "top-40" singer who presented with multiple medical/voice misuse factors causing hoarseness and reduction in singing ability.

CASE STUDY: PATIENT DD

Patient DD, a 27-year-old female singer, was self-referred to the professional voice clinic for complaints of diminished control of her singing voice, decreased vocal range for singing, and loss of "head register" (ability to focus her voice for high notes). In particular, she felt that she was unable to produce enough nasal resonance. She believed this inadequate nasal resonance was due to some sinus problem or nasal cavity deformity. She was seen in the multidisciplinary clinic on the same day by a speech-language pathologist, otolaryngologist, and voice teacher. She was planning to record a demonstration tape of her singing for distribution to record labels, and this was the impetus for seeking help now.

Patient DD gave the following voice history. She had been singing since she was very young. She was a cheerleader in high school. She sang in school choirs and began singing top-40 repertoire professionally in her late teens in night clubs. She typically sang six to seven nights per week, with multiple sets (at least three) per night. She often sang in smoky environments. At age 21 years she developed significant problems with her voice, particularly after one episode when she had prolonged voice loss after a "strep throat" infection. At that time she was diagnosed with vocal nodules. After a period of voice rest, the nodules persisted and she underwent a bilateral vocal fold stripping. She did not receive voice therapy at that time. Since then, her voice has been essentially the same.

Patient DD had formal voice training (for pop singing) at ages 18 and 21. She acknowl-

edged that she had difficulty at that time applying the knowledge from these lessons to her singing technique. She felt that she was an alto with an occasional ability to sing second soprano. She believed her singing style was most consistent with a "belting" technique. Her current singing range was approximately one-and-one-half octaves, which was significantly below her potential range when she was able to sing well. Any attempts to reach higher notes resulted in a "double sound."

The patient's medical history was remarkable for temporomandibular joint dysfunction with bruxism, hiatal hernia, and suspected allergies (which were not documented). Gastroesophageal reflux had not been demonstrated by barium swallow study or manometry. The patient described bulimic and anorexic behavior that had occurred approximately 8 years previously. This lasted for 1 year. She did not seek medical or psychiatric assistance. From her report, it was not clear whether she continued to be bulimic. The patient currently was taking no medications. She did not use antihistamines or aspirin. Fluid intake was adequate. She drank two to three beers per week. She occasionally drank a caffeinated beverage. She had a 5-year history of one pack per day cigarette smoking but had quit 6 years ago.

Patient DD was employed as a social activities director for an apartment complex. Job responsibilities included writing a weekly newsletter, organizing parties and events, and coordinating fund raisers for the community. She also modeled in clubs which were often smoky and dry. This job also involved speaking with people over noise and music. She described her daily voice use as moderate to heavy. At the time of assessment, she was involved in a relationship that was troublesome for her. Most of the yelling that she did was in arguments with her boyfriend. She described feeling her throat tighten during these episodes.

Otolaryngologic evaluation revealed slightly dry nasal mucosa. Oral cavity, oropharynx, and nasopharynx were normal. Indirect laryngoscopic examination was remarkable for a large posterior glottic chink with some erythema and edema of the arytenoid cartilages. There was also a small amount of irregularity along the free margin of the vocal folds. Palpation of the neck was unremarkable, although there was marked popping in her temporomandibular joints.

Objective voice analysis included videostroboscopy, which demonstrated a large posterior glottic chink, as noted on otolaryngologic examination. There was slight compression of the ventricular folds on phonation onset. This increased supraglottic activity was particularly apparent at the patient's register break, at the transition from her modal to head voice. During stroboscopy, it was noted that the mucosal wave was moderately decreased bilaterally. In addition, during phonation, vocal folds were open proportionately most of the time. All other vibratory parameters were essentially within normal limits. These videostroboscopic results indicated that the patient had a significant amount of air wastage during phonation and exhibited tension at selected points in her singing range. The patient's acoustic analysis is shown in Table 7–1. All acoustic measures, with the exception of low fundamental frequency at a comfortable pitch, were essentially normal. The

results of her aerodynamic analysis are shown in Table 7–2.

What appeared most striking about these results was that all measures were essentially normal except for high airflow rates at habitual pitch. Normally, we might expect that airflow values would be quite low at all pitches and even across all pitches for singers. Phonation times should be significantly longer than the average 18-20 seconds we expect for nonsingers. Results for this patient reflected inefficient laryngeal valving during phonation at her habitual pitch.

Perceptual analysis of the patient's voice revealed a mild dysphonia characterized by slight breathiness and slight dry hoarseness. Habitual pitch was perceived as being low. Habitual loudness in conversation was increased. There was a slight reduction in vocal fold compression when the patient shouted. Abusive voice production behaviors included throat clearing and hard glottal attacks. The patient was able to sustain /a/ for only 13 seconds. Her s/z ratio was 1.57 (normal = 1.4). An oral peripheral examination revealed normal oral structures for voice production. There

TABLE 7–1.

Acoustic Analysis for Patient DD

FO* (Hz)	Jitter (msec)	Shimmer (%)	Signal-to-Noise Ratio (dB)
Habitual pitch			
173.55	.020	2.045	21.50
High pitch			
624.50	.009	2.865	23.345
Low pitch			
148.30	.0325	3.025	18.485
Reading			
178.7	.075	4.06	14.17

*Mean values are shown. Semitone range = 33.4

TABLE 7–2.

Results of Aerodynamic Analysis for Patient DD

Flow Volume* (mL)	Maximum Phonation Time (sec)	Peak Flow Rate (mL/sec)	Airflow Rate (mL/sec)
Habitual pitch			
3,630	14.85	390	244.35
High pitch			
3,360	30.05	205	111.80
Low pitch			
3,245	25.0	225	130.25

*Mean values are shown.

was significant neck and jaw musculoskeletal tension on palpation and manipulation.

Assessment by the voice teacher was significant for reduced vocal range. There were some abnormal jaw and tongue postures observed during singing. In addition, the patient had some difficulty dissociating jaw and tongue movements while singing. Breath support appeared to be normal; however, the patient tended to fix the chest excessively during singing and especially on inhalation. Tension was quite apparent during all aspects of singing.

Consensus by the voice team was that the cause of the patient's voice disorder was multidimensional. There appeared to be influences from her speaking as well as her singing technique. Her medical and surgical history (bruxism, bulimia, vocal fold stripping) also contributed. At the time of assessment, it was not clear which was the most salient cause of her voice disorder. Consequently, it was decided to treat her from several different aspects. She was given anti-reflux regimen. This was the only medical intervention deemed necessary by the otolaryngologist at this time. Responsibility for day-to-day management was assigned to the voice pathologist and voice teacher.

Patient DD immediately began voice therapy and voice lessons. Coordination between the voice pathologist and voice teacher was quite close, and treatment goals were developed in such a fashion as to be parallel. We were quite struck by the patient's motivation and commitment to achieving improvement in her voice and felt that this reflected favorably on her prognosis and eventual outcome.

In voice therapy, treatment goals were established to improve vocal hygiene, in particular, to reduce yelling, throat clearing, and amount of time spent in aversive environments. Because the patient was not singing at this time, no restrictions were placed on singing. Voice production goals were to improve awareness of respiratory support of voice with a reduction in breath holding; change voice onset to a more breathy, more relaxed approach; reduce laryngeal area muscle tension; and change vocal focus for speech. In addition, to optimize vocal fold closure, a program of specific vocal exercise designed for vocal

strengthening and endurance (Vocal Function Exercises) was implemented to produce more vocal fold closure. As with many aspiring professional singers, this patient had no insurance. Therefore, treatment sessions were very focused and the patient followed a structured home program.

Weekly or biweekly visits were scheduled and the patient demonstrated compliance with vocal hygiene recommendations. Areas of treatment emphasis were coordinated with the voice teacher. For example, structured tasks specifically focused on reducing musculoskeletal tension were timed to correspond with work in relaxing jaw and tongue and increasing supraglottic "space" during voice lessons.

After four sessions, the patient's laryngeal status was monitored with videostroboscopy. At that time, there was a slight reduction in the size of her posterior glottic chink. Also evident at that time was an increase in the amplitude of vibration of the vocal folds. Subjectively, the patient was beginning to notice an increase in her vocal range. She remarked that she did not feel as though she had to "push" as much to produce voice for either speaking or singing. Perceptually, we noticed an increase in her habitual pitch.

Over the course of treatment, patient DD was able to increase times for sustaining notes C through G on Vocal Function Exercises. Gradually, she lost the breathy quality on a sustained tone, inferring increased vocal efficiency. In particular, the patient found these exercises to be most helpful for monitoring the status of her voice. If she had used her voice too strenuously on the previous night, then on the following morning she noticed a decrease in the amount of time she was able to produce a soft sustained tone. This served to reinforce her ability to self-monitor vocally abusive behaviors.

While most treatment goals were addressed using traditional techniques and methods, vocal fold closure was approached by using biofeedback. Utilizing the Phonatory Function Analyzer (Nagashima), the patient used the readout for airflow rate to monitor the relationship between vocal focus and laryngeal area tension and a more efficient vocal fold closure during production of sustained vowels. She was able to drop her airflow rate at habitual pitch into a more acceptable range below 150 mL/sec.

Progress in improvement of both speaking and singing voice was quite rapid. The patient reported that the coordinated focus of treatment goals in both voice therapy and voice lessons helped her to understand concepts more quickly, even though the vocabulary might be somewhat different. In voice therapy, the patient was asked to associate consciously techniques and principles for speaking with those for singing. Her voice teacher reported that as she worked during voice lessons; a soprano vocal range was emerging.

Voice therapy continued for eight sessions. At the end of that time, post-treatment objective measures were made as was a reanalysis of perceptual features. Significant changes were evident in airflow rate at habitual pitch, in fundamental frequency at habitual pitch and while reading, in vocal quality, and in perceived habitual pitch and loudness. Comparison of pretreatment and post-treatment measures are shown in Tables 7–3 and 7–4.

Perceptually, the patient's speaking voice was focused more appropriately. Loudness in conversation was at a suitable level. There was a reduction in laryngeal area muscle tension. Overall, the patient reported that producing a voice for speaking was easier. The effort to produce a well-focused voice was more automatic and less conscious.

The most telling result of treatment was demonstrated in comparison of recordings of her singing voice from 7 years ago, just prior

to treatment, and at the end of treatment. In the last recording, the patient observed a "brighter" sound with better resonance; better support of the voice throughout a phrase; notes produced on pitch; and stronger, clearer notes at the high end of her singing range. Voice therapy was ended with follow-up to be maintained by telephone contact. The patient continued to receive voice lessons.

HYPERFUNCTIONAL VOICE IN AN ACTOR

Contributed by Bonnie N. Raphael, Ph.D.

In the following case study, Bonnie N. Raphael, Ph.D., describes several excellent direct therapy techniques for retraining the hyperfunctional voice of an otherwise accomplished actor.

CASE STUDY: PATIENT EE

Among both students and long-time members of the acting profession, there is a high incidence of hyperfunctional voice production. In the case of the actress discussed, this hyperfunction led to the occurrence of vocal nodules, but the program of training she underwent would be basically the same even in their absence and would serve the needs of hyperfunctional actors and public speakers not yet exhibiting an organic change in the vocal folds.

TABLE 7–3.
Aerodynamic Analysis for Patient DD

Condition	Flow Volume (mL)	Maximum Phonation Time (sec)	Airflow Rate (mL/sec)
/a/	3,480	28.4	122.53
/i/	3,740	29.7	125.93
X	3,610	29.1	124.23

TABLE 7–4.
Airflow Rates (mL/sec) for Patient DD

Condition	Pretreatment	Following Treatment	% Change
/a/	235.4	122.5	52
/i/	253.3	125.9	49
X	244.3	124.2	51

History and Evaluation

When patient EE, a 26-year-old actor from Chicago, auditioned in February 1988, her acting skills and considerable talent were immediately apparent, as was her husky, hypernasal voice. When questioned, she volunteered that she had been diagnosed with vocal nodules 2 years earlier and had received some therapy at that time. She was accepted into the American Repertory Theatre Institute for Advanced Theatre Training at Harvard University, Cambridge, Massachusetts, on the condition that she put herself into the hands of the voice and speech coach and adhere to a specific program of remediation.

A preliminary voice and speech evaluation was done in September, 1988, during patient EE's first week of training. This assessment was based on a performance of two audition pieces, a background questionnaire, an interview, and a reading of a Shakespearian sonnet. I found that the location of major breathing activity was a bit too high, that ability to sustain phonation was poor, that conversational pitch level was a bit low, and that functional pitch range was a bit limited. Patient EE was not in the habit of linking words within the same phrase together and exhibited consistent hard glottal initiation, especially in performance and when reading aloud. The quality of her voice was hypernasal, husky, and breathy. Articulation was fairly close to standard, with the exception of a high degree of /r/ coloration (that is, an overly prominent /r/ sound following vowels and diphthongs) and enough habitual jaw tightness to lead to a substitution of [sI/aI]. Head posture was a bit stiff, and the head was thrust forward from the trunk of the body. Her upper spine and the chest were a bit collapsed, and her shoulders somewhat rounded as well. The characteristic position of the jaw was tight and held.

During the course of her diagnostic interview, the patient discussed the fact that she suffered from chronic allergies, had frequent upper respiratory infections and sinusitis, and had developed vocal nodules in May 1986, while performing in a show and teaching aerobics at the same time. She had had some voice therapy "to emphasize diaphragmatic breathing ('I use it so much that now sometimes my stomach hurts after I talk a lot'), to

adjust her neck position, to elevate pitch, and to decrease hard glottal attack," and she described herself as free of serious problems for the last 18 months. The patient said she had quit smoking in 1986, but I observed her smoking occasionally during the 2 years she spent at A.R.T.. At her initial interview, she stated two primary goals she wished to achieve during her training: to be able to do what she needs to as an actress without fear ("Right now, I feel okay for the first week or two, but then my voice breaks down"), and to develop a more extensive pitch range.

I was fortunate indeed to have a speech therapist interning with me at the time, and had her do a preliminary evaluation as well. In addition to corroborating my findings, the therapist classified this actress as an excessive talker, as having a rapid rate of utterance, as having an [s/z] ratio of 16 seconds to 10 seconds (a ratio of 1.4/1 or higher is considered indicative of voice disorder), and as having an ability to sustain phonation for 12 seconds (a normal voice should be able to sustain phonation for 20 seconds).

Patient EE was also examined at the Voice and Speech Laboratory at Boston University. Examination with a rigid endoscope, accompanied by videostroboscopy, produced a diagnosis of "mobile nodules — pliable and some thickening," which the consulting otolaryngological physician felt were "reversible with therapy."

Program of Study

On the basis of her history and evaluations, the following priorities were established for patient EE's vocal training program.

1. Information on vocal hygiene and preservation
2. Continued work on head posture in order to eliminate a habitual jaw thrust and to increase mobility
3. Lowering the location of major breathing activity and establishing a better isometric balance in the larynx
4. Releasing the jaw to allow more room for vocal production and articulation and also lessen the degree of /r/ coloration

5. Linking words within any phrase together in order not to break up the breathstream unnecessarily during speech (especially when projecting from on-stage) in order to eliminate hard glottal initiation
6. Enlivening the soft palate in order to lessen nasality
7. Developing the ability to focus vocal tone to get it out of the throat and into the mask.

(Note: We began to work on projection and range extension as well, but didn't get very far in these areas by the time the patient's training program came to an end.)

Patient EE was actively involved in a 2-year program of professional training, augmented by seventeen 30- to 45-minute individual therapy sessions with a consulting speech pathologist during the first half of her 1st year. Voice classes met three times each week for 75 to 90 minutes. During the 1st year of training, emphasis in class is placed on dynamic relaxation exercises, breathing, alignment, warm-up exercises, and warm-down exercises (for the whole body; for the shoulders, neck, jaw, tongue and face; and for the voice itself), resonation, range, and articulation. The text, and philosophy or technique, that forms the basis for the vocal work is Kristin Linklater's *Freeing the Natural Voice* (1976). In addition, one class per week is spent on text analysis, especially as it applies to the understanding of Shakespearian verse.

During the second year of training, facial posture, control of tonal sensations, and specificity and musicality of the consonant sounds are addressed through the work of Arthur Lessac, as discussed in his text, *The Use and Training of the Human Voice* (1967). In addition, one class per week is spent on stage dialects.

In addition, Patient EE had one singing class per week (12 students; 90 minutes) with another teacher during each of her 2 years of training.

Remediation of Hyperfunction

What follows is a selected number of specific exercises which I used with patient EE

in order to address the hyperfunction in her conversational and performing voice.

Isometric Exercise for Releasing Head Into Optimum Position

While sitting or standing easily and comfortably, intertwine the fingers of both hands so that they hold the back of your skull (not your neck). Allow the head to press backwards steadily into the palms of your hands as you pull the elbows forward with an equal, steady pressure. These two pressures should be firm and equal, strong enough to set up an isometric balance between the two forces but not strong enough to restrict the breath in any way or to cause any discomfort in the shoulders, the neck, the jaw or the spine. Continue this steady pressure for a full minute or so as you continue to breathe easily and freely. Release the shoulders as you press, so that they are not involved any more than is absolutely necessary. Then, drop your hands to your sides, releasing the head into a floating and weightless feeling atop your spine. Walk around a bit, turning your head, using your eyes and enjoying the freedom of a released cervical spine. (This exercise can be used as many times per day as you feel neck stiffness or fatigue.)

*Exercises to Release the Jaw**

Standing easily and comfortably, clasp one hand in the other in front of you in a "praying position" and, releasing the jaw, shake the hands to and fro in such a way that the resulting shimmer or shake spreads up the arms, through the shoulders and neck and into the jaw itself. See whether you can keep the jaw engaged in this passive or secondary shake as you inhale and exhale freely. If and when you can, vocalize on the outgoing breath while continuing the shake. If and when this becomes easy, move the voice up and down in pitch a bit and then more extensively, all the while continuing the hand shake. When you stop, you may notice a warmth or tingling in the muscles of the cheeks and jaw. Open the mouth a few times to see whether there is any difference in jaw mobility.

---

* For further information and exercises for releasing the jaw and tongue, see Kristin Linklater, *Freeing the Natural Voice*, New York, 1976, DBS Publications, pp. 57–71.

With your jaw hanging loosely and passively, place your thumbs together right under your chin and the knuckles of your forefingers in front of the chin. (Make sure you are grasping bone and not just flesh.) As you inhale and exhale easily, use your fingers (but not the muscles of your jaw) to gently shake the jaw, first slowly and easily and then, as you feel it letting go, more quickly and freely (but not extensively enough to hit your top teeth with your bottom ones.) If and when this becomes easy to do, vocalize on each outgoing breath. When this becomes easy to do, continue the shaking while moving the pitch higher and lower in your range. You'll know the exercise has accomplished what it was designed to do when you can sing any note in your range while freely shaking the jaw with your hand(s) at the same time.

Rules for Linking Together Words Within a Phrase*

If, as an actor speaks, words within phrases are connected together, this will save wear and tear on the throat by avoiding hard glottal initiation, especially when speaking over background noise or music. Linking also prevents the actor from sounding tense, angry, phony, overly careful, or choppy when speaking.

1. Whenever a word ends with /U/, or /OU/, or /aU/ (so that the lips are already rounded), and is followed by a word beginning with any vowel, a very light /w/ is used to connect them together: to (w)anybody, go (w)after, how amazing, two (w)animals, and so forth.

2. Whenever a word ends with /i/, or /eI/, or /oI/, or /aI/ (so that the lips are already gently spread), and is followed by a word beginning with any vowel, a very light /j/ ("y") is used to connect them together: be (y)able, stay over, toy animals, I (y)arrived, and so forth.

3. Whenever a word ends with a consonant and the next word begins with a vowel, they should be linked together directly: take action, live alone, call out, went over, less expensive, and so forth.

Kinesthetic Techniques for Getting the Vocal Tone Into the Mask†

If and when the actor can learn to sense the vibration of sound on the alveolar ridge during the production of the /i/ vowel, then he or she can use this as a referent or an anchor, first for the closely-related /eI/ diphthong and then, in a somewhat diluted form, for the other vowels as well.

1. Beautiful . . . Byyutiful . . . Byyyyutiful, and so forth. As you sustain the /i/ vowel for longer and longer periods of time, make whatever adjustments are needed (for example, in amount of air flow, pitch, amount of space between the teeth, shape of lip opening, tongue position) to maximize the sensation of vibration on the alveolar ridge.

2. YeeeYeeeYeeeYeee, and so forth, Each time you add a "Y" impulse to this vibration, let it serve as a reminder to you to allow the tongue to be forward in the mouth and to release sound vibration right into the alveolar ridge.

3. Pinch your nostrils shut, plug your ears and close your eyes as you continue to maximize the amount of buzzing vibration you can experience. When the buzz is rich and effortless, unplug ears and nose and enjoy the full power of this focused sound.

4. Explore the richness of this vibration over a range of about half an octave, from low in your range (but not fry) up into conversational pitches. Be sure to keep the sensation of vibration locked onto the alveolar ridge.

5. He sees me ski . . . We need steam heat immediately.

6. Move from a forward flowing /i/ vibration to the /eI/ diphthong and back to the /i/ again. As you alternate between the two sounds, take particular care to keep the vibration focused securely on the alveolar ridge: yyyyyyEyyyyyyEyyyyyEyyyyy.

7. Explore the range of this vibratory sensation by moving it up and down a bit in pitch while retaining the focus.

---

*For further information on and exercises for linking see Arthur Lessac, *The Use and Training of the Human Voice,* New York, 1967, DBS Publications, pp. 172–178.)

†For further information on and exercises in this area, see Arthur Lessac, *The Use and Training of the Human Voice,* New York, 1967, DBS Publications, pp. 79-94, especially the Carryover Exercise on p. 91.

8. create . . . berate . . . we ate . . . She creates extremely tame plays . . . Take the late train with me.

9. Intone the alphabet, finding as many opportunities as you can to incorporate the alveolar ridge sensations as you do so. If necessary, distort certain letters a bit, so that the sensations remain strong and specific. Repeat, this time allowing speech-like inflections to accompany the tonality; treat the alphabet like a language in itself, and use it to communicate thoughts and feelings without sacrificing tonal focus in the process.

Discussion

The training and therapeutic process were both augmented and undermined by the fact that patient DD was very much in demand as an actress in our company and played a number of major roles in an ongoing series of productions. Because of her level of talent, she was cast in both Equity company (professional) and Institute (student) productions, and she was often cast in vocally demanding roles or sizable understudy assignments as well. These included:

First Year

The Serpent Woman — Equity Company production directed by Andrei Serban. The patient played a major role very athletically and in a half mask. (Note: This show went into rehearsal 1 month after the patient's arrival in Cambridge.)

The Maids — Institute Production. Two-character play; a demanding role.

Talk to Me Like the Rain — Institute Production. Two-character play; a demanding role.

Second Year

Suburbia — Institute Production directed by Eric Bogosian. The patient played a rape victim, which involved highly emotional scenes.

Twelfth Night — Equity Production directed by Andrei Serban. The patient understudied the role of Viola and played a nonspeaking role.

Major Barbara — Equity Production directed by Michael Engler. The patient played the minor role of Sarah and understudied the title character.

Mirandolina — Institute Production. The patient played the title role.

Little Eyolf — Institute Production. The patient played the vocally demanding role of the Rat Wife.

Despite this excessive amount of casting throughout her 2 years at A.R.T., when patient EE was seen again at the Boston University Clinic during her second year of training, she was examined by the same consulting otolaryngological physician, who viewed her previous videotapes for purposes of comparison and noted "wide band nodules — less inflamed than previous examination — some reduction in size of nodules" despite the fact that the patient had been suffering "postnasal drip for the past 3 months — suspect allergies".

By the end of the 2-year training program at A.R.T., patient EE's voice was far more clear (had more tone, less wasted air, was more projectible) and less hypernasal. She was still using insufficient linking of words within phrases and exhibited too much hard glottal initiation, but this had improved as well. She was no longer losing her voice except for a rare occasion where she had a medical problem or abused it and suffered some temporary consequences.

Immediately after completing her training, the patient was cast in a major role in an A.R.T. production of *King Stag* which toured to Japan. Within 6 months of her graduation, she was hired to play a nonspeaking role and to understudy all the women's roles in *La Bete*, which opened in a commercial house in Boston and went on to play briefly on Broadway, and she did a voiceover for a nationally telecast commercial for a major brand of coffee. So it was incumbent on the actress, both throughout her training and at the beginning of a busy professional career, to practice and habituate the exercises, strategies, and techniques to which she had been introduced despite continuing acting challenges and severe restrictions on her time. In this respect, her circumstances are quite representative of those of many actors and public speakers.

The remediation of hyperfunctional vocal habits is a lifelong process, especially for professional actors working on the live stage (as opposed to film or television). It is only with an ongoing commitment to optimal vocal use that previously injured or damaged voices can be reclaimed to the extent that they become truly flexible and responsive to the actor's needs as well as sturdy and reliable.

LEVEL II PROFESSIONAL VOICE USER

Contributed by Bernice Gerdeman, Ph.D.

In the next case study, Bernice Gerdeman, Ph.D., describes methods she finds useful for improving the vocal technique of a lecturer.

CASE STUDY: PATIENT FF

Patient FF, a 45-year-old male college professor, was referred to the Institute for Voice Analysis and Rehabilitation, with a 1-year history of vocal fatigue, soreness in the throat, hoarseness, and a feeling of a "lump in the throat." An indirect laryngoscopy performed by his otolaryngologist revealed normal appearing vocal folds. The patient's past medical history was unremarkable. He was generally in good health, he never smoked, and was not taking any medications. He drank alcohol occasionally, had no known allergies, and was never hospitalized for any illnesses or had ever received surgery. He denied any symptoms of dysphagia or esophageal reflux. The otolaryngologist referred the patient for a voice evaluation, videolaryngostroboscopic examination, and therapy as needed.

History

A case history revealed that patient FF was engaged in moderate to heavy amounts of speaking throughout the day. He lectured weekly for two different courses and conducted a graduate seminar. He was actively involved with research and had several graduate students working in his laboratory. Six months prior to the otolaryngologic visit, he was asked to serve on two university-wide committees, for one of which he was the chairperson. The patient occasionally traveled to lecture or meet with collaborative researchers on combined projects. At least once a week he attended a reception or a dinner at the university, which called for him to engage in conversation with increased background noise

present. His office had no windows and was located off the laboratory.

This professor was married and enjoyed being actively involved with his two young children's school and sport activities. He reportedly experienced difficulty with his voice when reading to his children in the evenings. When reading, he stated that his voice felt "forced" and that at times the voice would just "give out." He also noted that he was unable to sing along with the radio or in church. His voice would "crack," and he had less flexibility when trying to sing.

The professor stated that his voice was very hoarse in the early morning, cleared somewhat by mid-morning, fatigued with use during the day, and became worse in the evening to the point that his throat felt sore. His hoarseness and soreness in the throat was particularly noticed after lecturing or when engaged in talking for an extended period of time. He cleared his throat often, trying to rid the "lump feeling" in his throat, but when questioned, he reported it had no positive effect. The throat clearing was usually nonproductive.

Patient FF drank six to eight cups of caffeinated beverages per day. Alcohol consumption was three to six glasses of wine per week. He had no training in public speaking.

During the case history intake, the professor was observed to speak with a back and throaty placement. Mandibular movement was restricted. He spoke rapidly and in long sentences with little breath support to sustain speech. His display of muscular tension was evident in his neck, and he often kept the shoulders raised.

Videolaryngostroboscopic Examination

An oral peripheral examination revealed normal structures and function. While sustaining the vowel /i/ under direct light, the patient presented with an anterior glottal chink with slight compression of the ventricular folds bilaterally. The vocal folds were on the same vertical plane, and the vocal fold edges appeared smooth and straight. While sustaining /i/, a large amount of thick, sticky mucus accumulated on the superior surface of the vocal folds. The vocal folds appeared slightly erythematous. Under stroboscopic light the amplitude of vibration and mucosal wave were slightly decreased bilaterally. During the vibratory cycle the closed phase predominated and symmetry of vibration was generally irregular during pitch and loudness changes. The video tape was reviewed by the clinician and the professor immediately following the examination. The result of this examination revealed laryngeal myasthenia, which was confirmed by the otolaryngologist.

Objective Voice Assessment

Acoustic analysis revealed increased frequency perturbation during sustained vowels in modal pitch. Maximum phonation times were decreased for modal, high, and low pitches. Speaking and reading fundamental frequency were at the lower end of his frequency range. Airflow measurements for modal, high, and low sustained vowels were within the normal range.

Voice Therapy

Voice therapy was initiated 1 week following the diagnostic examination. Goals for this patient were as follows: (1) to eliminate all vocally abusive behaviors, especially throat clearing; (2) to balance and restrengthen the laryngeal musculature through vocal function exercises (see Chapter 1); (3) to promote an open oral front focus when reading and speaking; (4) to establish an oral hydration program; (5) to establish a vocal hygiene program; and (6) to instruct in good public speaking skills.

During the initial therapy session, the diagnosis was reviewed, the goals were discussed, and all questions were answered. I felt it was very important to educate the patient about the anatomy and physiology of the larynx. The professor was given an explanation of the cover-body theory as well as the aerodynamic-myoelastic theory of phonation. The videolaryngostroboscopic examination, drawings, and a three-dimensional model of the larynx were used to help him achieve a clear understanding of phonation.

I have found that once the voice client has the basic understanding of how the vocal folds

function it is easier to explain the purpose and rationale behind the treatment goals. It is also necessary for the voice patient to recognize the importance of achieving these goals in order to maximize the results and improve the voice quality.

Patient FF was educated on the effects of the vocally abusive behavior of throat clearing. He was told to eliminate all throat clearing by substituting a hard swallow or taking a sip of water followed by a hard swallow. He was to inform his family that every time he cleared his throat they were to say to him "you cleared your throat" and he was to immediately perform a hard swallow. By the end of the 2nd week he reportedly eliminated all throat clearing.

The patient was counseled to eliminate all caffeinated products from his diet and to drink at least eight glasses of water or fruit juices per day. It was recommended that he use a sport bottle filled with ice water to have beside him throughout the day, especially in his office and laboratory where the air was reportedly dry. He was instructed to have water or a noncaffeinated beverage with him at the time of teaching or conducting his seminar. Since he traveled, he was to take a sport bottle or thermos filled with water or natural juices to keep himself well hydrated on the airplane. Humidity is very low in airplanes and can affect the voice by drying the tissue lining in the oral pharyngeal area.

Vocal function exercises were prescribed to be done twice daily, two times each. The exercises included the following: (1) holding a high pitch /i/, softly, at a comfortable pitch without strain for as long as possible; (2) pitch matching and holding the vowel /o/, softly, on the notes middle C, D, E, F, and G for as long as possible; (3) gliding up the scale slowly saying "whoop," and gliding down the scale slowly saying the vowel /o/.

The second voice therapy session introduced exercises to promote an open oral front focus. The tongue tip and voiced continuant words (Andrews and Summers, 1988) were initially used to elicit a forward tone or focus. I explained the concept of placement of the voice (nasal, throaty, forward, and back) (Boone and Macfarlane, 1988) and demonstrated the sound of each placement. The professor was told to be theatrical when reading the words. He was instructed to do the following:

1. Relax the jaw and open the mouth
2. Project the voice 15 to 20 inches from the nose
3. Elongate the vowels to gain control over voicing, such as tiiiiip (tip) or neeeeoooon (neon)
4. Take a breath before every word
5. Feel and listen to the voice.

In a very short time, the professor was able to feel when the voice dropped into the throat and could hear the hoarseness associated with the throaty placement. He became somewhat frustrated because he could not sustain a frontal focus when speaking. Subsequent therapy sessions focused on reading sentences, short paragraphs, long paragraphs, structured conversation, and conversational speech. At the sentence level the professor was trained to read the sentences with adequate breath support and pause to replenish the support at a natural break in the sentence. Initially the professor read the sentences rapidly without pauses and would always shorten the vowels and swallow the final word.

For several weeks the professor was given homework exercises to help improve and promote a forward focused voice. Each week he continued his hydration program and completed two sets of the vocal function exercises daily. At the end of 4 weeks, the patient reported that his throat did not feel dry and that he rarely experienced a "lump-in-the-throat" feeling. He stated that his voice was not fatiguing, especially in the evenings.

During conversational speech, the professor had a tendency to lower the pitch and drop the placement of "fillers" such as "oh, yeah, that's right" to the throat. It was recommended that he use notes taped to his telephone and write reminders in his daily organizer to help him remember to practice maintaining an open oral front focus. When the professor demonstrated a 90% accuracy rate in using proper focus with adequate breath support during conversational speech, he was subjected to background noise by use of headsets and audio tape. This forced him to increase the volume of his speech while maintaining proper vocal placement. Speaker-to-listener distance was varied to help him adjust the volume.

The 8th week of voice therapy concentrated on maintaining an open oral front focus while presenting a mock lecture in a classroom setting and in an auditorium (with and without a microphone). Both the hand-held and lavaliere microphones were used for practice. The following suggestions were given to help him maintain adequate volume and proper focus in these settings:

1. Project the voice to the middle of the room
2. Be aware of body presence in relationship to the audience
3. When using the hand-held microphone, be aware of mouth-to-microphone distance and when using the lavaliere microphone be aware of head position in relationship to the placement of the microphone
4. Maintain adequate projection and volume at the end of sentences
5. Be relaxed, move around the stage or classroom; if standing still or behind a fixed podium, then bend the knees slightly and place the body weight on the balls of the feet
6. Remember to breathe and support the voice.

After 10 weeks of voice therapy, a reexamination using videolaryngostroboscopy showed normal appearing vocal folds bilaterally. The closure of the glottis was complete, with normal amplitude of vibration and mucosal wave. The overall maximum phonation times improved from 8 seconds initially to 30 seconds. Remeasurement of the reading and conversational speech fundamental frequency showed an increase in the fundamental frequency, with an increase also in the dynamic range.

Direct vocal therapy proved successful in remediating functional misuse of this professional voice user.

REFERENCES

Andrews M, Summers A: *Voice therapy for adolescents,* Boston, 1988, College-Hill Publications.

Barker S: *The Alexander technique,* New York, 1978, Bantam Books.

Berry C: *Voice and the actor,* London, 1973, George G. Harrap.

Boone D, MacFarlane S: *The voice and voice therapy,* Englewood Cliffs, N.J., 1988, Prentice-Hall.

Eisenson J: *Voice and diction: a program for improvement,* ed 5, New York, 1985, Macmillan.

Feldenkrais M: *Awareness through movement,* New York, 1972, Harper & Row.

Fisher H: Improving voice and articulation, ed 2, revised, Boston, 1975, Houghton Mifflin.

Gould WJ: Caring for the vocal professional. In Paparella M et al., editors: *Otolaryngology,* vol III, *Head and Neck,* ed 3, 1991, Philadelphia, WB Saunders.

Khambato AS: Laryngeal disorders in singers and other voice users. In Ballantyne J, Groves J, editors: *Scott Brown's diseases of the ear, nose and throat,* vol 4, *Throat,* ed 4, London, 1979, Butterworths.

Koufman JA, Isaacson G: The spectrum of vocal dysfunction. In Koufman JA, Isaacson G, editors: *Voice Disorders,* Philadelphia, 1991, WB Saunders.

Lavorato A, McFarlane S: Treatment of the professional voice. In Perkins W (ed): *Current therapy of communication disorders: voice disorders.* New York, 1983, Thieme Medical Publishers.

Lessac A: *The use and training of the human voice,* ed 2 (revised). New York, 1967, DBS Publications.

Linklater K; *Freeing the natural voice,* New York, 1976, DBS Publications.

Sataloff RT: *Professional voice: science and art of clinical care,* New York, 1991, Raven.

Stemple JC: *Clinical voice pathology: theory and management,* Columbus, Ohio, 1984, Merrill.

Turner JC: *Voice and speech in the theatre,* ed. 3, revised, London, 1977, Malcolm Morrison.

CHAPTER 8

Successful Voice Therapy

The previous chapters of this text have focused on the successful management of a wide range of voice disorders by clinical, medical, and surgical methods. Each contributor demonstrated techniques and approaches that proved successful in improving voice quality of patients with various laryngeal disorders. These successful cases, however, may set an unrealistically high standard for the beginning voice clinician and may not adequately reflect the many management pitfalls that are encountered even by experienced voice clinicians. Such pitfalls may lead to delayed success in treatment, less than totally successful results, or failure to resolve the voice problem. In Chapter 1 and in many of the case studies it was shown that the clinician and the patient share equally in the success or failure of voice therapy. In this chapter some determinants of successful voice therapy are examined in detail.

CLINICAL PREPARATION

To manage voice disorders successfully, the voice pathologist must be well-grounded in anatomy, physiology, etiologic correlates, laryngeal pathology, and the psychodynamics of voice production. He or she must also possess outstanding skills in human interaction. Without a complete grasp of these areas of clinical knowledge, one's efforts in successful voice therapy may be sabotaged by some or all of the factors discussed in this chapter.

Poor Interview and Counseling Skills

The ability to talk to people — to skillfully and systematically divine the important aspects of the voice disorder and then to counsel appropriately — is a skill that must be mastered. For some, the skill is natural and is easily applied in clinical use. For others, it is a skill developed only with practice and experience. Most clinicians continue to hone this skill throughout their careers. The initial patient interview and subsequent counseling are the most important components of a voice evaluation. When these are conducted poorly, successful resolution of the patient's voice problem is in doubt. The following is but one example.

CASE STUDY: PATIENT GG

During her second year of graduate training, a student was assigned to intern at the voice center. Following appropriate observation, she was given her first case, in which she was to conduct the patient interview portion of the voice evaluation. Patient GG was a 38-year-old man who had been experiencing 6 weeks of persistent hoarseness. Laryngeal examination revealed only mild erythema of the bilateral folds. Voice quality was only mildly dysphonic, with a dry, strained hoarseness. The patient also complained of a "thickness" feeling in his throat that he tried to eliminate with throat clearing.

Other than throat clearing, the patient denied all aspects of voice abuse/misuse, and his medical history was unremarkable as related to this problem. The interview broke down when the intern began questioning the patient regarding his social history. It was obvious throughout the interview that the intern was nervous, which is certainly understandable in the new clinician. However, she became even more uncomfortable when asking questions regarding the patient's personal life. Every interview provides the clinician with either several little "aha's" or one big "aha" as the diagnosis becomes clearer; however, this intern was more attentive to her scripted questions than to the answers she received. The exchange between the student (S) and patient (P) went something like this.

> **S:** "Are you married, single, or divorced?"
> **P:** (Heavy sigh) "I was married until 2 months ago." (Tear in eye; face turned red.)
> **S:** (Assuming divorce, with face down in her prepared questions) "How many children do you have?"

She missed it! She missed the most important moment during the interview and moved right along to the next question. To that point, only one etiologic factor had been identified: throat clearing. Because of the intern's lack of experience, she had failed to "tune in" to the patient. She listened to **what** the patient said but not to **how** he said it. This breakdown was later pointed out to her as part of her internship training.

In a follow-up discussion with the patient, it was discovered that his wife had been fatally injured in an automobile accident just prior to the onset of his voice disorder. The patient was suffering from an emotional dysphonia. Learning this, the intern was then able to adequately explain the relationship of emotions to voice quality. In this patient, the voice problem was not resolved until he received psychological support along with voice therapy.

It is not adequate to simply ask the right questions. Successful voice evaluation, and thus choice of therapy, is determined by the clinician's ability to **apply** the questions appropriately during the interview, together with the ability to listen to what is said and how it is said, and to respond appropriately.

Lack of Clinical Understanding of the Problem

The clinician who does not fully understand all aspects of voice disorders may not grasp the less obvious nuances of various pathologic conditions. Certainly, if the clinician does not understand the problem, then successful resolution will either be by luck or will be doomed. I've received many secondary referrals from speech pathologists who obviously had not had a complete understanding of the clinical problem. These cases have included lack of recognition of conversion dysphonia, functional falsetto, and functional ventricular phonation among others. In all cases, the clinicians were attempting direct symptom modification without recognition of the true diagnosis.

Clinicians may also possess unrealistic expectations of therapy results if they do not grasp the effects of neurologic or surgical changes of the vocal folds. Vocal fold paralysis patients may become frustrated when effort closure therapy is continued for a lengthy period of time. Our experience has demonstrated that if this management approach is at all helpful, positive results are seen within 2 to 3 weeks of daily exercise. Continued exercise appears to yield little benefit, if any. Large glottic gaps do not often improve significantly, though we have secondarily seen patients in our clinic who have had months of voice therapy for "vocal fold compensation."

I recall also a postsurgical case in which, because of the clinician's lack of understanding regarding surgical treatment, both the patient's and clinician's expectations for improvement were unrealistically high. The patient was identified through indirect laryngoscopy as having bilateral polypoid degeneration with a suspicious lesion located on the superior surface of the middle third of the left true vocal fold. The patient underwent a microlaryngoscopy and biopsy of both vocal folds. The biopsy was positive for the suspicious lesion, but biopsies taken in a wide area around the lesion and on the right fold were negative. The decision was made to treat the lesion aggressively through "laser stripping" of the left true vocal fold. One month later the right vocal fold was surgically managed with a more conservative surgical approach. In 9 months of postsurgical voice therapy during which the patient stopped smoking, she had improved from a severe to a moderate dysphonia. The patient was very frustrated, however, because her presurgical voice, though low-pitched, was not nearly as dysphonic and "hard to push out." The clinician fed this frustration by indirectly accusing the patient of "doing something" to maintain the hoarseness.

The clinician should have understood that aggressive laser "stripping" might permanently damage the mucous membrane of the vocal fold. The trade-off for this conservative treatment of cancer would most likely be some level of permanent hoarseness. Indeed, stroboscopic examination of this patient's vocal folds revealed severe stiffness of the mucosal wave and amplitude of vibration of the left vocal fold. The clinician simply did not understand the consequences of surgery.

Countless examples could be given regarding the clinician's lack of understanding about some aspect of the voice disorder, thus, affecting treatment. Indeed, even the most experienced voice clinician is always learning new information to add to his or her bank of clinical knowledge. The most successful voice clinicians own the largest bank accounts of knowledge.

Misapplied Management Techniques

One of the problems in preparing a text similar to this is the fear that it will be used as a voice management "cookbook": Look up the recipe, stir in this and that ingredient, use this and that technique, practice for 8 weeks, and create a lovely normal voice. No! Voice therapy cannot be successful with the cookbook approach. Every patient is an individual with different problems requiring individual needs. People with similar voice disorders will not necessarily respond to the same management approaches. For example, some patients with vocal nodules may require and respond very well to a progressive relaxation therapy,

whereas this approach may be totally inappropriate for others. Some unilateral vocal fold paralysis patients may benefit from effort closure exercises while others are already spontaneously using too much effort closure. The voice clinician cannot and should not arbitrarily apply certain management techniques to certain voice disorders.

The successful voice clinician will be aware of and ready to use any and all management techniques as deemed appropriate. But, again, the appropriateness of the chosen techniques is dependent on the clinician's knowledge and expertise of all aspects of the voice disorder. Knowledge of the voice disorder will dictate the use of the various therapy techniques. The management technique does not dictate its own use.

Lack of Patient Education or Understanding of the Problem

Most patients have very little concept of why they sound dysphonic. Voice production, like speech production, is just one of those bodily functions that we all take for granted: that is, until a problem arises. Education is one key to successful management. The more information patients have regarding their voice disorders, the more likely it will be that they can successfully remediate the problem. For patients to "buy" the concept of voice therapy, they must understand why they were referred to a speech pathologist. Once this is adequately explained, the nuances of their particular disorder must be described in detail. With this information, the patient should be able to understand the purpose behind the management techniques (some of which seem very silly unless fully understood).

Without a full understanding of the problem, the total management burden remains on the clinician. The clinician must use education to shift the burden to the patient. The patient must become an equal, if not greater than equal, partner in the process of voice improvement. For patients to be motivated to change vocal behaviors, they must understand why the change is required. The successful voice clinician will take great care in educating the patient in all aspects of the voice disorder.

Recognition of One Philosophical Orientation or One Etiologic Factor

Successful voice therapy is eclectic. We need not say more regarding the folly of subscribing to one management philosophy. Another potential cause for a poor management result is failure to identify and treat all of the etiologic correlates. For example, much of the emphasis of management for children with vocal abuse problems is placed on eliminating or modifying shouting, screaming, and loud talking. The more subtle causes, such as throat clearing and noises of vocal play (mimicking cars, guns, and so on), may not be identified. I've had the experience of frustrated speech pathologists, consulting about children who they "know" are no longer shouting. But, "he's/she's not getting any better!" Without modifying or eliminating all contributing factors, then the voice disorder is likely to continue. The following is an example from my case files.

CASE STUDY: PATIENT HH

HH, a 36-year-old woman presented with small bilateral vocal fold nodules as well as mild bilateral vocal fold edema. The abusive behaviors of shouting at her three adolescent children, shouting at sporting events, straining her voice while singing in a gospel choir, and chronic throat clearing were identified. All of these problems were either modified or eliminated through therapy, and her voice quality improved. Except, during each Monday appointment patient HH was more dysphonic than when seen for a Thursday appointment. As a result of this quality fluctuation, the problem was not totally resolving. What was going on? What had I missed?

Though patient HH was not singing in the church choir at that time, she attended a church that apparently was verbally and vocally enthusiastic to the pastor's message. Patient HH admitted to many loud vocal outbursts over a period of 2 hours every Sunday. As it turned out, the patient chose not to control her vocal enthusiasm in church, and she remained mildly dysphonic.

The successful voice clinician realizes that voice problems do not just happen. There is always a reason for the dysphonia. Seeking and modifying all of the etiologic factors are essential for the successful remediation of the problem.

Premature Discontinuation of Therapy

One of the most difficult stages of therapy for any communication disorder is the carry-over phase. Voice therapy is no exception. Many aspects of the communication process are being modified during voice therapy. These aspects include the patient's own perception of vocal image, voicing habits, and behaviors, as well as the direct anatomic and physiologic modifications that often must occur in the laryngeal and respiratory systems. In addition, new skills acquired in the therapy setting will not automatically be applied outside of this setting. The carry-over phase of therapy must not be isolated from the changes demonstrated in the office. The new behaviors must occur in all situations.

I recall the difficulty I had with one young man who presented with the classic "pseudo-authoritative" voice.

The patient was a recent college graduate in business who in his new job had been made supervisor of a small auditing department. Being rather young, and even younger in appearance, he had affected a low-pitched voice with intermittent glottal fry phonation. This behavior had led to irritation (not yet ulcerated) of the vocal processes of the arytenoid cartilages. He was noticeably hoarse, with the chief complaint of voice fatigue.

Interestingly, the patient was readily able to modify the inappropriate vocal properties during the initial session. I assumed carry-over would be rather easy to accomplish. At one point (at about 4 weeks) he was discharged from therapy only to return 1 month later with recurring symptoms. This young man was so involved in his perceived need for a different vocal image at work that he continued his abusive vocal behaviors. As his clinician, I had not assured carry-over of his improved vocal habits to the offending environment and had prematurely discharged him from therapy. We then worked more diligently on his vocal image with the appropriate counseling, and the problem was successfully remediated.

The successful voice clinician will assure carry-over of the improved vocal condition to all environments before discharging the patient. Follow-up rechecks are also advisable to guarantee habituation of the vocal improvement.

The Poor Clinical Ear

Sometimes a clinician's clinical training cannot account for all the skills necessary to conduct successful voice therapy. In some instances, natural talent plays a role. One of these skills is the musical "ear." In a recent research project, we gave thirty speech pathology graduate students pretreatment and posttreatment phonatory function tests, including acoustic and aerodynamic analyses. During the post-test, subjects were required to match pretest frequency levels. I was amazed at the number of students who could not readily match pitch. Empirically the number exceeded 50%. Possession of a clinical/musical ear is necessary in voice therapy to recognize quality deviations and changes, to model inappropriate and appropriate voice productions, to recognize pitch deviations, and to work on pitch matching exercises. The successful voice clinician must possess a clinical/musical ear.

PATIENT REALITIES

Assuming adequate preparation of the voice clinician, failure to achieve success in voice therapy may be related to the patient. The patient must bring to the therapy process a level of cooperation necessary to permit change. Voice change and developing habits of good vocal hygiene are not always easy, and the process is often frustrating for the patient. Several situations, described in the following sections, may occur which could lead to therapeutic failure.

Lack of Patient Motivation

Any therapeutic change requires the individual to perceive that a problem exists and that the problem needs to be changed. The voice pathologist will determine the patient's level of motivation. Then, through education and counseling, induce the patient to have the incentive to follow through and comply with

the management suggestions. Most patients are motivated and require very little encouragement to improve their voices. Some patients, however, are simply not interested in voice therapy.

CASE STUDY: PATIENT II

Patient II was a 56-year-old male insurance agent who had become dysphonic 4 months prior to the laryngeal examination. He sought the opinion of a physician only after much encouragement from his wife. Because of the publicity regarding hoarseness as a sign of cancer, this patient, a smoker, was frightened, and delayed going to the doctor because of his fear. Examination by the laryngologist revealed the presence of diffuse polypoid degeneration. When informed that he did not have cancer, patient II was obviously relieved.

Patient II was referred to the voice center for laryngeal videostroboscopy, a phonatory function test, and a voice evaluation. During the interview, it became evident that the man was no longer concerned about the hoarseness. Though he submitted to the voice evaluation, he lacked the motivation to improve voice quality. He was satisfied that he did not have cancer and chose not to accept the argument that his current vocal condition was a sign of negative tissue change. II did not seek further treatment.

The voice clinician should always try to motivate the patient to seek improvement of the voice, but, as illustrated, will not always be successful. Successful voice therapy depends upon a well-motivated patient who has the incentive to work toward positive vocal change.

Resistance to Share Information

Information gathered during the patient interview is valuable only if it is complete and accurate. The patient must be willing to share all pertinent information. Even the most skilled clinician has experienced situations in which, several sessions into therapy, a patient finally releases information critical to management decisions. Some patients are reticent to talk about personal or family problems that may be directly related to the voice disorder (such as tension, shouting, or crying). Certain behaviors such as drug use, smoking, and alcohol consumption are inaccurately reported. An eating disorder, such as bulimia, or an emotional problem requiring medication may not be mentioned.

Successful voice therapy is dependent on an open and honest relationship between patient and clinician. The clinician must establish credibility and a positivie, relaxed therapeutic atmosphere. The patient must be made aware of the importance of answering all questions honestly and accurately. Ultimately, the patient has final control over the information he or she is willing to share.

Perceived Need for Negative Vocal Behavior

The young man previously described in this chapter as having a "pseudo-authoritative" voice perceived a need to produce a low-pitched voice with glottal fry phonation. He was resistant to vocal change, even though he was dysphonic and uncomfortable, and he maintained the inappropriate vocal symptoms in his work environment. He desired to project a more mature image and chose voice modification as a means of accomplishing this task.

The gospel-singing, vocally enthusiastic parishioner decided that her abusive vocal response to the pastor's message was more important than her vocal health. Her Sunday response was a deeply religious experience that she chose not to modify, and as a result she remained dysphonic.

Over the years, I have had several patients who had another motive for maintaining negative vocal behaviors. I recall the case of a woman who, during the evaluation, exhibited body language signaling that she did not want to participate in the process. She refused to remove her coat, gave monosyllabic responses, and gave little effort to produce her "best" voice during testing. We learned later that she was seeking disability for a work-related injury, inhaling toxic fumes, and that it was therefore in her best interest not to improve her negative vocal behavior. She did not.

Voice therapy is comprised of a series of choices by both the clinician and the patient.

One choice is to follow the management suggestions of the clinician. Successful voice therapy is dependent on the patient recognizing negative vocal behaviors and choosing the need to modify those behaviors.

Need to Identify With the Problem

Vocal image has a strong psychological influence on many people. Patients often find it difficult to modify even moderate to severe vocal disturbances because of the effect this change may have on their image. Individuals close to or related to the patient may also object to vocal change. For example:

"Matthew has always sounded a little husky. We think it's cute."

In this case, the parent so strongly identifies the voice problem with the child that cooperation for modification may prove difficult.

Occasionally patients may say, "My husband likes my voice; he thinks it's sexy," or "I don't want to change very much. I won't sound like me," or "But to me I'd sound like I'm shouting if I talk like that." All of these comments are legitimate concerns to the owners of these voices. Our auditory feedback systems dictate to us what we are **supposed** to sound like. The feedback system may become very accustomed to even the most dysphonic voice. Some patients become resistant to vocal change either because they like or approve of the dysphonic voice or they dislike the new feedback they are receiving. Occasionally this resistance is powerful enough to make the therapy program unsuccessful.

Many voice disorders may be a symptom of emotional or psychological disorientation. When this is the circumstance, the need to maintain a voice problem may far outweigh the benefits of vocal improvement. An obvious sign of emotional well-being is voice quality.

CASE STUDY: PATIENT JJ

Patient JJ, a 38-year-old woman, was identified as having an "emotional dysphonia" caused by a recent divorce and other rather serious family problems. As efforts were made to modify the problem, the patient continually sabotaged the proceedings. The sabotage came in the form of new ailments ("My chest hurts when I do these exercises") or lists of rather bizarre questions ("Do you think this all started when the horse bit my ear?") that monopolized much management time. At that moment in her life, this patient needed to sound ill. Family counseling was suggested, and voice therapy was postponed. Subsequent voice therapy was not needed, as II's vocal problem spontaneously cleared as her life's problems resolved.

Patients may feel the need to project poor voice quality as a means of subconsciously demonstrating emotional upheaval in their lives.

Successful voice therapy is therefore dependent on the patient's willingness and ability to identify with a different, hopefully improved voice quality. To accomplish this, the patient must often override the auditory feedback system and yield to a new vocal image.

Finances

Unfortunately, a patient's finances may play a role in the successful remediation of voice disorders. As with all medically related services, the costs of providing vocal rehabilitation are steadily rising. When prioritizing the use of funds, some patients will certainly find other areas for spending that they deem more important than voice therapy. When finances prove to be a factor in the patient's decision to participate in therapy, the clinician must be willing to provide the patient with a reasonable estimation of the number of sessions, time frame, and cost of services. Third-party payors are increasingly supporting the cost of voice therapy services, especially if the voice disorder has an "organic cause." Voice pathologists should learn as much as possible about funding services in order to assist patients in their decision to seek treatment. Successful voice therapy may be dependent on the patient's willingness to assume financial responsibility for the services provided.

PERSONALITY ISSUES

"He never met a person he didn't like."
In a Pollyanna world maybe this statement

could be made. But, I must admit, the statement does not apply to me. I have worked with a few patients with whom I had a difficult time appreciating their personalities. (To be blunt, I did not like them.) This being the case, I'm sure some of these patients, and others, did not necessarily appreciate my personality and skills. Being a professional, however, I have usually been able to recognize the problem and to work through it, and the patients have successfully remediated their voice disturbances.

When the occasional time arises that it becomes evident that a clinician and patient simply cannot work well together, then modifications must be made. With some patients, I always felt that we were on different pages of the same book. We could not communicate well, and progress was not being made. Successful voice therapy is dependent on excellent communication between clinician and patient. This may require constant adjustment in the mind-set of the clinician from patient to patient. When personality conflicts arise and communication breaks down, they must be handled with frank discussion of the problem, with referral to another clinician reserved as an option.

CAN ALL VOICES BE IMPROVED?

Most voice disorders can be improved. I certainly go out on the proverbial limb making this statement. I truly believe that through our many (as this text demonstrates) management approaches, most vocal systems, and the personalities that own them, can be manipulated, modified, medicated, and/or undergo surgical intervention, yielding voice quality improvement. The level of improvement will range from dramatic to subtle, but improvement is most often possible.

The patient must be given a realistic expectation of the level of improvement. With this information, informed decisions can be made regarding the advantages of various treatment approaches or whether to be treated at all. Some patients require dramatic change for the treatment to be considered worthwhile. Others relish subtle improvements that increase the effectiveness of their communication skills. This leads us to the final question we will address in this text: "Can we always expect success?"

CAN WE ALWAYS EXPECT SUCCESS?

What is successful voice therapy? Who determines a level of success? Is the clinician's definition of successful therapy equal to the patient's expectation? Obviously, answers to these questions must be clear in order for the success of therapy to be determined. As the clinician my goal is always that the patient should develop the best voice possible. This goal must be made clear to the patient. Otherwise, the patient's goal may be "normal voice" (whatever that is), when normal voice may not be attainable. Or the patient may be satisfied with mild improvement while the clinician continues to push hard to develop more vocal improvement. This added push may require more effort than the patient is willing to give.

As voice clinicians, we should always expect success, knowing that many pitfalls exist to sabotage our efforts. Our task is to limit the sabotage through our efforts, experience, and expertise.

INDEX